Telephone Triage Protocols for Nurses

Sixth Edition

Julie K. Briggs, RN, BSN, MHA
Portland, Oregon

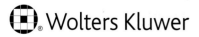 Wolters Kluwer

Philadelphia · Baltimore · New York · London
Buenos Aires · Hong Kong · Sydney · Tokyo

Acquisitions Editor: Nicole Dernoski
Development Editor: Maria M. McAvey
Senior Editorial Coordinator: Lindsay Ries
Marketing Manager: Linda Wetmore
Production Project Manager: Kim Cox
Design Coordinator: Elaine Kasmer
Manufacturing Coordinator: Kathleen Brown
Prepress Vendor: S4Carlisle Publishing Services

Sixth edition

9 8 7 6 5 4 3 2 1

Printed in China

Library of Congress Cataloging-in-Publication Data

Names: Briggs, Julie K., author.
Title: Telephone triage protocols for nurses / Julie K. Briggs, RN, BSN, MHA.
Description: Sixth edition. | Philadelphia: Wolters Kluwer Health, 2020. |
  Includes bibliographical references and index. | Summary: "Triage
  Protocols for Nurses is a resource to assist health care professionals
  make quick and effective decisions based on limited information using an
  algorithmic approach"— Provided by publisher.
Identifiers: LCCN 2020002058 | ISBN 9781975136871 (paperback)
Subjects: LCSH: Emergency nursing. | Triage (Medicine) |
  Telephone—Emergency reporting systems.
Classification: LCC RT120.E4 B75 2020 | DDC 616.02/5—dc23
LC record available at https://lccn.loc.gov/2020002058

RRS2003

Reviewers

Kathleen Baker, RN, BSN
Certified Ombudsman
State of Oregon Long Term Care
Portland, Oregon

Patricia Gabrielson, RN, BSN
Advice RN
Gastrointestinal & Minimally Invasive Surgery Division
The Oregon Clinic
Portland, Oregon

Pat Reder, RN, HHP, CCM
Holistic Health Practitioner
Chronic Disease Case Manager
Thornton, Colorado

John Zelko, MD
Gastrointestinal & Minimally Invasive Surgery Division
The Oregon Clinic
Portland, Oregon

Previous Edition Contributors

Gary Berg, RN, BSN, CEN
Telephone Triage Nurse
Emergency Department
Good Samaritan Community Healthcare
Puyallup, Washington

Shannon Fuller, RN
Obstetrics Department
Good Samaritan Community Healthcare
Puyallup, Washington

Sheila Graham, RN
Obstetrics Department
Good Samaritan Community Healthcare
Puyallup, Washington

Valerie G. A. Grossman, RN, BSN, CEN
Senior Nurse Telephone Triage Counselor
ViaHealth Call Center
Rochester, New York

Elaine Keavney, RN, BSN, CEN
Education
Nursing Education Department
MultiCare Health System
Tacoma, Washington

Laurie McGhee, RNC, ARNP
Obstetrics Department
Good Samaritan Community Healthcare
Puyallup, Washington

Linda Mercer, RN, CEN
Emergency Department
Good Samaritan Community Healthcare
Puyallup, Washington

Deborah Oakman, BSN, RN
Obstetrics Department
Good Samaritan Community Healthcare
Puyallup, Washington

Pat Reder, RN, CEN
Consulting Telephonic Nurse Case Manager
Boring, Oregon

Sandra Velliquette, BSN, RNC
Obstetrics Department
Good Samaritan Community Healthcare
Puyallup, Washington

Previous Edition Reviewers

Chris R. Andrews, MD, FACEP
Emergency Services
Providence Health System
Portland, Oregon

Coreen Arioto, MSN, RN
Former Advice Nurse Manager
Kaiser Metropolitan Los Angeles
Los Angeles, California

Meghan Arnold, RN, BSN, MHA
Quality Medical Management
Providence Health Plans
Portland, Oregon

Stephanie H. Asher, RN, MSN
Supervisor Quality Medical Management
Providence Health Plans
Banks, Oregon

Susan Barnason, PhD, RN, CEN, CCRN, CS
Associate Professor
College of Nursing
University of Nebraska Medical Center
Lincoln, Nebraska

Michelle Birge, RN, BSN, CCM
Quality Medical Management
Providence Health Plans
Portland, Oregon

Michael Brook, MD, FACEP
Emergency Medicine
Good Samaritan Community Healthcare
Puyallup, Washington
Clinical Assistant Professor of Medicine
University of Washington Medical Center
Seattle, Washington

Nancy Church, RN, BSN, MT, CIC
Manager, Infection Control
Providence St. Vincent Medical Center
Portland, Oregon

Shelley Cohen, RN, BS, CEN
Educator/Consultant
Health Resources Unlimited
Hohenwald, Tennessee

Mary Frances Condera, MS, RN, PMHNP-BC
Psychiatric Mental Health Nurse Practitioner
Northwest Catholic Counseling Center
Portland, Oregon

Sonja R. Dahl, RNC, BSN, IBCLC
Obstetric Department
Good Samaritan Community Healthcare
Puyallup, Washington

Timothy Dahlgren, MD
Emergency Medicine
Good Samaritan Community Healthcare
Puyallup, Washington

Margaret C. Dirienzo, BSN, RN, CEN
Director, Critical Care Services
North Austin Medical Center
Austin, Texas

Laura R. Favand, MS, RN
Chief, Education and Training
Army Trauma Training Center
Army Medical Department Center and School
Miami, Florida

Vickie K. Fieler, RN, MS, AOCN
Clinical Nurse Specialist, Oncology
Exeter Hospital
Exeter, New Hampshire

Laura Gernert Genovese, RN, MSN, APRN-BC
Assistant Clinical Manager
Network Telephone Care Program
Veterans Affairs Medical Center
Bronx, New York

Valerie Grossman, RN, BSN, CEN
Director of Nursing for Medical/Surgical Services
ViaHealth of Wayne
Newark, New York

Reneé S. Holleran, RN, PhD, CEN, CCRN, CFRN, FAEN
Nurse Manager
Adult Transport Services
Intermountain Life Flight
Salt Lake City, Utah

Elizabeth Jerabeck, RN, BSN
Senior Nurse Counselor
ViaHealth LINK
ViaHealth System
Rochester, New York

Diane Kamble, RNC, APRN
Network Telephone Care Program
Veterans Affairs Medical Center
Bronx, New York

Calvin A. Kierum, Jr., MD, FAAP
Pediatric Medicine
Good Samaritan Hospital
Puyallup, Washington

Bret Lambert, MD
Emergency Physician
President of Medical Staff
Good Samaritan Hospital
Puyallup, Washington

Eileen Westlake Lumb, MS, RN, CS, CEN, FNP
Adult Nurse Practitioner
Emergency Department
Strong Memorial Hospital
University of Rochester
Rochester, New York

Diane L. Mathews, RNC, MSN
Urgent Care/Telephone Care Service
William S. Middleton Memorial VA Hospital
Madison, Wisconsin

Judith McDevitt, PhD, RN, CS-FNP
Assistant Professor of Nursing
Coordinator, Family Nurse Practitioner Option
Department of Health Maintenance, School of Nursing
University of Wisconsin-Milwaukee
Milwaukee, Wisconsin

J. Michaelson, Jr., MD, FACOG
Obstetrics and Gynecology Medicine
Good Samaritan Hospital
Puyallup, Washington

Lyne Ouellet, MD
Emergency Medicine
Good Samaritan Community Healthcare
Puyallup, Washington
Clinical Assistant Professor of Medicine
University of Washington Medical Center
Seattle, Washington

Mary Beth Passauer, BSN
Clinical Coordinator
Saint Vincent Call Center
Erie, Pennsylvania

Iris Reyes, MD
Assistant Professor of Emergency Medicine
Department of Emergency Medicine
The Hospital of the University of Pennsylvania
Philadelphia, Pennsylvania

Patty C. Seneski
Emergency Preparedness Manager
Banner Desert Medical Center
Banner Children's Hospital at BDMC
Mesa, Arizona

Cynthia Smith, RN
Clinical Supervisor Specialty Clinics
Providence Medical Group
Providence Health and Services
Portland, Oregon

Danonne R. Smith
Project Consultant
Consumer Advocate
Portland, Oregon

Cecil Snodgrass, MD, FACEP, MRO
Family Practice
Good Samaritan Hospital
Puyallup, Washington

Leeta Stoughton, MPH, RN, BC, CEN
Regional Clinical Systems Manager
Providence Health System
Portland, Oregon

Phyllis Straight-Millan, SPHR, CSM, MA, MPA
Manager, Safety and Health, United States Postal
Service
Consultant
Workplace Violence Programs, Voluntary Protection
Programs (OSHA)
Portland, Oregon

Rebecca Sullivan, MD
Family Practice
Puyallup Valley Healthcare
Puyallup, Washington

Christina Terenzi, RN, MN, CEN
Clinical System Educator I
MultiCare Health System
Tacoma, Washington

Lisa Utter, RNC, ASN
Staff Nurse
Clarian Health
Indianapolis, Indiana

Steve Weinman, RN, CEN
Emergency Department
St. Luke's Northland Hospital
Kansas City, Missouri

Mark A. Whitaker, MD, MMM
Senior Medical Director
Quality and Medical Management
Providence Health and Services
Portland, Oregon

Addison Wilson, MD
Medical Director
Providence Health Plans
Providence Health Services
Portland, Oregon

Margaret Wilson, RN, MSN, EdD
Professor of Nursing
Cypress College
Cypress, California

Preface

The telephone has become a vital link in health care today. Heightened awareness of cost and access to health-care services has significantly increased the consumer's use of the phone to determine the urgency of a problem and the need for medical attention. Emergency departments, primary care providers, and other health-care providers receive numerous calls from individuals regarding the need to access medical care, often in an attempt to avoid spending unnecessary health-care dollars. Using organized, systematic telephone triage protocols, nurses can respond to these calls with confidence and consistency while minimizing subjectivity.

In this rapidly changing health-care environment, new medications, treatments, devices, and practice modalities are evolving daily. The number of FDA-approved over-the-counter medications has increased steadily and enabled individuals to effectively manage conditions at home rather than visit their primary care provider for a prescription. Many conditions are now treated in the outpatient setting or at home. Time-sensitive treatments such as thrombolytics for strokes and cardiac catheterization for heart attacks make rapid triage in an emergency care setting imperative. The sixth edition of *Telephone Triage Protocols for Nurses* has incorporated these considerations in the revision of existing protocols and the development of new ones.

New Features

- Protocols have been thoroughly reviewed, revised, and updated to reflect current practice and changes in access to medications and health care.
- Protocols address adult, pediatric, geriatric, and maternal/child and home health concerns.
- Protocols have been updated and expanded to ensure *pediatric* and the rapidly expanding *aging population*'s concerns and conditions are adequately addressed.
- Postoperative conditions and considerations have been added to numerous protocols.
- Expanded home care instructions provide more useful and timely information, list drug warnings whenever over-the-counter medications are suggested, and offer many home and alternative remedies.
- New protocols have been added to address current health issues and communicable disease outbreaks, including:
  - Arthritis problems
  - Chronic obstructive pulmonary disease (COPD)
  - Elder abuse
  - Stroke, Suspected
  - Zika virus
  - Mental health challenges in telephone triage
    - Altered mental status
    - PTSD
    - Suicide prevention
  - Emergency preparedness section
    - Tips for preparedness in telephone triage
    - START triage system
    - Mass casualty incidents
    - Active shooter incidents
- The **Other Protocols to Consider** section has been revised to reflect changes in protocol titles and new protocols to help the nurse select the

most appropriate protocol after asking the initial Key Questions. Additionally, page numbers have been included for each protocol to enhance the ability to rapidly locate a different protocol to complete the triage encounter.

- The **Nurse Alert** section has been enhanced and expanded to specific protocols to provide the nurse with additional important information to consider when choosing a protocol, recognizing potentially serious problems or when triaging the caller's concern. Referrals to additional resources are included to provide the nurse with Internet resources when appropriate or referrals to appendices to assist the nurse in gaining a better understanding of a specific condition.

- A number of key features have been added to make this book even more user-friendly and enhance the user's ability to quickly locate the appropriate protocol.
  - Several titles have been changed to more closely match what the caller may be describing.
    - "Altered Level of Consciousness" is changed to "Altered Mental Status."
    - "Nausea and Vomiting, Adult and Child" protocol is changed to "Vomiting, Adult" and "Vomiting, Child."
    - "Black and Bloody Stools" has been changed to "Rectal Bleeding."
  - Related protocols have been *combined* to minimize search time. The "Drug and Alcohol Problems" is included in the "Alcohol Problems" and "Substance Abuse, Use, or Exposure" protocols.
  - The **Table of Contents by Body System** has been updated and organizes the protocols by body system or part to help the user quickly identify the most appropriate protocol given a symptom or set of related symptoms. It includes separate sections for disease-related protocols, general problems, behavioral health problems, and pediatric-specific protocols.
  - The color tabs for each alphabetical section have been staggered, making it easier to locate

the appropriate section of the book. The reader may also wish to purchase alphabetical stick-on tabs, which can be found at most office supply stores.

- **Emergency home care instructions** are included in the action column of the protocol, providing the nurse with immediate access to important first aid actions to take while the caller is waiting for an ambulance or before going to the emergency department. Page numbers are included when the nurse is directed to a different page.

- The **Introduction** chapter has been reorganized to serve as a useful resource in establishing and maintaining an ongoing telephone triage program and includes Triage Roles and Responsibilities, Protocol Structure, Using Protocols Safely, Medical–Legal Considerations and case examples, Documentation Guidelines, and Strategies to Ensure Quality in a Telephone Triage Program.

Telephone Triage Protocols for Nurses assists health-care professionals in asking appropriate questions to quickly assess the severity of a problem and help the caller make an informed decision concerning health service utilization. The protocols are not designed to diagnose the caller's medical condition.

This manual contains more than 200 protocols that cover a wide range of common symptoms, disorders, and medical emergencies. Health problems unique to adults, children, pregnant women, the chronically ill, and the aged are included. While most of the protocols have "symptom-based" titles, a few have "diagnosis-based" titles for use with callers who have been previously diagnosed with a condition and are having concerns related to that condition (congestive heart failure, diabetes, sickle cell disease, asthma, etc.). Protocols are arranged alphabetically to help the health-care professional quickly locate the appropriate protocol. A team of experts has extensively reviewed all of the protocols to ensure accurate and up-to-date advice.

Key Features

- The format is easy to follow.
- Coverage of common symptoms and conditions is comprehensive.
- Age-specific considerations are built into the protocols, eliminating the need for several reference books.
- Questions and instructions are written in clear and concise language.
- All protocols are cross-referenced to additional protocols that could also be useful.
- Each protocol follows a standard design, which helps the nurse to utilize information efficiently.

Additional Features

- An expanded **Table of Contents** lists each protocol, directing the reader to the appropriate page.
- The **Appendices** include the following:
  - Abbreviations Chart
  - Sample Telephone Triage Protocol Forms
  - Community Resources Telephone List
  - Telephone Triage Quality Improvement Checklist
  - Telephone Triage Documentation Form
  - Telephone Triage "Call Back" Log
  - Consulting Nurse Call Tape Review Form
  - Consulting Nurse Call Documentation Review Form
  - Telephone Triage Training Guidelines, Course Outline, and Training Exercises
  - Communicable Diseases and Sexually Transmitted Diseases Tables
  - Temperature and Weight Conversion Charts
  - Teaching Self-Assessment Guide
  - Abdominal Pain, Chest Pain, and Headache Causes and Characteristics Charts
  - Additional Resources
  - Mental Health Challenges in Telephone Triage
  - Emergency Preparedness
- The **Bibliography** includes additional telephone triage and advisory resources.
- The **Index** includes all of the protocol titles as well as alternate terms to allow quick access to the correct protocol.

Telephone Triage Protocols for Nurses is a comprehensive resource that will benefit medical offices, emergency departments, urgent care centers, clinics, schools, home health agencies, occupational health departments, managed health-care providers, and all nurses who receive calls for advice. This quick reference manual can serve as:

- A systematic screening guide to assist callers in making informed decisions about when to access health-care resources.
- A ready resource for health-care professionals.
- A source for community referrals.
- A tool to help reduce inappropriate utilization of emergency services.
- A telephone service to triage patients with life-threatening problems.
- A mechanism to minimize risk management difficulties through consistency and documentation.
- A resource for additional website information to learn more about specific conditions, treatments, and prevention.

Acknowledgments

The efforts of many people are responsible for the successful completion of this book. I thank the reviewers for their consistent and thorough evaluation of the protocols for accuracy, safety, appropriateness, clarity, and completeness. Their ongoing efforts have been noteworthy and their comments invaluable.

Each revision brings challenges in balancing manuscript development, employment responsibilities, and relationships and activities with friends and family. A very special thank you goes to Patricia Reder, RN, CEN, who was instrumental in writing the first edition of *Telephone Triage Protocols for Nurses*, and now 20 years later is again instrumental in writing this book. Her insight into managing chronic disease, case and disease management, attention to detail, and contributions to the sixth edition were invaluable. I also thank Dr. John Zelko for his meticulous review of the manuscript and changes to ensure consistency with current medical practice. A special thank you to my husband, Worth, and to my family and friends, for their understanding of the time-consuming nature of this project. Additionally, I want to thank Kathleen Baker, RN, BSN who was invaluable in sharing her expertise in working with seniors and Patricia Gabrielson, RN, BSN for sharing her expertise in telephone triage and surgical procedures. I want to extend a very special thank you to Nicole Dernoski, acquisitions editor, for making this project possible and providing continuous support and encouragement for developing the vision for this sixth edition. Finally, I thank Lindsay Ries, editorial coordinator, for her assistance in moving this project smoothly through the production phase and her prompt responsiveness to my queries and concerns.

Julie K. Briggs

Contents

Protocols

Throughout this title, protocols with **Pediatric** or **Maternity** considerations are highlighted with the following icons:

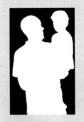

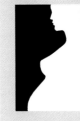

Table of Contents by Body System

Limb (Arm/Leg) Problems

Skin Problems

Chronic and Infectious Diseases

Behavioral Health Problems

General Problems

Pediatric-Specific Problems

Introduction: Practicing Telephone Triage Safely

Appropriate use of health-care resources is one of the biggest challenges in today's health-care environment. Effective telephone triage can help people access the right level of health care at the right time. The aging baby boomer population has become a significant consumer of health-care resources due to evolving chronic health conditions such as cardiac disease, diabetes, congestive heart failure, chronic obstructive pulmonary disease, cancer, degenerative neurologic disorders along with a rapidly rising increase in anxiety and depression. In an era of escalating health-care costs, corporate reorganization, and a surge in the number of managed care systems, consumers are forced to carefully evaluate whether and when to seek medical attention. They must contend with cost and access as key issues, and telephone triage nurses play a key role in helping consumers through this decision-making maze.

Primary care providers are increasingly called upon to control health-care costs and the use of health-care resources. However, most providers are too busy to personally answer the numerous calls from consumers who are seeking advice. The responsibility frequently falls on nurses. Standardized protocols help the nurse handle telephone questions efficiently, confidently, and in a safe and proficient manner. Telephone triage has become the entry point into the health-care system for many consumers. It is a tool to help improve access to health care, not to block access as some skeptics believe.

Nurses in a variety of settings, including emergency rooms, physician offices, clinics, home health, occupational health, urgent care centers, and crisis care centers, frequently find themselves in the position of giving telephone advice. It is important to recognize that not all nurses are equal in terms of education, experience, knowledge base, assessment skills, and communication skills. Therefore, advice based on what a nurse "thinks" is appropriate may in fact be harmful to the caller. The nurse may miss an important detail in the absence of a thorough, systematic assessment. A system for using organized, approved protocols helps to ensure that the assessment is thorough and that nothing significant is overlooked and that advice is consistent from one nurse to another.

Traditionally, hospital emergency departments (EDs) have been used as health-care information resources because of their availability 24 hours a day and because some patients are hesitant to disturb their primary care providers during evening and weekend hours. In the past, ED nurses have been told not to give advice over the telephone to avoid potential medical–legal problems. Although this practice may provide a perceived safety net for hospitals and their nursing staff, the nurse's refusal to give advice frustrates and angers callers. Many consumers believe it is the hospital's obligation to the community to provide health-care information upon request, and they will persist in asking questions until they receive advice. Unfortunately, in the absence of standardized protocols, the advice may be inaccurate or inconsistent. This haphazard approach is all too common and may increase liability risks. More and more EDs are providing their own telephone triage nurse to manage these calls or contract with a telephone triage call center to provide that service.

Telephone triage is a systematic process in which a nurse screens a caller's symptoms for urgency and advises the caller when to seek medical attention, based on the severity of the problem described. The nurse also helps direct the caller to the most appropriate health-care setting or gives advice about home care.

Despite the potential medical–legal risks of giving telephone advice, there has been considerable interest in telephone triage as a mechanism to help control costs and resource use while still responding to the consumer's need for information. Helping a caller to make an informed decision about health care will enhance the provider's image to a much greater extent than refusing to discuss health-care options over the telephone.

As health-care delivery systems evolve and formal relationships among physician groups, hospitals, and third-party payers are cultivated, telephone triage and advice programs are rapidly emerging as a necessary service. To be successful, they must be well-organized, protocol-driven, well-documented, and evaluated for quality, accuracy, and consistency.

Triage Roles and Responsibilities

Roles and responsibilities of staff in managing telephone calls must be defined and clarified to ensure that only trained and qualified staff is providing the triage function. Identify who can provide triage, health information, and make appointments. Clearly define the role of the receptionist, medical assistant, LPN (LVN), and RN. For example, some organizations have the receptionist take the initial call, then forward the call to the triage nurse. The triage nurse asks specific questions about a condition and advises home care, clinic appointment, or higher level of care. The organization needs to provide a list of conditions and situations that should be passed on to the nurse for triage, for example:

- Breathing problems
- Chest or abdominal pain
- Headaches
- Trauma
- Neurologic problems

- Psychiatric problems
- Drug and alcohol problems
- Symptoms that are sudden and severe
- Person sounds sick

Assign to the triage role experienced RNs who have a broad knowledge base, are trained in telephone triage, are excellent performers, and like telephone triage. Although there is some merit to training all RNs for greater flexibility within the setting, those who truly enjoy the role generally perform much better and promote better patient satisfaction and customer service. Provide a quiet environment that has the necessary resources for triage, documentation, and the discussion of sensitive issues in private.

Protocol Structure

- All the protocols in the book follow the same format and include the following:
  - Key Questions
  - Other Protocols to Consider
  - Nurse Alert (when appropriate)
  - Reminder for documentation
  - Assessment questions
  - Action for the nurse to take
  - Home Care Instructions
  - Section to write in additional instructions
  - Problems to report to provider
  - When to seek emergency care
  - Advice agreement reminder
- The **Key Questions** section prompts the nurse to ask for important information before proceeding through the protocol. This always includes asking for the caller's name, age, onset of symptoms, history, medication usage, and questions appropriate to the complaint, such as pain scale, immunization status, or frequency of symptoms. Disease-based protocols include questions about a known diagnosis, treatment, or known exposure to a disease.
- The **Other Protocols to Consider** section lists related protocols, serving as a quick resource for

multiple symptoms or related conditions. After asking key questions, the nurse may determine that a different protocol is more appropriate and can quickly select that protocol.

- A **Nurse Alert** section provides the nurse with additional important information to consider when choosing a specific protocol or when triaging the caller's concern. Referrals to additional resources are provided when appropriate to assist the nurse in gaining a better understanding of a specific condition. Background information is provided to give the nurse a better understanding of the condition and potential seriousness of that condition. It is not provided to diagnose a caller's concern.

- The **Reminder** text ("Document caller response to advice, home care instructions, and when to call back") prompts the nurse to document, per organizational policy, and ensure that the caller understands the advice provided.

- The **Assessment** section lists the symptoms, conditions, or combination of factors that should be assessed in determining urgency.

- **Action** is organized around yes-or-no answers to the assessment questions. If the caller answers "no" to the question, the nurse is directed to the next category of assessment questions. If the caller answers "yes," concrete advice is given regarding when and where to receive care. This advice is prioritized so that emergency actions always appear first. The terms used in the Action section instruct the nurse or the caller how to proceed. Actions the nurse should take appear in italicized type in the list below. Instructions to the caller appear in quotation marks. Action options are as follows:

  - *Go to [a related] protocol*: The nurse is directed to a related protocol that may address an emergent problem more appropriately.
  - "Call an ambulance" (911 in many areas): Emergency first aid instructions while waiting for the ambulance are also included in this section.
  - "Seek emergency care now": Refer caller to the nearest ED. Emergency first aid instructions

before going to the ED may also be included here as appropriate.

- "Seek medical care within 2 to 4 hours": Refer caller to usual care provider, clinic, or ED for urgent conditions.
- "Seek medical care within 24 hours": Refer caller to usual care provider, clinic, or ED for less urgent conditions. This may be a same-day appointment dependent upon the urgency of the condition, repeated calls, or time of day.
- "Seek medical care within 24 to 48 hours": Refer caller to usual care provider, clinic, or ED for nonurgent conditions.
- "Call back or call PCP for appointment if no improvement": Refer caller to primary care provider or clinic for nonurgent problems if no improvement occurs after following home care instructions.
- *Follow home care instructions*: The nurse is directed to explain the information described in the Home Care Instructions section, which follows the Assessment/Action columns.

- The **Home Care Instructions** section explains what care should be given in the home before emergency help arrives, while waiting for an appointment, or if the problem can be managed at home. These guidelines can provide symptom relief, prevent a condition from worsening, and reassure the caller. Home and alternative remedies are included and offer less-expensive options for symptom relief.

- An **Additional Instructions** section provides space in which the health-care professional can write customized health-care facility instructions.

- The **Report the Following Problems to Your PCP/Clinic/ED** section lists subsequent observations, symptoms, or conditions that should be reported wherever the caller generally receives ongoing health care.

- The **Seek Emergency Care Immediately** section lists subsequent observations, symptoms, or conditions that would require the caller to seek immediate emergency care. The caller is directed to watch for these symptoms and, if they occur, either call an ambulance or go directly to the ED.

- The **Advice Agreement** section prompts the nurse to ask whether or not the caller agrees with the advice given and encourages the caller to call back or follow up with the PCP, clinic, or ED if the problem persists or worsens. This warning should be given with every call. If the caller does not agree with the advice, the nurse should reassess the advice given.

Using Protocols Safely

Although protocol use does not replace nursing judgment, they do provide a quick, efficient, and safe way to communicate essential information. To ensure consistency and safe practice, policy should mandate that approved protocols be used for all telephone advice and then each call and advice provided documented. All protocols should be reviewed and approved by the medical provider or medical authority.

The importance of using protocols when giving telephone advice:

- Protocols are clinical rules for managing calls and provide structure and cues to ask specific questions, starting with the most emergent concerns.
- Protocols prompt the nurse to avoid missing important facts.
- Protocols provide validity and reliability. If followed, they lead to a reasonable and safe disposition, and if given the same set of data, another nurse would reach the same disposition.
- Protocols do not replace nursing judgment. Education, training, and experience affect the nurse's knowledge base and their ability to apply the protocols appropriately.
- When **selecting the appropriate protocol**, choose the protocol that:
  - best matches the symptom or condition;
  - will result in receiving care sooner when multiple symptoms are present;
  - is their most serious symptom or the most bothersome symptom.

- When overriding a protocol:
  - err on the side of caution;
  - upgrade rather than downgrade; do not downgrade without discussing with the provider or supervisor;
  - document the reason for choosing a different resource or overriding a protocol;
  - ensure caller is comfortable with the advice; if not, then reassess.
- **Disease-based protocols** are designed to address already diagnosed problems and should not be used to diagnose a condition. They should be used when a caller has a known diagnosis and has questions about managing his symptoms or treatment regimen, or a known exposure to a communicable disease. Examples of diagnosis-based protocols are diabetes problems, chickenpox, arthritis, congestive heart failure, or a history of an allergic reaction or a communicable disease exposure.
- **Closure to the call** is extremely important and can significantly help to reduce liability. Each protocol includes a reminder to ensure the caller understands the advice, home care instructions, and when to call back. It is important to understand that this critical step helps to ensure that the caller:
  - verbalizes understanding of the directions and information;
  - expresses intent to comply or not comply with the advice;
  - establishes agreement with the plan of care;
  - has the opportunity to ask additional questions or address concerns;
  - addresses any concerns about appropriate transportation to the referred care center;
  - is directed to call back if condition worsens, new symptoms develop, or there is no improvement.

Following this important step helps the nurse to determine nonunderstanding or noncompliance and provides the opportunity to reassess before ending the call.

Medical–Legal Safeguards

A variety of methods can be used to reduce the risks of giving medical advice over the telephone. Experts in the telephone triage field agree that the use of approved protocols substantially reduces risk. Protocols establish a standard of care, and they provide a mechanism to address potentially serious conditions in a consistent manner when the nurse cannot see or touch the person.

Once telephone contact is made and the nurse has offered to help, a patient–nurse relationship has been established. Failure to follow through and provide advice could be considered abandonment, according to some experts.

Although no assurances can be made that all medical–legal problems associated with telephone triage and advice can be avoided, using the following guidelines will help in preventing them.

Tips for Practicing Safe Telephone Triage

- Consider all calls life-threatening until proven otherwise so that all emergent questions are asked and help to prevent missing emergent problems.
- Err on the side of caution to avoid the risk in delaying treatment for potentially serious problems.
- Recognize knowledge deficits and use protocols to supplement knowledge to make appropriate triage decisions.
- Document the call and the advice given. If a lawsuit is filed a few years later claiming that the nurse did not advise a caller appropriately, the nurse's position is much more defensible if documentation shows that protocols were followed and appropriate advice was given, the caller's response to the advice, and the caller was advised to call back if no improvement or condition worsens. (See Appendix E1 (**679**) for sample documentation forms.) Documentation may include a log, a note in the patient's chart, or a recording of the call.

- Establish a positive, helping relationship at the onset of the call. Good initial contact can greatly influence the caller's trust in, and satisfaction with, the telephone interaction. The average call lasts only about 6 minutes, and the effectiveness of this brief encounter depends on skillful communication.
- Use terminology the caller can understand. Avoid medical jargon as much as possible.
- Encourage the caller to briefly describe the problem and its duration, onset, and location. Be sure to obtain the age, medical history, medications, and allergies of the person with the problem. Always ask about allergies before giving medication advice.
- When advising the caller to take over-the-counter medication, give the appropriate drug warnings:
  - Do not give aspirin to a child or to anyone who is also taking blood-thinning medication. Avoid aspirin-like products if age is <20 years.
  - Do not take anti-inflammatory medications if stomach problems or kidney disease is present or in the case of pregnancy.
  - Avoid acetaminophen if liver disease is present.
  - Avoid taking antihistamines if the prostate is enlarged.
  - Avoid taking decongestants if hypertension is present.
- Know how to elicit a description of a petechiae-type rash—flat, purple or dark red dots that do not blanch with pressure. Teach the caller how to test for blanching. Be on the alert for signs of meningitis: headache, stiff neck, fever, petechial rash, vomiting, irritability, altered mental status.
- Listen carefully to the caller and avoid jumping to conclusions. Callers may mask their real concern because of embarrassment, particularly regarding sensitive issues, such as sexually transmitted diseases, drug or alcohol problems, or mental health issues.

  Case example: A young man called an ED asking to reserve a room for the weekend. A busy nurse hurriedly answered the call, told the patient that the ED does not reserve rooms, and put him on hold for the secretary to handle. In further questioning, the caller revealed that he had attempted suicide in the past, was feeling suicidal again, and was asking for help and protection from himself. He wanted to be in a safe place where he could not harm himself.

- Try to talk directly to the person with the problem, if possible. Direct communication usually is more reliable and inclusive than secondhand information.

- Thoroughly assess the problem before determining an action plan. The caller may underplay the symptoms and want reassurance that the problem is insignificant. Consider the case of a 50-year-old man who states that his wife is making him call, but that he does not think his neck and jaw pain is anything to worry about. A thorough assessment is essential to identify potential cardiac symptoms.

- Do not try to diagnose the caller, or let the caller self-diagnose. Assess the symptoms to determine a disposition. Chest pain, diaphoresis, and weakness may very well signal a heart attack, but they also may indicate pneumonia or some other condition.

- Condition-/diagnosis-specific protocols are to be used only on callers with a previously diagnosed condition or suspected or known exposure to a specific contagious condition. *Do not* try to diagnose the problem and give advice, which is outside the scope of practice for a licensed RN in most states. The focus of triage is the assessment and management of symptoms and referral to the appropriate level of care at the right time.

- You may override a protocol, but do not downgrade without discussing the case with the primary care provider. Although experience will enhance your telephone triage skills, you must always use the protocols to ensure an appropriate and safe disposition or to document the rationale for deviating from a protocol.

    Case example: A 45-year-old man called with concerns about anxiety, a bad taste in his mouth, and profuse sweating. The patient was taking medication for anxiety and hypertension. The nurse had personal experience with antianxiety medication and advised the patient to rest, as he was probably experiencing the side effects of his fairly new medication. He died of a heart attack at home several hours later.

- Pay attention to the degree of anxiety and concern expressed by the caller. Remember, the telephone triage nurse has the disadvantage of not being able to see or touch the person. If the caller is emphatic that the person he or she is talking about is ill, encourage the caller to seek medical attention sooner than the protocols may recommend. If the caller thinks it is an emergency, it probably is. Let the EMS or ED staff determine otherwise. It is better to err on the side of caution than to miss a serious condition, such as meningitis, a stroke, or heart attack, which can result in permanent impairment or death.

- Triage is the practice of exclusion. It is permissible to be conservative and overreact.

- When telling a parent to report specific signs and symptoms, give him or her a time period, for example, to report a change in behavior within 4 hours of onset.

- When directing the caller to call an ambulance, several avenues may be most appropriate based on the circumstances: (Ambulance, EMS, 911 = emergency services for that area of the country)
  - Caller hangs up and calls the ambulance or 911.
  - Caller stays on the line but calls the ambulance on a cell phone or other device.
  - Triage nurse calls 911 for the caller and gives address, cross streets, and telephone number.
  - EMS dispatch centers are trained in providing specific emergency procedure directions while waiting for an ambulance and often have GPS capability to locate the caller's location.
  - When there is a contagious communicable disease in question, advise not to use public transportation. Depending on the lethality of the potential contagious disease, advise to

call 911 and tell dispatchers of potential contagiousness so they can prepare appropriately with personal protective equipment and transport to the appropriate facility that can manage the contagion.

- When referring a caller to the ED, give a time frame, such as "now" or "within the next 1 or 2 hours." How are they going to get there?

- When advising a caller to seek emergency care now, consider the caller's condition and circumstances. Is there a risk of deterioration that could compromise the airway or limb, or loss of life (myocardial infarction, stroke, or allergic reaction)?

- Calls that often require emergent/urgent referral to medical care:
  - Confused or too weak to stand
  - Signs of meningitis: fever, confusion, headache, vomiting, stiff neck, or rigid body in an infant, red or blood-colored flat rash
  - Signs of stroke: sudden-onset numbness or tingling, difficulty walking, talking, swallowing, or thinking

- When there are repeated calls within a 12-hour period (two or more), the caller's needs may remain unmet. Ask for more information than the standard protocol. What advice was given, what has changed, get specifics and reassess. Either the caller is not satisfied with the advice or the person is sicker than described.

- Consider the time of day. If the advice is to seek medical care in 2 to 4 hours and it is 11 pm, refer the caller to the ED. If it is Friday evening and the advice is to seek medical care in 24 hours, refer the caller to a clinic or ED that is open and available within 24 hours.

  Case example: At 1 am on a Saturday, a caller with a severe sore throat, fever, and difficulty managing secretions was told to keep his doctor's appointment on Monday morning. He did keep his appointment and was immediately sent to the ED, where he was found to be critically ill from a peritonsillar abscess and sepsis.

- Treat young mothers, teenagers, and young adults cautiously.

  Case example: A 17-year-old mother called in hysterics because her baby had a fever (felt warm) and was constipated (making grunting noises as though he needed to go to the bathroom but couldn't). She was uncooperative and wouldn't answer questions. The nurse talked to her sister and recommended a bath with baking soda to stimulate a bowel movement. The child expired from meningitis within 8 hours.

- Treat calls at the end of the day cautiously. Do not rush through them.

- Do not give advice without an opportunity for follow-up. Determine whether the caller agrees with the advice. If the caller does not agree or is not satisfied with the advice given, reassess. You may have missed something important to the caller.

- Ask the caller what he or she is going to do.

- Provide callers with an option to seek medical attention sooner if they do not agree with the advice or if their condition persists or worsens. Make sure callers know what "worse" means.

Documentation

The purpose of documentation is to provide a clear picture of the interaction and patient condition. It provides a permanent record that serves as a resource if the caller calls back or there is a lawsuit and the call needs to be reviewed. As the saying goes, if it was not documented, it was not done, was not important, or was not considered, and this would make it difficult to recall the encounter and support the decision-making process. Use the caller's own words as much as possible, applying "quotation marks." Show evidence that questions were asked, and document denials to rule out serious conditions. Documentation policy should describe whether the documentation process is by exception, omitting negatives, or by inclusion, including negatives.

Documentation elements should include the following whether it is an electronic record or handwritten document (See Appendix E1 (**679**) for sample documentation form.):

- Caller name and relation to the patient
- Date and time of call
- Demographics per policy
- Chief complaint
- Provider
- Description of signs and symptoms, onset, and duration
- Associated symptoms
- Relevant medical history
- Medications
- Disposition and advice given
- The protocol followed and recommended time frame to seek care
- Your name and title
- Time frame to call back if no improvement

Strategies to Help Ensure a Quality Telephone Triage System

- The top priority should always be patient safety.
- Use the medically approved protocols to establish a standard of care. Do not deviate from the protocols unless changes are made in writing and approved by the appropriate medical authority.
- Orient and train staff in telephone triage protocols, policies, and procedures; telephone encounter techniques; dealing with difficult callers; and documentation. (See Appendix I (**684**) for a sample training outline and Appendices J (**687**), K (**691**), and L (**693**) for training exercises.)
- Develop a mechanism to regularly review documentation and advice for consistency, accuracy, and quality. (See Appendices G (**682**) for a sample tape review and H (**683**) for documentation review forms.)
- Measure outcomes. Conduct regular consumer satisfaction surveys. Follow up promptly on problems and quality issues. (See Appendix D (**678**)

Through Direct Listening and Observation the Nurse Will Learn How to:

- elicit the caller's concern to select the appropriate protocol;
- recognize serious symptoms that should be directed to an urgent/emergent disposition;
- ask appropriate assessment questions to reach an appropriate disposition;
- review home care instructions to help callers manage their problems at home or before going to the doctor or ED;
- advise the caller when to call back or seek treatment;
- assure caller understanding and agreement with the advice and plan and what action the caller will take. If not in agreement, reassess;
- document the call.

for a sample survey form and Appendix L (**693**) for a skills assessment tool.)

- Use telephone triage to improve access to care, not to impede it. Follow up on all complaints concerning limited access to care.
- Follow up and review calls where staff fails to use protocols and relies only on nursing knowledge. Review caller concern, advice given, reason for deviating from a protocol, and outcome.
- Know your State Board of Nursing laws regarding medication advice. Laws vary from state to state.
- Research and review current events, such as local outbreaks of communicable diseases like pertussis, influenza, SARS, Ebola, and meningitis. Callers may hear about them on the news and have questions or be worried that they have been exposed. Telephone triage nurses can be the first to recognize an outbreak from the frequency and types of calls received.

Abdominal Pain, Adult

 Key Questions Name, Age, Onset, Medications, Pain Scale, Associated Symptoms, Date of Last Menstrual Period, Prior Medical History

 Other Protocols to Consider Abdominal Swelling (18); Constipation (160); Diarrhea, Adult (192); Food Poisoning, Suspected (262); Menstrual Problems (404); Rectal Bleeding (510); Urination, Difficult (624); Urination, Painful (628); Vomiting, Adult (642).

> *Nurse Alert:* Many conditions can cause abdominal pain, and some can be potentially life-threatening. Err on the side of caution when triaging callers with abdominal pain. Abdominal Pain: Causes and Characteristics: Appendix R (709) is provided to help the nurse gain a better understanding of the many conditions causing abdominal pain. It is NOT to be used to try and diagnose a caller's condition.

Reminder: Document caller response to advice, home care instructions, and when to call back.

ASSESSMENT	ACTION

A. Are any of the following present?

- Faint (unconsciousness) or unresponsiveness
- Severe weakness and inability to stand
- Cold, pale skin, or profuse sweating
- Severe, sudden pain radiating to back or legs

YES "Call ambulance"

NO Go to B

B. Are any of the following present?

- Lightheadedness
- Vomiting blood or dark coffee-ground–like emesis
- New onset of rapidly worsening symptoms and age >60 years
- Bloody or black stools unrelated to hemorrhoids or iron supplements
- Sudden abdominal and shoulder pain in a woman with menses >4 weeks late
- Age >30 years, heavy smoker, high blood pressure, high cholesterol, or obesity
- History of diabetes, heart disease, blood clotting problems, or CHF

YES "Seek emergency care now"

NO Go to C

C. Are any of the following present?

- Rapidly increasing pain
- Pregnancy
- Unusually heavy vaginal bleeding and possibility of pregnancy
- History of recent abdominal surgery, frequent falls, or injury to the abdomen
- RLQ pain with poor appetite, nausea and/or vomiting, or fever
- Ingestion of plant, drug, or chemical
- Temperature >101°F (38.3°C) and age >60 years, bedridden, or weakened immune system
- Temperature >103°F (39.4°C)
- Severe nausea and vomiting
- Persistent nausea and vomiting, and decreased oral intake and urination
- Pain worsens with coughing
- Taking antibiotics for diverticulitis or other abdominal condition and pain and fever worsens

YES "Seek medical care within 2 to 4 hours"

NO Go to D

D. Are any of the following present?

- History of hepatitis or exposure
- Continuous pain >1 hour
- Unexplained progressive abdominal swelling
- Painful or difficult urination
- Blood in urine
- Pain interferes with activity
- Age >60 years
- Nausea, vomiting, or diarrhea >24 hours

YES "Seek medical care within 24 hours"

NO Go to E

E. Are any of the following present?

- Vaginal or urethral discharge
- History of abdominal pain, and usual treatment is ineffective
- Constipation
- History of nervous stomach or irritable bowel syndrome
- Significant increase in stress level
- Intermittent mild pain associated with an empty stomach, eating certain foods, or use of pain, antibiotic, or anti-inflammatory medications
- Mild, infrequent diarrhea
- Other family members ill
- Recently started taking antibiotics for diverticulitis or other abdominal condition and abdominal pain persists for a few days

YES "Call back or call PCP for appointment if no improvement"
and
Follow **Home Care Instructions**

NO Follow **Home Care Instructions**

Home Care Instructions
Abdominal Pain, Adult

- Rest.
- Consume clear liquids (broth, tea, ginger ale, apple juice, flavored ice, gelatin) in frequent small amounts (sips) until vomiting or diarrhea subsides.
  - After 12 hours without vomiting or diarrhea, introduce a bland diet (rice, potatoes, bread, crackers, bananas, cereal).
- Take medications as directed by the pharmacy. Some should be taken on an empty stomach and others with food. Avoid aspirin, ibuprofen, and naproxen. Do not take acetaminophen if liver disease is present. Follow the instructions on the label, or as directed by the PCP in the elderly or those with liver or kidney problems.
- Apply heat (moist hot towel or heating pad) to the abdomen for cramping or discomfort, or take a warm bath. Do not sleep on a heating pad. Do not apply heating pad directly to the skin without a cloth barrier between heating pad and skin. Use caution in the elderly as the thinning skin burns easily.
- For gas relief, try Maalox or Mylanta, and follow the instructions on the label. Ask the pharmacist for other suggestions.
- Avoid alcohol, caffeine, and greasy or spicy foods.
- If taking antibiotics for diverticulitis 7 to 14 days:
  - Anticipate continued abdominal pain first 1 to 3 days.
  - Consume clear liquids (broth, tea, ginger ale, apple juice, flavored ice, gelatin) in frequent small amounts (sips) to give the bowel a chance to rest.
  - After 3 to 4 days, introduce a bland diet (rice, potatoes, bread, crackers, bananas, cereal).
  - Some antibiotics will decrease appetite or cause nausea with eating. Follow pharmacy instructions when taking meds with foods or fluids.
  - If abdominal pain not resolved within 4 to 5 days after starting antibiotics, follow up with PCP.
  - Once diverticulitis resolved, start high-fiber diet to prevent constipation as prescribed by PCP.
- If known GERD exists, encourage consumption of smaller, more frequent meals, and avoid spicy or greasy food, caffeine, and chocolate.
- Try herbal teas, such as peppermint or chamomile, to soothe an upset stomach.

Additional Instructions

Report the Following Problems to Your PCP/Clinic/ED

- Severe pain >2 hours
- Temperature >101°F (38.3°C) and age >60 years, bedridden, or weakened immune system
- Temperature >103°F (39.4°C)
- Persistent vomiting or diarrhea and decreased oral intake or urination
- Pain worsens with heat or activity

Seek Emergency Care Immediately If Any of the Following Occur

- Unusually firm or hard abdomen
- Persistent vomiting
- Severe persistent pain
- Fainting/lightheadedness
- Bloody or black stools or emesis

If the caller agrees with the advice given, document the call and encourage the caller to call back or see PCP if the problem worsens. If the caller does not agree with the advice given, reevaluate and advise the caller to follow up with PCP, Clinic, or ED.

Abdominal Pain, Child

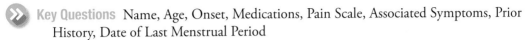

>> **Key Questions** Name, Age, Onset, Medications, Pain Scale, Associated Symptoms, Prior History, Date of Last Menstrual Period

>> **Other Protocols to Consider** Abdominal Swelling (16); Constipation (160); Diarrhea, Child (195); Food Poisoning, Suspected (262); Menstrual Problems (404); Urination, Difficult (624); Urination, Painful (628); Vomiting, Child (645).

> *Nurse Alert:* Many conditions can cause abdominal pain, and some can be potentially life-threatening. Err on the side of caution when triaging callers with abdominal pain. Abdominal Pain: Causes and Characteristics: Appendix R (709) is provided to help the nurse gain a better understanding of the many conditions causing abdominal pain. It is NOT to be used to try and diagnose a caller's condition.

Reminder: Document caller response to advice, home care instructions, and when to call back.

ASSESSMENT	ACTION

A. Are any of the following present?

- Severe persistent pain >2 hours
- Rapidly increasing pain
- RLQ pain with poor appetite, nausea and/or vomiting, fever, grasping abdomen, walking bent over, screaming, grunting respirations, or lying with knees drawn toward chest
- Unusually heavy vaginal bleeding and possibility of pregnancy
- Ingestion of unknown chemical substance, plant, or medication
- Recent abdominal trauma
- Black, bloody, or jellylike stools unrelated to hemorrhoids or iron supplements
- Weight loss
- Vomiting blood or dark coffee-ground–like emesis
- Weakness and inability to walk
- Severe pain and swelling in testicle(s) or scrotum

YES "Seek emergency care now"

NO Go to B

B. Are any of the following present?

- Severe nausea and vomiting
- Continuous pain >2 hours and unresponsive to home care
- Unexplained progressive abdominal swelling
- Painful or difficult urination
- Age <2 years and intermittent pain
- Pain interferes with activity
- Decreased urine output
- Nausea, vomiting, or diarrhea >24 hours and unresponsive to home care
- Known hernia or hydrocele and pain or crying >2 hours

YES "Seek medical care within 2 to 4 hours"

NO Go to C

C. Are any of the following present?

- Vaginal or urethral discharge
- History of abdominal pain, and usual treatment is ineffective
- Significant increase in stress level
- Blood in urine
- Temperature >101°F (38.3°C), cough, or weakness

YES "Seek medical care within 24 to 48 hours"

NO Go to D

D. Are any of the following present?

- Constipation
- History of a nervous stomach and increased stress level
- Intermittent mild pain associated with an empty stomach, eating certain foods, or use of pain, antibiotic, or anti-inflammatory medications
- Mild infrequent diarrhea
- Other family members are ill
- Persistent sore throat >24 hours

YES "Call back or call PCP for appointment if no improvement"
and
Follow **Home Care Instructions**

NO Follow **Home Care Instructions**

Home Care Instructions
Abdominal Pain, Child

A

- Rest.
- Consume clear liquids (fruit juice diluted with ½ water, weak tea, broth, sports drinks, flavored ice, gelatin, clear soft drink) or bland diet (rice, potatoes, soda crackers, pretzels, dry toast, applesauce, bananas) for 12 to 24 hours. Recommend electrolyte/mineral supplement or other rehydrating fluid solution (such as Pedialyte) for small children or infants.
- If diarrhea is present, avoid fruit juice or full-strength sports drinks.
- Take medications as directed by the pharmacy. Some should be taken on an empty stomach and others with food. Avoid ibuprofen and other anti-inflammatory medications. Do not give aspirin to a child. Avoid aspirin-like products if age <20 years. Avoid acetaminophen if liver disease is present. Avoid ibuprofen if kidney disease or stomach problems exist or in the case of pregnancy. Follow the directions on the label. Use the dosing device that comes with the medication, a measuring device, or a medicine syringe from the pharmacy. Household teaspoons often do not give the correct amount of medication.
- Apply a moist, hot towel or heating pad to the abdomen for cramping. Do not sleep on a heating pad. Do not apply heating pad directly to the skin without a cloth barrier between heating pad and skin.

Additional Instructions

Report the Following Problems to Your PCP/Clinic/ED

- Severe pain >1 hour
- Fever
- Pain worsens with heat or activity

Seek Emergency Care Immediately If Any of the Following Occur

- Unusually firm or hard abdomen
- Persistent vomiting
- Bloody or black stools or emesis
- Weakness and inability to walk
- Severe pain and swelling in testicle(s) or scrotum

If the caller agrees with the advice given, document the call and encourage the caller to call back or see PCP if the problem worsens. If the caller does not agree with the advice given, reevaluate and advise the caller to follow up with PCP, Clinic, or ED.

Abdominal Swelling

Key Questions Name, Age, Onset, Medications, Prior History, Pain Scale

Other Protocols to Consider Abdominal Pain, Adult (9), Child (13); Constipation (160); Diarrhea, Adult (192), Child (195); Gas/Belching (287); Gas/Flatulence (289); Rectal Bleeding (510); Swelling (597); Vomiting, Adult (642), Child (645).

Reminder: Document caller response to advice, home care instructions, and when to call back.

ASSESSMENT	ACTION

A. Is abdominal pain present?

YES Go to Abdominal Pain protocols; Adult (9), Child (13)

NO Go to B

B. Are any of the following present?

- History of recent trauma or abdominal surgery
- Vomiting blood
- New onset of black or bloody stools

YES "Seek emergency care now"

NO Go to C

C. Are any of the following present?

- Swelling developed suddenly within past 24 hours and is unrelieved by passing gas or vomiting
- Fever
- Painful or tender area does not disappear with pressure

YES "Seek medical care within 2 to 4 hours"

NO Go to D

A

D. Are any of the following present with no prior history?

- Swollen ankles
- Difficulty breathing, especially at night
- Decreased urine output
- Swelling decreases after passing urine
- New onset of yellow skin and eyes
- Painful or tender area disappears with pressures or enlarges with coughing

YES "Seek medical care within 24 hours"

NO Go to E

E. Are any of the following present?

- Persistent constipation
- Possibility of pregnancy and tender enlarged breasts, morning nausea, missed period >2 months
- Abdominal swelling in a female 1 to 5 days before or during menstruation
- Swelling associated with cramping, diarrhea, or constipation
- Swelling is slowly increasing throughout a 1-week period
- Rapid weight gain
- Increased flatus or gas

YES "Call back or call PCP for appointment if no improvement" and Follow **Home Care Instructions**

NO Follow **Home Care Instructions**

Home Care Instructions
Abdominal Swelling

- Drink an adequate amount of fluid each day as tolerated.
- Include fruits and high-fiber foods in daily diet.
- Establish a daily routine for bowel elimination.
- Avoid gas-producing foods such as onions, cabbage, and beans.
- Exercise regularly as tolerated.
- Eat more slowly.
- Take antacids for increased gas. Follow instructions on the label.
- Consider mild OTC laxatives, and follow the instructions on the label. Ask your local pharmacist for OTC laxative or stool softener product suggestions.

Additional Instructions

Report the Following Problems to Your PCP/Clinic/ED

- Problem persists >1 week
- Sharp or severe abdominal pain
- Abdominal pain, diarrhea, constipation, vomiting, or urinary retention
- Fever

Seek Emergency Care Immediately If Any of the Following Occur

- Black or bloody stools or emesis

If the caller agrees with the advice given, document the call and encourage the caller to call back or see PCP if the problem worsens. If the caller does not agree with the advice given, reevaluate and advise the caller to follow up with PCP, Clinic, or ED.

Abrasions

>> **Key Questions** Name, Age, Onset, Cause, Other Injuries, Medications, Pain Scale, Prior History

>> **Other Protocols to Consider** Foreign Body, Skin (278); Laceration (395); Puncture Wound (496); Skin Lesions: Lumps, Bumps, and Sores (556); Wound Healing and Infection (664).

Nurse Alert: Wounds are defined as clean or dirty. A wound is considered dirty if it is contaminated with dirt, feces, saliva, or soil; puncture wounds; avulsions; caused by flying or crushing objects, animal bites, burns, or frostbite.

Reminder: Document caller response to advice, home care instructions, and when to call back.

ASSESSMENT	ACTION
A. Are any of the following present?	
• Difficulty controlling bleeding • History of hemophilia • Large area of the body is affected	**YES** "Seek emergency care now" **NO** Go to B
B. Are any of the following present?	
• Unable to remove dirt or other foreign material from the wound • Source is dirty, and last tetanus shot was >5 years ago	**YES** "Seek medical care within 2 to 4 hours" **NO** Go to C
C. Are any of the following present?	
• History of diabetes • Difficulty moving affected part • Wound is 24 to 48 hours old, and signs of infection are appearing: redness, swelling, pain, warm to touch, red streaks extending from site, drainage or pus, or fever	**YES** "Seek medical care within 24 hours" **NO** "Call back or call PCP for appointment if no improvement" Follow **Home Care Instructions**

Home Care Instructions
Abrasions

- Apply direct pressure over the wound with a clean bandage or cloth to control the bleeding.
- Clean the wound daily with a soapy wash cloth and rinse thoroughly with water.
- Apply antibiotic ointment 2 to 3 times daily for several days. Follow instructions on the label.
- Cover wound with dry, clean dressing for 1 to 2 days.
- Check wound daily for signs of infection (redness, swelling, pain, warm to touch, red streaks extending from site, drainage or pus, or fever).
- If dressing sticks to the wound, soak with water.
- If wound is moist looking, allow wound to air dry for 5 to 10 minutes, then redress each day to promote healing.

Additional Instructions

_____

_____

_____

Report the Following Problems to Your PCP/Clinic/ED
- Signs of infection
- Delayed healing >1 week

If the caller agrees with the advice given, document the call and encourage the caller to call back or see PCP if the problem worsens. If the caller does not agree with the advice given, reevaluate and advise the caller to follow up with PCP, Clinic, or ED.

Alcohol Problems

>> **Key Questions** Name, Age, Onset, Drinking Habits (amount and frequency), Hours/Days Since Last Drink, Medications, Prior History, Other Ingested Substances, Street Drugs or Pills, History of Alcohol Withdrawal, Pain Scale (If injury occurred, see appropriate injury protocol.)

>> **Other Protocols to Consider** Anxiety (36); Confusion (150); Depression (184); Diarrhea, Adult (192), Child (195); Headache (308); Heart Rate Problems (320); Vomiting, Adult (642), Child (645); Seizure (531); Substance Abuse, Use, or Exposure (582).

Nurse Alert: Alcohol withdrawal can be life-threatening. Assess for signs of withdrawal, and refer for medical care urgently before symptoms worsen if there is a history of heavy drinking and a cessation of alcohol use >48 hours.

Reminder: Document caller response to advice, home care instructions, and when to call back.

ASSESSMENT	ACTION

A. Are any of the following present combined with a history of heavy drinking?

- Seizures
- New onset of auditory (voices, buzzing, clicks), sensory (bug crawling), or visual hallucinations or delusions
- Vomiting blood or coffee-ground–like emesis
- 24 to 48 hours after alcohol cessation and signs of withdrawal such as rapid or irregular heart rate, sweating, difficulty breathing, shakiness or tremors
- Extreme anxiety, sense of terror, agitation, or paranoia
  - Altered mental status (AMS)
  - Apnea or difficulty breathing
  - Pale, diaphoretic, and light-headed or weak
  - Suicidal or homicidal ideation
  - Unresponsive
  - Face, lips, or tongue blue or gray

YES "Call ambulance" or "Seek emergency care now"

NO Go to B

B. Are any of the following present combined with a history of heavy drinking?

- History of seizures or DTs with withdrawal in the past
- Desire to hurt self or other
- New black or bloody stools
- Acute anxiety
- Distorted perceptions
- Persistent vomiting >24 hours and unresponsive to home measures

 "Seek medical care within 2 to 4 hours"

NO Go to C

C. Are any of the following present combined with a history of heavy drinking?

- Upset stomach, diarrhea, heartburn, or difficulty sleeping
- Recent abrupt cessation of alcohol
- Request for help to stop drinking

YES "Seek medical care within 24 hours"
and
Follow **Home Care Instructions**

NO Go to D

D. After consuming a large quantity of alcohol, are any of the following present?

- Nausea, vomiting, or diarrhea
- Fatigue
- General ill feeling
- Headache
- 12 hours after alcohol cessation and mild tremors or anxiety, anorexia, nausea or vomiting, weakness, or body aches

YES "Call back or call PCP for appointment if no improvement"
and
Follow **Home Care Instructions**

NO Follow **Home Care Instructions**

Home Care Instructions
Alcohol Problems

- Keep the intoxicated person safe, do not allow to drive or prevent the person from engaging in risky behavior that could result in a fall or injury.
- Increase intake of fluids (nonalcoholic beverages) until urine is pale yellow, which is an indicator of proper hydration (may take as long as 2 days).
- Increase intake of fruit, vegetables, potatoes, rice, cereal, whole grains, eggs, meat, poultry, and dairy products.
- Take antacids as needed for indigestion. Follow instructions on the label.
- Take vitamin B complex supplements, and follow the directions on the label.
- Exercise daily.
- Get an adequate amount of sleep.
- Do not give aspirin to a child. Avoid aspirin-like products if age <20 years. Avoid acetaminophen if liver disease is present. Avoid ibuprofen if kidney disease or stomach problems exist or in the case of pregnancy. Follow the directions on the label. Do not take acetaminophen products with alcohol; doing so can lead to liver problems.
- If the caller requests a referral or help to stop drinking, provide telephone numbers of local resources for alcohol treatment programs, counseling, detoxification programs, inpatient and outpatient treatment programs, AA, and Al-Anon.

A

Referral Phone Numbers

Additional Instructions

Report the Following Problems to Your PCP/Clinic/ED

- No improvement or condition worsens
- Increased anxiety, agitation, or depression
- Persistent tremors

Seek Emergency Care Immediately If Any of the Following Occur

- Seizures
- Desire to harm self or other
- Black or bloody stools
- Vomiting blood or coffee-ground–like emesis
- Signs of withdrawal: rapid or irregular heart rate, sweating, difficulty breathing, shakiness or tremors
- Extreme anxiety, sense of terror, agitation, or paranoia
- Auditory, sensory, or visual hallucinations or delusions
  - AMS
  - Apnea or difficulty breathing
  - Pale, diaphoretic, and light-headed or weak
  - Suicidal or homicidal ideation
  - Unresponsive
  - Face, lips, or tongue blue or gray

If the caller agrees with the advice given, document the call and encourage the caller to call back or see PCP if the problem worsens. If the caller does not agree with the advice given, reevaluate and advise the caller to follow up with PCP, Clinic, or ED.

Allergic Reaction

 Key Questions Name, Age, Onset, Suspected Cause, Allergies, Prior History, Medications

 Other Protocols to Consider Bee Stings (72); Bites, Insect (79); Breathing Problems (106); Food Allergy (260); Hay Fever Problems (305); Hives (337); Itching (382); Piercing Problems (445); Rash, Adult (500), Child (505); Swelling (596); Tattoo Problems (604); Wheezing (657).

Nurse Alert: Signs of anaphylaxis, a severe life-threatening allergic reaction, can occur within seconds to an hour after exposure to the offending substance such as food, medication, and a bee sting. An anaphylactic reaction involves the respiratory, cardiovascular, and central nervous systems. Sudden onset of symptoms may include difficulty breathing, feeling faint, swelling of the tongue, throat or lips, hives, wheezing or coughing, or a feeling of impending doom. The sooner symptoms occur after exposure to the antigen, the more severe the anaphylaxis.

Reminder: Document caller response to advice, home care instructions, and when to call back.

ASSESSMENT	ACTION
A. Are any of the following present?	
• Difficulty breathing • Difficulty swallowing • Swelling of tongue, back of mouth, or throat • Inability to speak • Chest pain • Used EpiPen or epinephrine injection as instructed by the provider and symptoms have not resolved	**YES** "Call ambulance" **NO** Go to B
B. Are any of the following present?	
• Faintness or dizziness • History of previous anaphylaxis to same allergen • Change in vision • Confusion • Rapid progression of symptoms • Speaking in short words • Sudden onset of hoarseness • Swelling of the lips • Fast heartbeat • Used EpiPen or epinephrine injection as instructed by the provider and symptoms have resolved	**YES** "Seek emergency care now" **NO** Go to C

C. Are any of the following present?

- Swelling in face/extremities
- Persistent nausea, vomiting, diarrhea, or abdominal pain
- Persistent rash, fever, fatigue, or headache
- Speaking in partial sentences

YES "Seek medical care within 2 to 4 hours"

NO Go to D

D. Are any of the following present?

- Cause of reaction unknown
- Controlled nausea, vomiting, or diarrhea
- Mild rash/itching
- No respiratory problems
- Normal breathing
- Suspicion of medication reaction

YES "Call back or call PCP for appointment if no improvement" and
Follow **Home Care Instructions**

NO Follow **Home Care Instructions**

Home Care Instructions
Allergic Reaction

- Use prescribed inhalers, medications, or EpiPen for known allergic reaction as directed by PCP. If EpiPen used, should seek emergency care now as symptoms may return after the medication wears off.
- If symptoms occurred shortly after taking an OTC medication, discontinue use.
- Rest. Try to sleep in a cool room. Limit exercise or overheating to prevent increased itching.
- If hives are widespread, try baking soda or oatmeal baths, or OTC preparations (such as Benadryl, Caladryl, Cortaid, Cortizone, and Claritin) for the itching. Follow instructions on the label. Ask your local pharmacist for OTC product suggestions.
- Avoid hot showers. Heat can increase itching.
- Apply cold cloth or ice to small area of itchy hives to help reduce swelling.

A

Additional Instructions

Report the Following Problems to Your PCP/Clinic/ED

- Symptoms occurred after taking a prescription medication
- Symptoms persist after taking Benadryl and following **Home Care Instructions**
- Rash worsens
- Fever

Seek Emergency Care Immediately If Any of the Following Occur

- Difficulty breathing or swallowing
- Change in vision
- Confusion
- Chest pain
- Sudden onset of hoarseness and unable to speak
- Swelling of the lips, tongue, back of mouth, or throat
- Fast heartbeat
- Used EpiPen or epinephrine injection as instructed by the provider and symptoms have resolved

If the caller agrees with the advice given, document the call and encourage the caller to call back or see PCP if the problem worsens. If the caller does not agree with the advice given, reevaluate and advise the caller to follow up with PCP, Clinic, or ED.

Altered Mental Status (AMS)

 Key Questions Name, Age, Onset, Cause If Known, Medications, Prior History

Other Protocols to Consider Alcohol Problems (21); Breathing Problems (106); Chest Pain (123); Confusion (150); Dehydration (180); Diabetes Problems (187); Dizziness (199); Fainting (237); Fever, Adult (250), Child (253); Headache (308); Heart Rate Problems (320); Seizure (531), Seizure Febrile (533); Stroke, Suspected (576); Substance Abuse, Use, or Exposure (582); Urination, Difficult (624).

Nurse Alert: Signs of AMS may include confusion; irritability; less responsive to voice or touch; drowsiness; combative; uncooperative; nonsensical verbalizing; sudden change in behavior, thinking process, or ability to communicate; auditory (voices, buzzing, clicks), sensory (bug crawling), or visual hallucinations.

- AMS may be one of the first indicators of a UTI, dehydration, or a stroke in the elderly.
- In a child, AMS may be one of the first indicators of rapidly progressing meningitis or a head injury after trauma.

Reminder: Document caller response to advice, home care instructions, and when to call back.

ASSESSMENT	ACTION

A. Is the following present?

• Unconsciousness, not breathing	**YES** "Call ambulance and begin CPR"
	NO Go to B

28

A

B. Are any of the following present?

- Loss of consciousness more than once during the day
- Unresponsive at the time of the call
- Drug/alcohol overdose
- Difficulty breathing
- AMS and any of the following:
  - severe headache
  - chest pain/discomfort
  - rapid heartbeat
  - diabetic and unresponsive to home care measures
  - pregnancy, vaginal bleeding, or abdominal pain
  - severe abdominal pain
  - pain worsens upon sitting or standing
  - child with fever and rigid or flaccid body
- Persistent AMS
- Drowsiness and difficulty in arousing

YES "Call ambulance" and "Give person with diabetes and AMS immediate source of sugar" and
See **Home Care Instructions**

NO Go to C

C. If person arouses easily, are any of the following present?

- Headache, fever, or stiff and painful neck
- Recent head injury or trauma
- New seizure or prolonged postictal state
- Persistent high fever
- New onset of auditory (voices, buzzing, clicks), sensory (bug crawling), or visual hallucinations or delusions

YES "Seek emergency care now"

NO Go to D

D. Is the following present?

- Brief episode of loss of consciousness

YES Go to Fainting protocol (237)

"Seek medical care within 2 to 4 hours if no improvement" and

NO Follow **Home Care Instructions**

Home Care Instructions
Altered Mental Status (AMS)

- Keep person safely lying down until fully awake and responsive.
- Turn person on side if vomiting.
- Do not leave the person unattended.
- If a person has diabetes and experiences a sudden change in level of consciousness, give source of sugar immediately but only if the person is awake enough to eat or drink. Good sources of fast acting sugar include orange juice or other fruit juice, flavored drink mixes (such as Kool-Aid), regular cola, candy such as Life Savers or gummies, or a tsp of sugar or jelly.
- If event is alcohol or drug related, see also Alcohol Problems protocol (22) and Substance Abuse, Use, or Exposure protocol (581). For future assistance, contact local resources for assistance: counseling, detoxification programs, inpatient/outpatient treatment programs, AA, or Al-Anon.

Additional Instructions

Report the Following Problems to Your PCP/Clinic/ED

- No improvement or condition worsens

Seek Emergency Care Immediately If Any of the Following Occur

- Loss of consciousness >1 time during the day
- Difficulty breathing
- AMS and any of the following:
  - severe headache
  - chest pain/discomfort
  - rapid heartbeat
  - severe abdominal pain
  - pain worsens upon sitting or standing
  - child with fever and rigid or flaccid body
  - persistent AMS
  - drowsiness and difficulty in arousing
  - headache, fever, or stiff and painful neck

If the caller agrees with the advice given, document the call and encourage the caller to call back or see PCP if the problem worsens. If the caller does not agree with the advice given, reevaluate and advise the caller to follow up with PCP, Clinic, or ED.

Ankle Injury

A

>> **Key Questions** Name, Age, Onset, Cause, Medications, Prior History, Pain Scale

>> **Other Protocols to Consider** Ankle Problems (33); Bone, Joint, and Tissue Injury (95); Extremity Injury (222); Joint Pain/Swelling (390); Swelling (597).

Reminder: Document caller response to advice, home care instructions, and when to call back.

ASSESSMENT	ACTION

A. Are any of the following present?

- Bone is protruding through the skin
- Obvious deformity
- Foot is cold or blue
- Difficulty controlling bleeding

YES "Seek emergency care now"

NO Go to B

B. Are any of the following present?

- Severe pain
- Unable to bear weight
- Immediately unable to walk after injury

YES "Seek medical care now"

NO Go to C

C. Is the following present?

- Swelling, pain, or bruising continues to increase after 24 hours, despite use of ice, elevation, compression, and rest

YES "Seek medical care within 2 to 4 hours"

NO Go to D

D. Is the following present?

- Swelling, discomfort, bruising, limited movement, which occurred sometime after the injury

YES "Call back or call PCP for appointment if no improvement"
and
Follow **Home Care Instructions**

NO Follow **Home Care Instructions**

31

Home Care Instructions
Ankle Injury

- Apply ice pack to the injured area for 20 to 30 minutes every 2 hours for the first 24 to 48 hours after the injury. Do not place ice directly on the skin. Place a thin towel or sock between the ice pack and the skin. Unopened packages of frozen vegetables work well, as does crushed ice in a sealed plastic bag.
- Elevate the ankle as often as possible for the first 24 to 48 hours.
- When the person is up and active, the ankle should be wrapped with an elastic bandage or an air splint. If the toes begin to swell or tingle or become cold, numb, or painful, remove the bandage and rewrap loosely.
- Begin to exercise ankle after 24 hours or as tolerated.
- 48 hours after injury, apply heating pad or heat pack for 10 minutes, 3 times a day. Do not apply heating pad directly to the skin without a cloth barrier between heating pad and skin.
- Take usual pain medication for discomfort. Do not give aspirin to a child. Avoid aspirin-like products if age <20 years. Avoid acetaminophen if liver disease is present. Avoid ibuprofen if kidney disease or stomach problems exist or in the case of pregnancy. Follow the directions on the label. Use the dosing device that comes with the medication, a measuring device, or a medicine syringe from the pharmacy. Household teaspoons often do not give the correct amount of medication.
- Pain should improve within 3 days, swelling within 7 days. It may take up to 2 weeks to resolve.

Additional Instructions

Report the Following Problems to Your PCP/Clinic/ED
- Pain becomes intolerable
- Pain, swelling, or bruising worsens after 24 to 48 hours, despite home care measures
- Moving the joint or bearing weight becomes increasingly difficult after 24 to 48 hours
- No resolution after 1 to 2 weeks

Seek Emergency Care Immediately If Any of the Following Occur
- Foot becomes numb, cold, blue, or symptoms persist after removing bandage

If the caller agrees with the advice given, document the call and encourage the caller to call back or see PCP if the problem worsens. If the caller does not agree with the advice given, reevaluate and advise the caller to follow up with PCP, Clinic, or ED.

Ankle Problems

>> **Key Questions** Name, Age, Onset, Cause, Prior History, Medications, Pain Scale (If pain and swelling are related to a recent injury, see Ankle Injury protocol [32].)

>> **Other Protocols to Consider** Arthritis Problems (48); Bone, Joint, and Tissue Injury (95); Breathing Problems (106); Congestive Heart Failure (157); Extremity Injury (222); Foot Problems (265); Leg Pain/Swelling (398).

Reminder: Document caller response to advice, home care instructions, and when to call back.

ASSESSMENT	ACTION

A. In addition to ankle swelling, are any of the following present?

- Chest pain
- Coughing up blood
- Sudden onset of severe shortness of breath
- Ankle or foot is cold or blue

YES "Call ambulance" or "Seek emergency care now"

NO Go to B

B. Are any of the following present?

- Swelling and pain in thigh/calf
- Severe pain
- Inability to walk
- Fever
- Area over the ankle, calf, or thigh is hot or warm to touch or is red
- Sudden swelling in single leg/ankle

YES "Seek medical care within 2 to 4 hours"

NO Go to C

C. Are any of the following present?

- History of heart, liver, or kidney disease; cancer; recent illness; sore throat; skin infection; or leg surgery
- Use of new prescription medication
- Bilateral ankle swelling
- Severe pain in the joint or base of the big toe
- Skin over the joint is red and shiny
- Pregnancy with sudden weight gain

YES "Seek medical care within 24 hours"

NO Go to D

D. Are any of the following present?

- No improvement with home care
- Pregnancy
- Recent weight gain of >10 pounds
- Pain in other joints
- General ill feeling

YES "Call back or call PCP for appointment if no improvement" and Follow **Home Care Instructions**

NO Follow **Home Care Instructions**

Home Care Instructions
Ankle Problems

- Elevate legs on pillows so that the feet are higher than the heart. Do not place anything under the knees. Place pillows under the calves.
- Reduce salt in diet.
- Rest.
- Apply heat to area. Do not sleep on a heating pad. Do not apply heating pad directly to the skin without a cloth barrier between heating pad and skin.
- Do not massage area.
- Avoid sitting or standing for long periods of time. If such activity is unavoidable, move toes and calf muscles frequently, and wear full-length support stockings.
- Avoid tight clothing.

Additional Instructions

Report the Following Problems to Your PCP/Clinic/ED

- No improvement or condition worsens
- Increased pain
- Decreased mobility
- Fever

Seek Emergency Care Immediately If Any of the Following Occur

- Chest pain
- Shortness of breath
- Coughing up blood
- Ankle or foot becomes cold or blue

If the caller agrees with the advice given, document the call and encourage the caller to call back or see PCP if the problem worsens. If the caller does not agree with the advice given, reevaluate and advise the caller to follow up with PCP, Clinic, or ED.

Anxiety

 Key Questions Name, Age, Onset, Triggers, Medications, Prior History, Recent Drug or Alcohol Use or Cessation

 Other Protocols to Consider Alcohol Problems (21); Altered Mental Status (28); Appetite Loss, Adult (39), Child (42); Chest Pain (123); Confusion (150); Depression (184); Heart Rate Problems (320); Hyperventilation (350); Mental Health Challenges in Telephone Triage (720); Substance Abuse, Use, or Exposure (5); Suicide Attempt, Threat (585).

Reminder: Document caller response to advice, home care instructions, and when to call back.

ASSESSMENT	ACTION
A. Is chest pain present?	
	YES Go to Chest Pain protocol (123)
	NO Go to B
B. Are any of the following present?	
• Hallucinations (auditory, tactile, or visual) • Paranoia (unfounded distrust in others), new onset • Confusion, new onset • Suicidal threat or gesture	**YES** "Seek emergency care now" **NO** Go to C
C. Are any of the following present?	
• Palpitations • Inability to function • Extreme anxiety • Hyperventilation unresponsive to home care measures	**YES** "Seek medical care within 2 to 4 hours" For palpitations, see Heart Rate Problems protocol (317) **NO** Go to D

D. Are any of the following present?

- Profuse sweating
- Persistent upset stomach that interferes with activity
- Lightheadedness
- Drug or alcohol use/abuse
- Recent abrupt cessation of drugs (OTC or prescription), alcohol, or caffeine

 YES "Seek medical care within 24 hours"

 NO Go to E

A

E. Are any of the following present?

- Difficulty sleeping
- History of anxiety episodes
- Chronic history of drug/alcohol abuse
- Recent onset
- Intermittent episodes
- Contributing cause, such as stress; weight loss; use of medication (including decongestants or OTC herbal preparations), caffeine, or tobacco; or change in job, relationships, or finances
- No physiologic or psychological symptoms

YES "Call back or call PCP for appointment if no improvement"
and
Follow **Home Care Instructions**

NO Follow **Home Care Instructions**

Home Care Instructions
Anxiety

- If the cause is known, explore ways to eliminate or reduce causative factor.
- Reduce or eliminate caffeine, tobacco, alcohol, illicit drugs, or inappropriate use of stimulants, prescription medications, or OTC herbal teas or supplements.
- Increase sleep, rest, and relaxation time. Rest in a dark, quiet room.
- Take a long hot bath, shower or soak in a hot tub.
- Picture yourself successfully facing and resolving the concern or conflict.
- Increase exercise and regular activity, relaxation or visualization exercises, and deep breathing.
- Eat regular meals and a healthy diet. Focus on fruits, whole grains, and fish (or fish oil) as they may all help to reduce anxiety.
- Distract yourself watching television, a movie, reading a book, or other pleasant activity.
- Talk with a supportive person.

Additional Instructions

Report the Following Problems to Your PCP/Clinic/ED

- Symptoms related to prescribed medication
- Condition persists or worsens

Seek Emergency Care Immediately If Any of the Following Occur

- Risk of hurting self or other
- Hallucinations, paranoia, disorientation, or confusion

If the caller agrees with the advice given, document the call and encourage the caller to call back or see PCP if the problem worsens. If the caller does not agree with the advice given, reevaluate and advise the caller to follow up with PCP, Clinic, or ED.

Appetite Loss, Adult

 Key Questions Name, Age, Onset, Medications, Prior History

 Other Protocols to Consider Abdominal Pain, Adult (9); Alcohol Problems (21); Anxiety (36); Depression (184); Dizziness (199); Fever, Adult (250); Heart Rate Problems (320); Postoperative Problems (457); Substance Abuse, Use, or Exposure (5); Vomiting, Adult (642).

Reminder: Document caller response to advice, home care instructions, and when to call back.

ASSESSMENT	ACTION

A. Are any of the following present?

- AMS
- Fainting
- Abdominal pain
- Thoughts of suicide
- Hallucinations (auditory, tactile, or visual)

YES "Seek emergency care now" If abdominal pain, go to Abdominal Pain, Adult, protocol (9).

NO Go to B

B. Are any of the following present?

- Palpitations
- Fever >101°F (38.4°C) and weakened immune system or advanced age
- Known or suspected eating disorder, and persistent increase in dizziness and heart rate with sitting or standing

YES "Seek medical care within 2 to 4 hours"

NO Go to C

C. Are any of the following present?

- Sudden weight loss >5 to 10 pounds
- History of cardiac failure, extremity swelling, edema, cancer, viral illness, gastroenteritis, parasites, hyperthyroid, or bowel disease
- Lethargy
- Yellowing of the skin or whites of the eyes
- Fever >101°F (38.4°C) and unresponsive to fever-reducing measures
- Sudden weight gain >5 pounds
- Inadequate fluid intake
- Unexplained weight loss during a period of several weeks
- Severe depression
- Abrupt cessation of drugs (including prescription or OTC), alcohol, or caffeine

YES "Seek medical care within 24 hours"

NO Go to D

D. Are any of the following present?

- Poor eating habits
- Recent surgery
- Depression
- Increased stress/anxiety
- Recent onset of appetite loss
- No other symptoms
- Decrease in activity

YES "Call back or call PCP for appointment if no improvement" and Follow **Home Care Instructions**

NO Follow **Home Care Instructions**

Home Care Instructions
Appetite Loss, Adult

A

- Eat a balanced meal.
- Slowly increase amount of food after surgery or illness.
- Exercise regularly.
- May try liquid diet supplements (ensure, Boost). Ask your PCP or pharmacist for additional OTC liquid diet supplements.
- Try to identify the cause of the appetite loss, and take appropriate action to address the problem (poorly fitting dentures, mouth sores, nausea, depression, swallowing difficulties, recent surgery, chemotherapy, etc.).
- Provide reassurance that appetite loss is not unusual following surgery involving anesthesia, antibiotics, and multiple other medications. Talk to your surgeon or PCP about ways to improve appetite and slow down weight loss.
- Take usual medication for discomfort and fever. Avoid acetaminophen if liver disease is present. Avoid ibuprofen if kidney disease or stomach problems exist or in the case of pregnancy. Follow the directions on the label.

Additional Instructions

Report the Following Problems to Your PCP/Clinic/ED
- Nausea and vomiting
- Failure to improve

Seek Emergency Care Immediately If Any of the Following Occur
- AMS
- Fainting
- Hallucinations
- Thoughts of suicide
- Known or suspected eating disorder, and persistent increase in dizziness and heart rate with sitting or standing

If the caller agrees with the advice given, document the call and encourage the caller to call back or see PCP if the problem worsens. If the caller does not agree with the advice given, reevaluate and advise the caller to follow up with PCP, Clinic, or ED.

Appetite Loss, Child

 Key Questions Name, Age, Onset, Allergies, Weight, Medications, Prior History, Eating Disorder Treatment

 Other Protocols to Consider Abdominal Pain, Child (13); Altered Mental Status (28); Anxiety (36); Dehydration (180); Depression (184); Dizziness (199); Fever, Child (253); Heart Rate Problems (320); Vomiting, Child (645).

Reminder: Document caller response to advice, home care instructions, and when to call back.

ASSESSMENT	ACTION
A. Is the following present?	
• Abdominal pain	**YES** Go to Abdominal Pain, Child, protocol (13)
	NO Go to B
B. Are any of the following present?	
• AMS	**YES** "Seek emergency care now"
• Fainting	**NO** Go to C
• Vomiting, drowsiness, irritability, and headache or stiff or painful neck	
C. Are any of the following present?	
• Child refuses to eat or drink and looks ill	**YES** "Seek medical care within 2 to 4 hours"
• Known or suspected eating disorder, and persistent increase in dizziness and heart rate with sitting or standing	**NO** Go to D
• Signs of dehydration:	
• decreased urination	
• no urine for >8 hours in child <1 year of age	
• no urine for >12 hours in child >1 year of age	
• crying without tears	
• sunken fontanels	
• excessive thirst, dry mouth	

D. Are any of the following present?

- Unusual frequent urination or bed-wetting
- Nausea at sight of food, vomiting, yellow skin, fever, and fatigue
- Skin persistently pale
- Dark urine and pale stools
- Persistent decrease in appetite, swollen glands, and fatigue
- Poor weight gain
- Sudden weight loss
- Severe dieting or excessive exercise and distorted body image in a teenager
- Rash or fever

YES "Seek medical care within 24 hours"

NO Go to E

E. Are any of the following present?

- Poor eating habits
- Increased stress/anxiety
- Dry skin, brittle hair
- Recent onset of appetite loss

YES "Call back or call PCP for appointment if no improvement"
and
Follow **Home Care Instructions**

NO Follow **Home Care Instructions**

Home Care Instructions
Appetite Loss, Child

- Encourage a balanced meal.
- Do not force child to eat when sore throat makes swallowing difficult. Encourage consumption of ice cream, flavored ice, and cold fluids.
- Avoid putting too much emphasis on food when child is ill.
- Understand that it is normal for the child's appetite to decrease around 2 years of age.
- Slowly increase amount of food after surgery or illness.
- Give acetaminophen for fever. Do not give aspirin to a child. Avoid aspirin-like products if age <20 years. Avoid acetaminophen if liver disease is present. Avoid ibuprofen if kidney disease or stomach problems exist or in the case of pregnancy. Follow the directions on the label.

Additional Instructions

Report the Following Problems to Your PCP/Clinic/ED

- Nausea and vomiting
- Persistent appetite loss
- Persistent weight loss

Seek Emergency Care Immediately If Any of the Following Occur

- AMS
- Fainting
- Vomiting, drowsiness, irritability, and headache or stiff or painful neck
- Known or suspected eating disorder, and persistent increase in dizziness and heart rate with sitting or standing

If the caller agrees with the advice given, document the call and encourage the caller to call back or see PCP if the problem worsens. If the caller does not agree with the advice given, reevaluate and advise the caller to follow up with PCP, Clinic, or ED.

Arm or Hand Problems

 Key Questions Name, Age, Onset, Cause, Location, Medications, Prior History, Pain Scale

 Other Protocols to Consider Arthritis Problems (48); Bone, Joint, and Tissue Injury (95); Bruising (109); Chest Pain (123); Extremity Injury (222); Hand and Wrist Problems (301); Joint Pain/Swelling (390); Laceration (395).

Reminder: Document caller response to advice, home care instructions, and when to call back.

ASSESSMENT	ACTION
A. Are any of the following present?	
• Sudden onset of arm pain during or immediately after exertion • Chest pressure, chest pain • Pain radiates to the neck, jaw, and shoulder	**YES** Go to Chest Pain protocol (123) **NO** Go to B
B. Are any of the following present?	
• Deformity • Arm, hand, or fingers cold or blue • No pulse in affected arm • Sudden onset of weakness in one arm • Deep cut • Inability to move part of arm or hand beyond deep cut	**YES** "Seek emergency care now" **NO** Go to C

C. Are any of the following present?

- Inability to move joint above or below the injured area
- Severe pain
- Inability to use that affected part of the body
- Suspicious explanation, particularly in children
- Affected area is red, hot, painful, or swollen, but has no known injury

 "Seek medical care within 2 to 4 hours"

NO Go to D

D. Are any of the following present?

- Joint is painful or swollen, and movement is limited
- Swelling or bruising increased after 48 hours
- Pain, swelling, or discoloration occurred within 30 minutes of the injury
- Stiff neck and arm or hand pain, numbness, or tingling
- Pain in elbow, wrist, or finger joint when bending arm or hand
- Numbness or tingling in the hand, especially at night
- Following amputation of hand or arm 1 to 6 months after surgery, and new pain is below the site of the amputation

YES "Seek medical care within 24 hours if no improvement" and Follow **Home Care Instructions**

NO Follow **Home Care Instructions**

Home Care Instructions
Arm or Hand Problems

- Apply ice pack to injured area for 20 to 30 minutes every 2 hours for the first 24 to 48 hours after the injury. Do not place ice directly on the skin. Place a thin towel or sock between the ice pack and the skin. Unopened packages of frozen vegetables work well, as does crushed ice in a sealed plastic bag.
- Elevate the affected part higher than the level of the heart to help reduce swelling.
- Talk with provider about phantom pain after an amputation. There are a variety of treatment options, including medications, acupuncture, spinal stimulator, mirror box therapy, injections, implanted devices, biofeedback, and massage therapy.
- Rest the affected part.
- If there is no known injury, apply heat pack or towel soaked in hot water to the affected area. Wait 48 hours after an injury before applying heat.

Additional Instructions

Report the Following Problems to Your PCP/Clinic/ED

- Increased pain
- No improvement in pain or swelling after 48 hours
- No improvement in ability to use the affected part after 48 hours

Seek Emergency Care Immediately If Any of the Following Occur

- Arm, hand, or fingers are cold or blue
- No pulse in affected arm
- Sudden onset of weakness in one arm
- Chest pressure
- Pain radiates to the neck, jaw, and shoulder

If the caller agrees with the advice given, document the call and encourage the caller to call back or see PCP if the problem worsens. If the caller does not agree with the advice given, reevaluate and advise the caller to follow up with PCP, Clinic, or ED.

Arthritis Problems

Key Questions Name, Age, Onset, Cause, Location of Pain, Allergies, Medications, History, History of Arthritis, Type of Arthritis, Pain Scale

Other Protocols to Consider Ankle Injury (31); Ankle Problems (33); Back Pain (62); Bone, Joint, and Tissue Injury (95); Extremity Injury (222); Finger and Toe Problems (257); Hand/Wrist Problems (301); Hip Pain/Injury (334); Joint Pain/Swelling (390); Knee Pain/Swelling/Injury (393); Leg Pain/Swelling (398); Neck Pain (415); Pregnancy Problems (481); Shoulder Pain/Injury (549); Sickle Cell Disease Problems (551).

Nurse Alert: Use this protocol only if previously diagnosed and under treatment for arthritis and have questions about arthritis, or arthritis symptoms not responding to usual medications or treatment. The most common forms of arthritis include:

- **Degenerative Arthritis or Osteoarthritis:** progressive disease found mostly in the elderly. Affects the fingers, neck, hips, knees, and lower back. Generally caused by wear and tear or post-traumatic injury to the joints.

- **Juvenile Idiopathic Arthritis:** persistent arthritis not caused by trauma or infection for a period >6 weeks in children <16 years of age. Initially systemic onset with intermittent spikes of fever >39°C (102.2°F) for >12 weeks followed by a rash and joint pain up to four joints. Initial signs include limping and flulike symptoms.

- **Rheumatoid Arthritis (RA):** gradual onset of swollen, painful joints and fatigue for weeks to months. Symptoms are worse in the morning, start in small joints of hands and feet, then progresses to the elbows, and finally weight-bearing joints.

- **Septic Arthritis:** abrupt onset of pain, swelling, warmth, fever, and severe pain with movement of a single joint. Usually affects the knee, hip, shoulder, or ankle. Also common in IV drug users (IVDUs), animal and human bites, steroid use, bacterial, viral, or fungal infections. Septic arthritis requires emergent evaluation.

Reminder: Document caller response to advice, home care instructions, and when to call back.

ASSESSMENT	ACTION

A. Are any of the following present?

- Ankle swelling with chest pain, coughing up blood, or shortness of breath
- Dislocation or deformity
- Fingers or toes of affected part are cold or blue

 YES "Call ambulance" or "Seek emergency care now"

NO Go to B

B. Are any of the following present?

- Traumatic injury to arthritic joint with pain and impaired ROM
- Fever spike >102.2°F (39.0°C) >2 weeks, and rash or joint pain unrelieved by current prescribed medications
- Joint becomes unusable
- Sudden joint, calf, or thigh painful, swollen, warm, or red with no known injury
- Sudden onset of severe pain, fever, swelling, and warmth in a single joint

 YES "Seek medical care within 2 to 4 hours"

NO Go to C

C. Are any of the following present?

- Skin around the joint is red and warm
- Pain, swelling, or stiffness for 3 days or several times a month
- Joints tender to touch and difficult to move
- Fever and chills

YES "Seek medical care within 24 hours"

NO Go to D

D. Are any of the following present?

- Pain in other joints
- General ill feeling
- Sudden onset with no known injury
- Mild swelling
- Chronic pain unrelieved with home care measures

 YES "Call back or call PCP for appointment if no improvement" and Follow **Home Care Instructions**

NO Follow **Home Care Instructions**

Home Care Instructions
Arthritis Problems

- For relief of hand pain, try dipping hands in hot wax (paraffin) dips in the morning. Wax and warming devices can be found at pharmacies and medical supply stores. Warm water soaks and wearing cotton gloves at nighttime are also helpful in relieving discomfort.
- For newly swollen joint, apply cold pack or compress to area for 20 minutes. Place a towel or cloth barrier between the cold pack and the skin to prevent burning the skin. Cold packs may include purchased cold packs, bag of frozen vegetables, or bags of ice cubes.
- Apply heat to stiff joints to promote blood flow and relax muscles. Soak in hot shower or apply hot water bottle or heating pad to stiff joint. Use caution when applying heat and are diabetic. Do not fall asleep on a heating pad. May place a moist wash cloth in a plastic bag and heat in a microwave for 1 minute. Remove warm cloth from the plastic, wrap in a towel, and cover swollen or painful joint.
- Follow your PCP instructions for taking anti-inflammatory medications, such as ibuprofen, naproxen, and celecoxib as well as corticosteroids. These medications can help to slow the progress of joint damage, ease pain and stiffness, reduce inflammation, and prevent deformity.
- Some topical pain relievers are helpful with fewer complications affecting the digestive system. They may have a cold or hot sensation after application.
- Rest.
- Lose weight if overweight.
- Stay active with light-to-moderate exercise and stretch daily.
- Eating fish 2 times a week or more or taking fish oil (omega-3 fatty acid supplements) may help reduce RA symptoms.
- Ensuring adequate amounts of vitamin C each day through citrus fruits, strawberries, red peppers, and so on may help prevent RA and maintain healthy joints with degenerative arthritis or osteoarthritis.
- Consider an anti-inflammatory diet that may help to reduce RA symptoms: whole plant, low-fat, low-animal protein foods.
- Practice mind–body pain relief through creative visualization, meditation, aromatherapy, and daily stretching for a reduction in pain and stress.

Additional Instructions

Report the Following Problems to Your PCP/Clinic/ED

- No improvement or condition worsens
- Increased pain
- Decreased mobility
- Fever
- Fever spike >102.2°F (39.0°C) >2 weeks, and rash or joint pain unrelieved by current prescribed medications
- Joint becomes unusable
- Sudden joint, calf, or thigh painful, swollen, warm, or red with no known injury
- Sudden onset of severe pain, fever, swelling, and warmth in a single joint

Seek Emergency Care Immediately If Any of the Following Occur

- Ankle swelling with chest pain, coughing up blood, or shortness of breath
- Fingers or toes of affected part are cold or blue

If the caller agrees with the advice given, document the call and encourage the caller to call back or see PCP if the problem worsens. If the caller does not agree with the advice given, reevaluate and advise the caller to follow up with PCP, Clinic, or ED.

Asthma

 Key Questions Name, Age, Onset, Prior Asthma History, Severity, Peak Flow Measurement, Prior Treatment, Medications, Prior History, Suspected or Known Triggers

 Other Protocols to Consider Breathing Problems (106); Choking (135); Congestion (153); Fever, Adult (250), Child (253); Hay Fever Problems (305); Wheezing (657).

> *Nurse Alert:* Use this protocol only if previously diagnosed with asthma. Peak flow meters measure how well air is moving out of the lungs and help to gauge the severity of an asthma attack. Peak flow values are divided into three zones:
>   Green: 80% of baseline or higher (mild attack)
>   Yellow: 50% to 80% of baseline (moderate attack)
>   Red: <50% of baseline (severe attack)

Reminder: Document caller response to advice, home care instructions, and when to call back.

ASSESSMENT	ACTION

A. Are any of the following present?

- Persistent wheezing after a treatment
- Difficulty breathing or shortness of breath
- Inability to breathe lying down; must sit up to breathe
- Pain or tightness in the chest
- Dusky or blue lips, tongue, or face
- Sudden onset of wheezing after medication, food, bee sting, or exposure to known allergen or asthma triggers
- Weakness, listlessness, and restlessness
- Speaking in short words
- Peak flow rate < 50% of baseline
- Severe wheezing or cough, and nebulizer or inhaler not available

YES "Seek emergency care now" "If breathing difficulty is severe, call ambulance"

NO Go to B

B. Are any of the following present?

- Vomiting and inability to retain medication
- Upper respiratory infection symptoms and history of:
  - steroid treatment
  - prior hospitalization for same symptoms
  - intubations
- Speaking in partial sentences
- Peak flow rate 50% to 80% of baseline and no improvement using nebulizer or inhaler
- Nebulizer or inhaler used < every 4 hours

YES "Seek medical care within 2 to 4 hours"

NO Go to C

C. Are any of the following present?

- Fever >100.5°F (38.1°C)
- Cough unresponsive to medication
- Minimal or temporary relief of asthma symptoms with current medications
- Yellow or green sputum
- Peak flow rate >50% to 80% of baseline

YES "Seek medical care within 24 hours"

NO Follow **Home Care Instructions**

A

Home Care Instructions
Asthma

- Increase fluid intake; consume water and clear fluids.
- Treat symptoms early to decrease the severity of asthma attack. Use preventive medication as prescribed by PCP.
- Use a vaporizer, steamy bathroom, or cool damp air to help relieve symptoms.
- Follow treatment plan or management plan as prescribed by PCP for the use of peak flow meters, medications, and inhalers to best control asthma.
- Avoid aspirin products and decongestants.
- Shower every night to reduce pollen exposure.
- Limit exposure to pets, particularly in sleeping areas.
- Avoid smoky and dusty areas. Encourage smokers in the home to smoke outside.
- Avoid known triggers, such as, animal dander, body and hair products, perfumes, strong odors, tobacco smoke, air pollution, pollen, and cleaning solvents.
- If asthma symptoms are induced by strenuous exercise, take medication 90 minutes before activity (use inhaler 30 minutes before activity).

Additional Instructions

_____

_____

_____

_____

Report the Following Problems to Your PCP/Clinic/ED

- No improvement after medication
- Difficulty breathing
- Prescribed treatment plan is unclear
- Peak flow rate 50% to 80% of baseline
- Nebulizer or inhaler used < every 4 hours

Seek Emergency Care Immediately If Any of the Following Occur

- Breathing difficulty worsens
- Face, tongue, or lips become dusky or blue
- Pain or tightness in the chest
- Weakness, listlessness, restlessness
- Peak flow rate <50% of normal baseline

If the caller agrees with the advice given, document the call and encourage the caller to call back or see PCP if the problem worsens. If the caller does not agree with the advice given, reevaluate and advise the caller to follow up with PCP, Clinic, or ED.

Avian Influenza ("Bird Flu") Exposure

>> **Key Questions** Name, Age, Onset, Travel Within Past 10 Days to Suspect Location (known avian influenza infection in poultry or humans), Recent Contact With Poultry or Domestic Birds (poultry farm, a household raising poultry, or a bird market), Frequent Exposure to Dead Poultry, Recent Outbreak in Current Location and Possible Exposure, Medications, Prior History

>> **Other Protocols to Consider** Breathing Problems (106); Common Cold Symptoms (146); Congestion (153); Cough (170); Dehydration (180); Eye Problems (228); Fever, Adult (250), Child (253); Sore Throat (564).

> *Nurse Alert:* Use this protocol if exposure to avian influenza is suspected. Incubation period is 3 to 5 days. Bird flu normally infects birds, less commonly pigs and humans.

Reminder: Document caller response to advice, home care instructions, and when to call back.

ASSESSMENT	ACTION

A. Are any of the following present?

- Diaphoresis and lightheadedness or weakness
- Severe difficulty breathing
- Pale or gray face and prior diagnosis of viral pneumonia
- Confusion, delirium, or difficulty in arousing

YES "Call ambulance" or "Seek emergency care now"

"Notify caregiver of potential exposure"

NO Go to B

B. Are any of the following present?

- Probable or possible exposure to contaminated birds, including surfaces contaminated with secretions/excretions, and symptoms of conjunctivitis and fever, cough, sore throat, body aches
- Nonblanching dark red or purple rash
- Conjunctivitis after caring for a person with known avian influenza
- Child with fever >105°F (40.6°C)
- Adult with fever >103°F (39.4°C)
- History of immunosuppression, age >60 years, sickle cell anemia, diabetes, or bedridden and fever >101°F (38.3°C)
- Infant <3 months of age and fever >100.4°F (38°C)
- Signs of dehydration in the elderly or persons who are immunosuppressed

YES "Seek medical care immediately" and "Notify caregiver of potential exposure"

NO Go to C

C. Are any of the following present?

- Caretaker of person with known avian influenza and flulike symptoms or conjunctivitis
- Sore throat or fever >2 days
- Fever and history of asthma, cancer, COPD, CHF, diabetes, heart disease, or renal disease
- Green, brown, or yellow sputum or nasal discharge >72 hours
- Signs of dehydration

YES "Seek medical care within 24 hours"

NO Go to D

D. Are any of the following present?

- Green, brown, or yellow sputum or nasal discharge <72 hours
- Blood streaks in sputum
- Concern about potential exposure to avian influenza and no other (or mild) symptoms

YES "Call back or call PCP for appointment if no improvement" and Follow **Home Care Instructions**

NO Follow **Home Care Instructions**

Home Care Instructions
Avian Influenza ("Bird Flu") Exposure

- Individuals with flulike symptoms should stay home for 24 hours after last fever (except for doctor appointments).
- Caregivers should frequently wash their hands with soap and water or an alcohol-based hand rub after contact with the person or his or her environment, including laundry.
- Cover mouth and nose when coughing and sneezing, and dispose of tissue in a bag.
- Soiled dishes and utensils should be washed in the dishwasher or with warm water and soap.
- Take medications as prescribed.
- Take usual medication for discomfort and fever. Do not give aspirin to a child. Avoid aspirin-like products if age <20 years. Avoid acetaminophen if liver disease is present. Avoid ibuprofen if kidney disease or stomach problems exist or in the case of pregnancy. Follow the directions on the label.
- Cook all poultry to 180°F (70°C) throughout.
- Thoroughly cook all poultry (no pink parts) and eggs (no soft, runny parts of egg after cooking).
- Clean any surfaces exposed to raw poultry immediately with soap and water.
- Minimize exposure of other family members who are not ill.
- Be aware that there is antiviral medication to prevent or treat for low pathogenic avian influenza (H9N2).
- Avoid handling dead birds or touching surfaces contaminated with secretions/excretions.

A

Additional Instructions

_____

_____

_____

Report the Following Problems to Your PCP/Clinic/ED

- Caretaker develops flulike symptoms
- Sore throat or fever >2 days
- Green, brown, or yellow sputum or nasal discharge >72 hours
- Signs of dehydration
- No improvement or condition worsens

Seek Emergency Care Immediately If Any of the Following Occur

- Diaphoresis and lightheadedness or weakness
- Severe difficulty breathing
- Pale or gray face and prior diagnosis of viral pneumonia
- Confusion, delirium, or difficulty in arousing
- Chest pain

If the caller agrees with the advice given, document the call and encourage the caller to call back or see PCP if the problem worsens. If the caller does not agree with the advice given, reevaluate and advise the caller to follow up with PCP, Clinic, or ED.

Back/Neck Injury

 Key Questions Name, Age, Onset, Mechanism of Injury, Medications, Pain Scale, History

 Other Protocols to Consider Back Pain (62); Breathing Problems (106); Headache (308); Incontinence, Stool (364), Urine (366); Numbness and Tingling (431); Weakness (649).

B

Nurse Alert: Use caution with victims of high-risk mechanisms of injury; MVA, MCA, bicycle, and trampoline accidents; falls >10 feet; and skiing and snowboarding accidents. Spinal precautions should be taken and maintained until cleared by the hospital. If a victim needs to be moved for safety reasons, log roll, while protecting the head and neck from moving.

A neck injury should always be considered whenever there is a head injury or blow to the head. Look for weakness, incoordination, numbness, and neck pain. Altered mental status may be one of the first signs of a head injury after trauma, particularly in the elderly and children, and needs prompt medical attention.

Reminder: Document caller response to advice, home care instructions, and when to call back.

ASSESSMENT	ACTION

A. Did the injury result from a new traumatic event, and are any of the following present?

- Difficulty breathing
- Severe back or neck pain
- Inability to move fingers or toes
- Numbness, tingling, or weakness in arms, legs, fingers, or toes
- Incontinence of stool or urine
- Difficulty controlling bleeding
- Gunshot, knife, or other penetrating wound
- Signs of shock: lightheadedness, skin pale, cold or moist, excessive thirst, rapid pulse

 YES "Call ambulance"
"Support breathing"
"Do not move person"
Follow **Emergency Home Care Instructions**

NO Go to B

B. Are any of the following present?

- Traumatic event within past week and the following:
  - Worsening pain
  - Weakness or incontinence
  - Increasing or persistent numbness or tingling
  - Urinary retention >4 hours and bladder feels full
  - New onset of numbness around the rectum and groin

 YES "Seek emergency or medical care now"

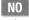 **NO** Go to C

C. Are any of the following present?

- Age >65 years
- History of cancer or bleeding disorder
- Pain interferes with activities

YES "Seek medical care within 24 hours" and
Follow **Home Care Instructions**

NO Go to D

D. Are any of the following present?

- Continued mild-to-moderate neck or back pain unresponsive to rest, heat, ice, and pain medications
- Mild-to-moderate neck or back pain and home care measures not initiated

YES "Call back or call PCP for appointment if no improvement" and
Follow **Home Care Instructions**

NO Follow **Home Care Instructions**

Home Care Instructions
Back/Neck Injury

Emergency Instructions

- Do not move injured person; keep the person warm.
- Apply sandbags, books, rolled magazines, sheets, or towels to both sides of the neck if a neck injury is suspected. Secure with tape from one support, across the forehead, to the opposite support.
- If the victim is in the water, support the body and neck as 1 unit until medical help arrives. Positioned at the head of the victim, the rescuer should extend his or her arms under the victim's head, neck, and shoulders, keeping the back and neck in a straight line. Do not allow the neck to bend forward, backward, or side to side.
- Do not remove penetrating object. Leave in place until evaluated by the hospital.
- Apply ice packs to the affected area for 20 minutes every 2 to 4 hours for as long as 48 hours after injury. Do not place ice directly on the skin; place a cloth barrier between the ice and the skin.
- After 48 hours, apply heat to the area for discomfort.
- Take your usual pain medication. Do not give aspirin to a child. Avoid aspirin-like products if age <20 years. Avoid acetaminophen if liver disease is present. Avoid ibuprofen if kidney disease or stomach problems exist or in the case of pregnancy. Follow the directions on the label.
- Use a heating pad on the affected area 20 to 30 minutes every 2 to 4 hours. Do not sleep on a heating pad. Do not apply heating pad directly to the skin without a cloth barrier between the heating pad and the skin.
- Rest. Limit activities until medically evaluated or pain subsides.

Additional Instructions

_____

_____

_____

Report the Following Problems to Your PCP/Clinic/ED

- Shooting pain into leg, buttocks, or arms
- Pain worsens
- No improvement in 3 days

Seek Emergency Care Immediately If Any of the Following Occur

- Severe headaches
- Tingling, weakness, or numbness in the extremities
- Bowel or urine incontinence of stool or urine
- Difficulty controlling bleeding
- Gunshot, knife, or other penetrating wounds
- Signs of shock: lightheadedness, skin pale, cold or moist, excessive thirst, rapid pulse
- Urinary retention >4 hours and bladder feels full
- New onset of numbness around the rectum and groin

If the caller agrees with the advice given, document the call and encourage the caller to call back or see PCP if the problem worsens. If the caller does not agree with the advice given, reevaluate and advise the caller to follow up with PCP, Clinic, or ED.

Back Pain

 Key Questions Name, Age, Onset, Cause, Location, Medications, Pain Scale, History

 Other Protocols to Consider Abdominal Pain, Adult (9); Back/Neck Injury (59); Chest Pain (123); Numbness and Tingling (431); Pregnancy Problems (481); Urination, Painful (628), Abnormal Color (631); Weakness (649).

Nurse Alert: Use caution triaging persons with back pain and no known injury. Back pain may be a symptom of a more serious condition such as infection in the spinal area, a pathologic fracture, disk herniation and cord compression, cancer in the spine, or a bleeding problem.

Reminder: Document caller response to advice, home care instructions, and when to call back.

ASSESSMENT	ACTION

A. Are any of the following present?

- Progressive weakness in legs
- New sudden onset of numbness or tingling in legs or feet or loss of bladder or bowel control
- New onset of numbness in the groin or rectal area
- New-onset, rapidly increasing pain, and age >60 years
- Dizziness, lightheadedness, or abdominal fullness
- Inability to urinate for >4 hours and bladder feels full
- Cool, moist skin
- Pain radiates to neck, shoulders, jaw, or arm

YES "Seek emergency care now" See Back/Neck Injury protocol (59) if recent back injury or traumatic accident has occurred

NO Go to B

B. Are any of the following present?

- Severe pain with blood in the urine
- Difficulty moving legs, feet, or toes
- Fever with nausea or vomiting in a female
- Sudden pain after a prolonged period of time in bed or a wheelchair, or if age >60 years
- New-onset, rapidly increasing pain, and age <60 years
- Pain radiates to the groin or genitals
- Known cancer and sudden onset of new back pain

YES "Seek medical care immediately"

NO Go to C

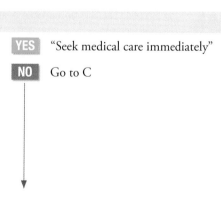

C. Are any of the following present?

- Pain radiates to buttocks or limbs
- Persistent severe pain
- Frequent urination or pain with urination
- Some difficulty walking because of discomfort
- No relief with OTC medications
- Fever with nausea or vomiting in a male
- History of trauma >48 hours
- History of diabetes, a weakened immune system, or steroid use
- History of cancer or unexplained weight loss
- Intravenous drug abuse
- Pain worsens at night or when lying down
- Blisters or rash and pain in same area
- Persistent loss of bowel or bladder control
- Persistent numbness or tingling in legs or feet

YES "Seek medical care within 24 hours"

NO Go to D

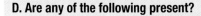

B

D. Are any of the following present?

- History of chronic back pain, back problems, back surgery, kidney stones, or renal disease
- Mild pain without radiation or limited movement
- Fever with flulike symptoms

YES "Call back or call PCP for appointment if no improvement" and
Follow **Home Care Instructions**

NO Follow **Home Care Instructions**

Home Care Instructions
Back Pain

- Restrict to light activities for 2 to 3 days.
- Use a firm mattress or place a board under a soft mattress.
- Avoid activities such as prolonged sitting, lifting, or jumping until the pain is resolved (do not stay in bed).
- Take your usual pain medication for discomfort. Do not give aspirin to a child. Avoid aspirin-like products if age <20 years. Avoid acetaminophen if liver disease is present. Avoid ibuprofen if kidney disease or stomach problems exist or in the case of pregnancy. Follow the directions on the label.
- If pain is related to an injury, apply ice packs for the first 24 hours, then moist heat. Do not place ice directly on the skin; place a cloth barrier between the ice and the skin.
  - Use moist heat (shower, tub, or moist hot towels) for 20 to 30 minutes every 2 hours for 48 hours, but only while the person is awake.
- Sleep in a fetal position with a pillow between your knees or on the back with one to two pillows under the knees to help reduce discomfort.
- For intermittent or chronic back discomfort, use a heating pad on the affected area 20 to 30 minutes every 2 to 4 hours. Do not sleep on a heating pad. Do not apply heating pad directly to the skin without a cloth barrier between the heating pad and the skin.
- May take a warm bath or shower or sit in a hot tub or whirlpool to help ease discomfort.

Additional Instructions

Report the Following Problems to Your PCP/Clinic/ED

- No improvement in 3 days
- Pain worsens
- Pain radiates into a limb, groin, or genitals
- Painful urination, frequent urination, fever, or blood in the urine

Seek Emergency Care Immediately If Any of the Following Occur

- New onset of persistent numbness or tingling in legs, feet, groin, or rectal area; loss of bowel or bladder control; or inability to urinate for >4 hours, and bladder feels full
- Persistent weakness in the limbs
- New-onset cool, moist skin, or pain radiates to neck, shoulders, jaw, or arm

If the caller agrees with the advice given, document the call and encourage the caller to call back or see PCP if the problem worsens. If the caller does not agree with the advice given, reevaluate and advise the caller to follow up with PCP, Clinic, or ED.

Bad Breath

 Key Questions Name, Age, Onset, Medications, History

 Other Protocols to Consider Diabetes Problems (187); Gas/Belching (287); Indigestion (368); Mouth Problems (407); Swallowing Difficulty (591); Tongue Problems (610); Toothache (613).

B

Reminder: Document caller response to advice, home care instructions, and when to call back.

ASSESSMENT	ACTION
A. Are any of the following present?	
• Breath smells fruity or ammonia like • Foul odor, accompanied by abdominal swelling and pain • Fever and sores in the mouth or throat • Severe pain in the mouth or tongue	**YES** "Seek medical care within 24 hours" **NO** Go to B
B. Are any of the following present?	
• Persistent gum bleeding or swelling • Persistent cough with foul-smelling sputum • Loose, missing, or decayed teeth • Frequent use of cast iron cooking utensils or dishes • Recent ingestion of a large dose of vitamins or minerals • History of gastrointestinal or chronic lung disease • History of chronic allergies or sinus problems	**YES** "Call PCP or dentist for appointment if no improvement" and Follow **Home Care Instructions** **NO** Follow **Home Care Instructions**

Home Care Instructions
Bad Breath

- Rinse mouth with antiseptic mouthwash, such as Listerine.
- Brush teeth or dentures, gums, and tongue twice a day and floss regularly.
- Remove and soak bridges and dentures daily.
- Decrease dosage of vitamins and mineral supplements if they are believed to be the cause of bad breath.
- Reduce use of cast iron cooking utensils (unless recommended by physician).
- Reduce ingestion of garlic, onions, alcohol, or coffee.
- See dentist regularly and as dental problems occur.

Additional Instructions

_____

_____

_____

Report the Following Problems to Your PCP/Clinic/ED

- Severe pain or fever
- No improvement or condition worsens
- Breath smells like fruit or ammonia

If the caller agrees with the advice given, document the call and encourage the caller to call back or see PCP if the problem worsens. If the caller does not agree with the advice given, reevaluate and advise the caller to follow up with PCP, Clinic, or ED.

Bedbug Exposure or Concerns

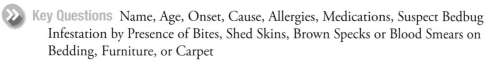

Key Questions Name, Age, Onset, Cause, Allergies, Medications, Suspect Bedbug Infestation by Presence of Bites, Shed Skins, Brown Specks or Blood Smears on Bedding, Furniture, or Carpet

Other Protocols to Consider Allergic Reaction (25); Itching (382); Lice (401); Rash, Adult (500), Child (505).

B

Reminder: Document caller response to advice, home care instructions, and when to call back.

ASSESSMENT	ACTION
A. With bedbugs visible, are any of the following also present?	
• Severe itching, blisters, or hives • Persistent rash and itch that interfere with sleep • Rash persists after 1 week of treatment • Sores spread or show signs of infection • Rash clears, then returns • Fever, malaise, or enlarged nodes • Allergic reaction to OTC or prescribed treatment medication	**YES** "Seek medical care within 24 hours" See Allergic Reaction protocol (26) if suspected allergic reaction to medication **NO** Go to B
B. With no bedbugs visible, are any of the following present?	
• Red or brown spots with darker or red center • Itching • Multiple spots on the skin in a line or cluster • New onset of flat or raised spots on the face, neck, arms, or hands • Undergoing treatment for bedbugs and has questions regarding medication or preventing the spread of bedbug exposure to others • Known or suspected exposure to bedbug infestation	**YES** "Call back or call PCP for appointment if no improvement" and Follow **Home Care Instructions** **NO** Follow **Home Care Instructions**

Home Care Instructions
Bedbug Exposure or Concerns

- If bedbug bites are suspected:
  - Inspect for insects at night when they are most active. Examine cracks or crevices in the walls, look between the mattress and box spring, and inspect upholstered furniture and behind the headboard of the bed.
  - Look for dark specks (bedbug excrement), empty light brown skins (shed before becoming an adult), and bloody smears on sheets (after bites).
- Treating the itch:
  - Apply hydrocortisone cream for short periods of time. Do not use longer than 3 days. Ask your pharmacist for product suggestions.
  - Apply cool compresses to the area. Soak cloth in ice water.
  - Take OTC antihistamine (Benadryl, Chlor-Trimeton) for severe persistent itching. Follow the instructions on the label. Ask pharmacist for additional product suggestions.
  - Apply baking soda paste, calamine lotion, or Aveeno to the affected area.
- Treating the home environment:
  - Hire a professional exterminator. More than one treatment may be necessary as bedbugs disappear into their hiding places after consuming a blood meal.
  - Vacuum furniture, carpets, mattresses, and box springs. Vacuum thoroughly all cracks and crevices in rooms and immediately throw away the vacuum bag in a sealed plastic bag and dispose of it outside in the trash.
  - Wash clothing and linens in hot water >120°F (49°C) to kill the bedbugs. Dry the wash on medium-to-high heat for 20 minutes to kill bedbugs and their eggs.
  - During warm weather months, place clothing and items that cannot be washed in a plastic bag outdoors or in a car parked in the sun with the windows closed for 24 hours.
  - Place infected items in a bag in the freezer or outside when temperature is below freezing for several days.
  - Consider discarding heavily infested items such as mattress, box spring, or couch.
- Preventing bedbug infestation:
  - Cover up as much skin as possible when sleeping.
  - Inspect second-hand items before bringing them into the home.
- Take hotel precautions: check the mattress seams for dark specks, bloody smears, and shed skins. Check the back of the headboard and cracks in the walls. Keep unneeded clothes in zipped luggage placed on top of dressers. Do not put luggage or clothes on the floor. For further protection, zipped luggage can be kept in the bathtub overnight since bedbugs cannot climb over the side of the tub.
- Remember that bedbugs are most commonly found in crowded lodgings with high turnover such as dormitories, hotel rooms, homeless shelters, and military barracks.
- Provide reassurance that there is no known evidence that bedbugs can transmit disease.

Additional Instructions

Report the Following Problems to Your PCP/Clinic/ED

- The rash disappears and then returns
- Signs of infection: redness, pain, drainage, or fever
- Questions concerning the medication for the ill, elderly, infants, children, or pregnant women
- Mild allergic reaction to the medication
- Rash itching >1 week after treatment

Seek Emergency Care Immediately If the Following Occur

- Severe allergic reaction to medication

If the caller agrees with the advice given, document the call and encourage the caller to call back or see PCP if the problem worsens. If the caller does not agree with the advice given, reevaluate and advise the caller to follow up with PCP, Clinic, or ED.

B

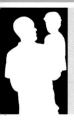

Bed-Wetting

 Key Questions Name, Age, Onset, Frequency, Medications, History

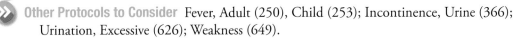 **Other Protocols to Consider** Fever, Adult (250), Child (253); Incontinence, Urine (366); Urination, Excessive (626); Weakness (649).

Reminder: Document caller response to advice, home care instructions, and when to call back.

ASSESSMENT	ACTION

A. New onset of bed-wetting in an adult or child and are any of the following present?

- Temperature >101°F (38.3°C)
- Pain or burning sensation with urination
- Urgency or frequency with urination
- Abdominal pain or back pain
- Blood or pus in the urine
- Nausea or vomiting

YES "Seek medical care within 24 hours"

NO Go to B

B. Are any of the following present?

- Bed-wetting has become more frequent
- The child has previously been dry for several months or years
- Child >3 years of age has daytime bladder control problems
- Child >3 years of age soils underwear with stool during bed-wetting
- Family history of bed-wetting

YES "Call back or call PCP for appointment if no improvement" and Follow **Home Care Instructions**

NO Follow **Home Care Instructions**

Home Care Instructions
Bed-Wetting

- Encourage daytime fluids, but limit what the child drinks 2 hours before bedtime.
- Do not punish child or force child to wear diapers at night. Use waterproof underwear and thick pads or plastic cover to protect the mattress.
- Reward the child verbally or by use of a "dry night" calendar or chart.

B

Additional Instructions

Report the Following Problems to Your PCP/Clinic/ED

- Bed-wetting occurs more frequently or becomes more severe
- Child is older than 6 years and shows no improvement after following Home Care Instructions for 1 month
- Temperature >101°F (38.3°C)
- Urgency, frequency, or pain/burning sensation with urination
- Abdominal or back pain
- Blood or pus in the urine
- Nausea or vomiting

If the caller agrees with the advice given, document the call and encourage the caller to call back or see PCP if the problem worsens. If the caller does not agree with the advice given, reevaluate and advise the caller to follow up with PCP, Clinic, or ED.

Bee Stings

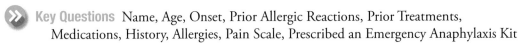

>> **Key Questions** Name, Age, Onset, Prior Allergic Reactions, Prior Treatments, Medications, History, Allergies, Pain Scale, Prescribed an Emergency Anaphylaxis Kit

>> **Other Protocols to Consider** Allergic Reaction (25); Bites, Insect (79); Itching (382); Rash, Adult (500), Child (505); Wound Healing and Infection (664).

> *Nurse Alert:* Signs of anaphylaxis, a severe life-threatening allergic reaction, can occur within seconds to an hour after exposure to the bee sting. Sudden onset of symptoms may include difficulty breathing; feeling faint; swelling of the tongue, throat, or lips; hives; wheezing or coughing; or a feeling of impending doom. The sooner the symptoms occur after exposure to the antigen, the more severe the anaphylaxis.
>
> - If prescribed an emergency anaphylaxis kit (EpiPen), instruct to use as directed by provider. Injections into outer upper thigh are usually most effective. See Emergency Home Care Instructions for additional information.

Reminder: Document caller response to advice, home care instructions, and when to call back.

ASSESSMENT	ACTION

A. Is the person unconscious or collapsed after a bee sting?

YES	"Call ambulance"
NO	Go to B

B. Is there difficulty breathing or swallowing?

YES	"Call ambulance" and Follow **Emergency Home Care Instructions**
NO	Go to C

C. Are any of the following present?

- A history of a serious bee sting reaction, such as difficulty breathing or loss of consciousness
- Bee sting in the mouth
- Swelling of the tongue, throat, or lips
- Used epinephrine injection as instructed and symptoms have improved

YES "Seek emergency care now" and
Follow **Emergency Home Care Instructions**

NO Go to D

D. Are any of the following present?

- Generalized hives unresponsive to home care measures
- Itching or a rash on parts of the body other than the area surrounding the sting site, and condition is unresponsive to home care measures
- Nausea, vomiting, or weakness
- >10 stings
- Signs of infection (drainage, fever, red streaks, or pus) >24 hours after the sting

YES "Seek medical care within 2 to 4 hours" and
Follow **Home Care Instructions**

NO Go to E

E. Is there a localized reaction, such as swelling, pain, or itching, around the sting site?

YES Follow **Home Care Instructions**

NO Follow **Home Care Instructions**

B

Home Care Instructions
Bee Stings

Emergency Instructions

- Use emergency bee sting kit if previously instructed in use.
  - Go to the emergency department even if symptoms improved.
  - After the medication wears off, the symptoms may return requiring additional medication.
- Take OTC antihistamine (Benadryl) to reduce allergic reaction and itching. Follow instructions on the label.
- Remove all jewelry on the affected extremity.
- If hands or feet swell because of a local sting, keep the extremities elevated to help decrease swelling.
- If stinger is still present, remove quickly to minimize exposure to venom in the stinger. Removal methods include the following:
  - Scrape the site until all of stinger is removed using a credit card, finger nails, or other flat surface.
  - Apply adhesive tape over the site and quickly pull up and off.
  - DO NOT squeeze the stinger and push more venom into the wound.
  - Wash the site with soap and water.
- May try folk home remedy. Make a paste of water and meat tenderizer and apply to the wound for 10 minutes. Do not apply meat tenderizer near eyes.
- Apply cold or ice pack to the sting site for the first 24 to 48 hours, then apply warm soaks. (Swelling may be worse on the second day.) Do not place ice directly on the skin; place a cloth barrier between the ice and the skin. Pain, redness, swelling, and warmth are expected immediate reactions.
- Take your usual pain medication and follow instructions on the label. Do not give aspirin to a child. Avoid aspirin-like products if age <20 years. Avoid acetaminophen if liver disease is present. Avoid ibuprofen if kidney disease or stomach problems exist or in the case of pregnancy. Follow the directions on the label.
- Take OTC antihistamine (Benadryl) for itching, rash, or hives and follow instructions on the label. May cause drowsiness. Ask pharmacist for additional product suggestions.
- Apply underarm deodorant or witch hazel to the site to help reduce itching.
- Watch for signs of infection during the next few days.

Prevention: To help keep bees away from outdoor dining areas, place fabric softener towels or wasp or yellow jacket traps around the perimeter of the area.

Additional Instructions

Report the Following Problems to Your PCP/Clinic/ED

- Nausea, vomiting, or weakness occurs within 24 hours
- Fever, headache, hives, swollen glands, spreading or streaking redness, or joint pain occur after 24 hours
- Persistent pain and swelling at the sting site or foul-smelling drainage from wound after 48 hours
- No tetanus immunization, immunization status unknown, or last tetanus immunization >5 years ago
- Itching or a rash on parts of the body other than the area surrounding the sting site occurs within 24 hours

B

If the caller agrees with the advice given, document the call and encourage the caller to call back or see PCP if the problem worsens. If the caller does not agree with the advice given, reevaluate and advise the caller to follow up with PCP, Clinic, or ED.

Bites, Animal/Human

Key Questions Name, Age, Onset, Cause, Location of Bite, Tetanus Status, Type of Animal, Immunization Status of the Animal, Medications, Pain Scale, History

Other Protocols to Consider Bleeding, Severe (90); Blood/Body Fluid Exposure (93); Domestic Abuse (202); HIV Exposure (340); Immunization, Tetanus (355); Laceration (395); Puncture Wound (496); Wound Healing and Infection (664).

Nurse Alert: Large dogs can inflict the most serious wounds, resulting in a crushing-type wound causing damage to vessels, tendons, muscles, nerves, and bones. Cat bites are at high risk for infection due to puncture wounds caused by sharp pointed teeth pushing bacteria deep into the tissue. Hand bites have the highest rate of infection due to the relatively poor blood supply of many structures in the hand. Local infections and cellulitis are the leading causes of morbidity from bite wounds and can potentially lead to sepsis, particularly in immunocompromised individuals. Unprovoked bites from wild or sick-appearing animals (dogs, cats, skunks, bats, and raccoons) raise concern for rabies exposure.

Reminder: Document caller response to advice, home care instructions, and when to call back.

ASSESSMENT	ACTION

A. Is the following present?

- Difficulty breathing

YES "Call ambulance"

NO Go to B

B. Are any of the following present?

- Difficulty controlling bleeding with direct pressure
- Deformity or inability to use affected limb
- Head, face, neck, or hand laceration
- History of hemophilia

YES "Seek emergency care now"

NO Go to C

C. Are any of the following present?

- Animal is not immunized for rabies
- Animal is not available for observation
- Laceration to arms, legs, or trunk
- Signs of infection: redness, pain, swelling, red streaks from the wound, drainage, or pus
- Cat bite
- Puncture wound

YES "Seek medical care within 2 to 4 hours"

NO Go to D

D. Are any of the following present?

- No tetanus immunization, immunization status unknown, or last tetanus immunization >5 years ago
- Fever
- History of diabetes or immunosuppression

YES "Seek medical care within 24 hours"

NO Go to E

E. Are any of the following present?

- Small laceration/abrasion/puncture wound

YES "Call back or call PCP if no improvement within 24 to 48 hours"
and
Follow **Home Care Instructions**

NO Follow **Home Care Instructions**

B

Home Care Instructions
Bites, Animal/Human

- Clean the area daily with a soapy cloth and rinse well with water.
- Apply your usual antibiotic ointment (e.g., Mycitracin Triple Antibiotic [bacitracin, neomycin, and polymyxin B], Neosporin, Polysporin) 3 times a day, following instructions on the label. Ask pharmacist for additional product suggestions.
- Cover the wound with a clean, dry dressing for 2 days, then leave the wound open to the air, unless it is oozing blood.
- If the dressing sticks to the wound, rinse with water.
- If the wound looks moist, allow the wound to air-dry for 5 to 10 minutes, then redress it to promote healing.
- Apply ice pack for swelling during the first 24 hours. Apply heat to the area after 24 hours. Do not place ice directly on the skin; place a cloth barrier between the ice and the skin.
- Check wound daily for signs of infection. Cat and human bites become infected easily.
- Observe animal for 2 weeks for signs of rabies or illness.
- Report animal bites to animal control or appropriate authority.
- Report bat and skunk bites.
- Report dog and cat bites when the following occurs:
  - Animal is sick
  - Bite is unprovoked
  - Animal is a stray
  - There is no indication of rabies vaccination
  - Circumstances surrounding the injury are suspicious or unclear/uncertain

Additional Instructions

Report the Following Problems to Your PCP/Clinic/ED

- Signs of infection: increased pain, redness, swelling, fever, red streaks from wound, or drainage
- No improvement in 24 to 48 hours
- Sensation of foreign matter in the wound

If the caller agrees with the advice given, document the call and encourage the caller to call back or see PCP if the problem worsens. If the caller does not agree with the advice given, reevaluate and advise the caller to follow up with PCP, Clinic, or ED.

Bites, Insect

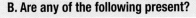 **Key Questions** Name, Age, Onset, Type of Insect, Allergies, Location of Bite, Medications, Pain Scale, History, Prescribed an Emergency Anaphylaxis Kit

 Other Protocols to Consider Allergic Reaction (25); Bedbug Exposure or Concerns (67); Bee Stings (72); Bites, Tick (87); Hives (337); Itching (382); Rash, Adult (500), Child (505); West Nile Virus (653); Wound Healing and Infection (664).

Nurse Alert: Signs of anaphylaxis, a severe life-threatening allergic reaction, can occur within seconds to an hour after a sting/bite and include difficulty breathing; feeling faint; swelling of the tongue, throat, or lips; hives; wheezing or coughing; or a sense of impending doom. The sooner the symptoms occur after exposure to the antigen, the more severe the anaphylaxis.

- If prescribed an emergency anaphylaxis kit, instruct to use as directed by provider. Injections into outer upper thigh are usually most effective. See Emergency Home Care Instructions for additional information.
- If stinger is present, remove as quickly as possible to decrease toxin exposure.

Reminder: Document caller response to advice, home care instructions, and when to call back.

ASSESSMENT	ACTION
A. Are any of the following present?	
• Chest tightness or difficulty breathing or swallowing	**YES** "Call ambulance"
	NO Go to B
B. Are any of the following present?	
• History of severe allergic reaction to same insect • Bite is from a brown recluse or black widow spider • Altered mental status • Sudden onset of sweating and pale skin after the bite or sting • Swollen tongue, throat, or lips • Bee sting in the mouth • Scorpion bite	**YES** "Seek emergency care now" or "If the person has collapsed, is unconscious, or is in severe respiratory distress, call ambulance" and Follow **Emergency Home Care Instructions**
	NO Go to C

C. Are any of the following present?

- Sudden onset of hives, rash, itching, or swelling in areas other than the sting site
- Muscle stiffness, abdominal pain, and restlessness
- Nausea, vomiting, or abdominal cramping
- Multiple stings
- Drainage, fever, red streaks, or pus in addition to redness and swelling
- Severe pain

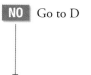 "Seek medical care within 2 to 4 hours"

NO Go to D

D. Are any of the following present?

- Headache, chills, fever, or sweating
- Unable or unwilling to remove stinger or tick
- Peeling skin at or near the site
- Increasing redness/swelling at the site >48 hours after bite
- Diabetic and bite or sting on foot

 "Seek medical care within 24 hours"

NO Go to E

E. Are any of the following present?

- Persistent discomfort, itching, redness, swelling, or rash
- No tetanus immunization, immunization status unknown, or last tetanus immunization >5 years ago

YES "Seek medical care within 24 to 48 hours"
and
Follow **Home Care Instructions**

NO Follow **Home Care Instructions**

Home Care Instructions
Bites, Insect

Emergency Instructions for Known Allergic Reaction

- Use emergency epinephrine kit if previously instructed in use of kit and take OTC antihistamine (Benadryl).
- Go to the emergency department even if symptoms improved.
- After the medication wears off, the symptoms may return requiring additional medication.
- Remove entire tick promptly. Avoid crushing or squeezing. (See Bites, Tick (87), for tick removal instructions.)
- If stinger is still present, quickly remove by scraping the site until all of stinger is removed, applying adhesive tape and pulling up and off the site, or using fingernails to grasp and pull the stinger out. Wash the site with soap and water. Do not pluck or squeeze the stinger.
- Apply meat tenderizer paste to the site for 10 minutes. Do not use meat tenderizer near the eyes.
- Wash the site with mild soap and water.
- Expect initial swelling at the site. Apply cold compresses or ice packs for the first 24 hours, then warm soaks as needed. Do not place ice directly on the skin; place a cloth barrier between the ice and the skin.
- Apply underarm deodorant or witch hazel to the site to help decrease itching.
- Try home remedy for itching: apply baking soda paste mixed with white vinegar to the itchy area.
- Take usual OTC pain reliever (aspirin, acetaminophen, ibuprofen) for discomfort. Do not give aspirin to a child. Avoid aspirin-like products if age <20 years. Avoid acetaminophen if liver disease is present. Avoid ibuprofen if kidney disease or stomach problems exist or in the case of pregnancy. Follow the directions on the label.
- Take an OTC antihistamine (Benadryl) for itching, rash, or hives and follow instructions on the label. Ask pharmacist for additional product suggestions.
- Observe for signs of allergic reaction, such as increased rash, swelling in other areas of the body, difficulty breathing, or swelling of the throat.
- Watch for signs of infection: increased pain, redness, swelling, warmth, red streaks, drainage, or fever occurring approximately 48 hours after the bite or sting.
- Remember that pain, redness, swelling, and warmth immediately after the bite or sting are usually a reaction to the venom and should be expected.
- If black widow or brown recluse spider bite is suspected, collect the spider in a jar and present it for proper identification.
- If black widow or scorpion bite is suspected, apply ice pack to site for 20 minutes to reduce the spread of venom. Do not place ice directly on the skin; place a cloth barrier between the ice and the skin.

B

Additional Instructions

Report the Following Problems to Your PCP/Clinic/ED

- No improvement or condition worsens
- Signs of infection or allergic reaction
- Rash, fever, headache, or joint pain after a tick bite
- Hives, muscle spasms, muscle weakness, or abdominal cramping

Seek Emergency Care Immediately If Any of the Following Occur

- Altered mental status
- Difficulty breathing or swallowing (call ambulance)
- Chest tightness
- Swollen lips/tongue/throat

If the caller agrees with the advice given, document the call and encourage the caller to call back or see PCP if the problem worsens. If the caller does not agree with the advice given, reevaluate and advise the caller to follow up with PCP, Clinic, or ED.

Bites, Marine Animal

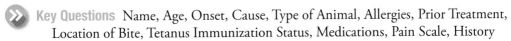

>> **Key Questions** Name, Age, Onset, Cause, Type of Animal, Allergies, Prior Treatment, Location of Bite, Tetanus Immunization Status, Medications, Pain Scale, History

>> **Other Protocols to Consider** Allergic Reaction (25); Laceration (395); Puncture Wound (496); Wound Healing and Infection (664).

Reminder: Document caller response to advice, home care instructions, and when to call back.

ASSESSMENT	ACTION

A. In addition to a jellyfish or other marine animal sting, are any of the following present?

- Faintness, dizziness, or confusion
- Changes in vision
- Chest tightness, difficulty breathing or swallowing, and swollen lips or tongue
- Previous history of severe systemic allergic reaction to the same animal sting or bite
- Sudden onset of sweating and pale skin after the bite or sting
- Fast/irregular heartbeat

YES "Seek emergency care now"
or
"If the person has collapsed, is unconscious, or is in severe respiratory distress, call ambulance"

NO Go to B

B. Are any of the following present?

- Sudden onset of hives
- Stung by a Portuguese man-of-war jellyfish or stingray
- Entire arm or leg is swollen
- Severe pain interferes with activity
- Dirty or serious wound and tetanus immunization status >5 years

YES "Seek medical care within 2 to 4 hours"

NO Go to C

C. Are any of the following present?

- Pain, redness, swelling at the sting site
- Stinger still present
- No tetanus immunization, immunization status unknown, or last tetanus immunization >5 years ago

YES "Call back or call PCP if no improvement"
Follow **Home Care Instructions**

NO Follow **Home Care Instructions**

Home Care Instructions
Bites, Marine Animal

- For the following marine spine punctures, immerse injured part in hot water for 30 to 90 minutes for pain relief:
  - catfish, cone shells, scorpion fish, sea urchins, sharks, stingrays, certain starfish, stone fish, and surgeonfish.
- Man-of-war and jellyfish: do not scrape stingers off or use ice. Douse stingers with vinegar and pluck off with tweezers. Use sting-no-more. Heat is effective at minimizing damage. Do not rinse with sea water.
- Leeches: apply salt, alcohol, or vinegar to remove.
- Do not rub area.
- Apply to the sting site a solution of vinegar, baking soda, or meat tenderizer dissolved in water.
- Do not touch stinger with bare hand.
- Apply calamine lotion or hydrocortisone cream to help relieve pain and itching. Follow instructions on the label.

Additional Instructions

Report the Following Problems to Your PCP/Clinic/ED

- Signs of infection, including increased or spreading redness, pain, swelling, drainage, or warmth
- No improvement or condition worsens

Seek Emergency Care Immediately If Any of the Following Occur

- Faintness, dizziness, or confusion
- Changes in vision
- Chest tightness or difficulty breathing or swallowing
- Sudden onset of sweating and pale skin after the bite or sting
- Fast/irregular heart beat

If the caller agrees with the advice given, document the call and encourage the caller to call back or see PCP if the problem worsens. If the caller does not agree with the advice given, reevaluate and advise the caller to follow up with PCP, Clinic, or ED.

Bites, Snake

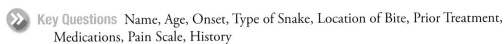 **Key Questions** Name, Age, Onset, Type of Snake, Location of Bite, Prior Treatment, Medications, Pain Scale, History

Other Protocols to Consider Allergic Reaction (25); Laceration (395); Puncture Wound (496); Wound Healing and Infection (664).

B

Reminder: Document caller response to advice, home care instructions, and when to call back.

ASSESSMENT	ACTION

A. Are any of the following present?

- Bite from a poisonous snake: rattlesnake, copperhead, water moccasin, or coral snake
- Chest tightness or difficulty breathing or swallowing
- Purple rash, fever, numbness and tingling around the mouth, pale skin, or sweating after the bite

YES "Call ambulance"

NO Go to B

B. Are any of the following present?

- Puncture wound or fang marks from an unidentified snake
- History of a reaction to a snake bite
- Change in mental status

YES "If the person has collapsed or is unconscious, call ambulance"
or
"Seek emergency care now"
and
Follow **Home Care Instructions**

NO Go to C

C. Are any of the following present?

- Sudden onset of hives, rash, itching, or swelling in areas other than the bite site
- Multiple bites from a nonpoisonous snake
- Signs of infection at the bite site: redness, swelling, drainage, fever, red streaks, or warmth
- Severe pain and swelling around the wound
- No tetanus immunization, immunization status unknown, or last tetanus immunization >5 years ago

YES "Seek medical care within 2 to 4 hours"
and
Follow **Home Care Instructions**

NO Follow **Home Care Instructions** and call PCP now

Home Care Instructions
Bites, Snake

- Use emergency snake bite kit per instructions if in a remote area and medical attention is unavailable.
- Remain calm. Do not run.
- Identify snake if possible.
- Elevate and splint the affected part and seek emergency care immediately.
- Restrict movement of the affected part.
- Remove jewelry or other constricting items.
- Take your usual pain medication (aspirin, acetaminophen, ibuprofen) for discomfort. Do not give aspirin to a child. Avoid aspirin-like products if age <20 years. Avoid acetaminophen if liver disease is present. Avoid ibuprofen if kidney disease or stomach problems exist or in the case of pregnancy. Follow the directions on the label.
- Do not apply ice or a tourniquet to area.
- Expect initial swelling and pain at the site. Apply cold compresses the first 24 hours, then warm soaks as needed.
- Watch for signs of infection: increased pain, redness, swelling, warmth, red streaks, drainage, or fever.

Additional Instructions

Report the Following Problems to Your PCP/Clinic/ED

- No improvement or condition worsens
- Signs of infection or allergic reaction
- Purple rash, fever, headache, numbness and tingling around the mouth, bruising, or excessive sweating

Seek Emergency Care Immediately If Any of the Following Occur

- Altered mental status
- Chest tightness
- Difficulty breathing or swallowing

If the caller agrees with the advice given, document the call and encourage the caller to call back or see PCP if the problem worsens. If the caller does not agree with the advice given, reevaluate and advise the caller to follow up with PCP, Clinic, or ED.

Bites, Tick

 Key Questions Name, Age, Onset, Type of Tick If Known, Location of Tick Bite, Allergies, Medications, History

 Other Protocols to Consider Allergic Reaction (25); Foreign Body, Skin (278); Rash, Adult (500), Child (505).

B

Reminder: Document caller response to advice, home care instructions, and when to call back.

ASSESSMENT	ACTION

A. Are any of the following present?

- Sudden onset of hives, rash, itching, or swelling in areas other than the bite site
- Chest tightness or difficulty breathing or swallowing

YES "Seek emergency care now"

NO Go to B

B. Are any of the following present?

- Widespread rash and flulike symptoms such as fever, chills, sore throat, or headache 2 to 14 days after tick bite
- Signs of infection such as redness, pain, swelling, drainage from the wound, or warmth
- History of allergic reaction to tick bites

YES "Seek medical care within 2 to 4 hours"

NO Go to C

C. Are any of the following present?

- Unwillingness or inability to remove tick, and tick head is embedded in the skin
- No tetanus immunization, immunization status unknown, or last tetanus immunization >5 years ago
- Rash or flulike symptoms such as fever, chills, sore throat, or headache >14 days after tick bite
- Bull's-eye rash develops around tick bite

YES "Seek medical care within 24 hours" and
Follow **Home Care Instructions**

NO Go to D

D. Is the following present?

- No attempt to remove the tick

YES "Call back or call PCP for appointment if no improvement" and
Follow **Home Care Instructions**

NO Follow **Home Care Instructions**

Home Care Instructions
Bites, Tick

- Using tweezers, apply steady upward traction until the tick releases its grip (try to get a grip on its head as close to the skin as possible). If tweezers are unavailable, use fingers, plastic wrap, or paper in the same manner or tie a thread around the tick jaws and firmly pull upward.
- Tiny ticks may be removed by scraping them off with a knife edge or credit card.
- Try to avoid crushing the tick during removal or afterward. Crushing increases the chance of disease transmission.
- If the tick body is removed but the head remains, remove it with a sterile needle.
- Wash the wound and hands with soap and water and apply antibiotic ointment.
- Watch for signs of infection such as redness, swelling, pain, warmth, drainage, or fever.
- Recent studies show that ticks do not back out with the application of a hot match or when covered with petroleum jelly, fingernail polish, or rubbing alcohol.
- If a rash develops within several weeks of removing a tick, follow up with PCP. Explain when the tick bite occurred and where you were when you acquired the tick bite.

B

Additional Instructions

Report the Following Problems to Your PCP/Clinic/ED

- Unable to remove the tick or its head
- Rash or flulike symptoms >14 days and up to 4 weeks after the tick bite
- Deer tick, from areas where Lyme disease is prevalent, attached >18 hours
- Signs of wound infection such as redness, swelling, pain, warmth, drainage, or fever
- Sudden onset of hives, rash, itching, or swelling in areas other than the bite site

If the caller agrees with the advice given, document the call and encourage the caller to call back or see PCP if the problem worsens. If the caller does not agree with the advice given, reevaluate and advise the caller to follow up with PCP, Clinic, or ED.

Bleeding, Severe

 Key Questions Name, Age, Onset, Cause, Location, Medications, Pain Scale, History

 Other Protocols to Consider Bites, Animal/Human (76); Chest Trauma (127); Extremity Injury (222); Vomiting, Adult (642), Child (645); Nosebleed (425); Rectal Bleeding (510); Rectal Problems (513); Shock, Suspected (547); Vaginal Bleeding (633).

Nurse Alert: With the significant increase in mass casualty events and violent incidents around the world, hemorrhage control has been key to saving lives. Many public areas are making hemorrhage control kits readily available and may be stored with fire extinguishers, automatic defibrillators, and with first kits maintained by fire and police personnel. See Home Care Instructions for applying a tourniquet and first aid for bleeding.

Reminder: Document caller response to advice, home care instructions, and when to call back.

ASSESSMENT	ACTION

A. Are any of the following present?

- Gunshot, knife, or other penetrating wound and difficulty controlling bleeding
- Signs of shock include:
  - lightheadedness, confused
  - unresponsive
  - skin is pale, cold, or moist
  - thirst
  - rapid pulse
- Blood is spurting from the wound and cannot be controlled with direct pressure
- Clothing and bandages soaked with blood
- Blood pooling on the ground
- Penetrating wound to abdomen, chest, or neck
- Exposed bone or deformity at injury site

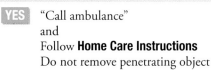 **YES** "Call ambulance"
and
Follow **Home Care Instructions**
Do not remove penetrating object

NO Go to B

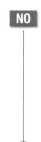

B. Are any of the following present?

- Persistent bleeding >10 minutes after application of direct pressure
- Gaping bleeding wounds
- History of bleeding disorder and difficulty controlling the bleeding
- Taking a blood thinner medication
- Unable to move limb or digit beyond the injury site

YES "Seek emergency care now" and
Follow **Home Care Instructions**

NO Follow **Home Care Instructions**

B

Home Care Instructions
Bleeding, Severe

- Lay the person down and elevate the injured part.
- Apply pressure directly over the area for at least 10 minutes.
- If wound is spurting blood, apply pressure with palm of hand and sterile or clean bandages directly over the wound.
- If wound is deep and large, pack it with bandages or cloth. Avoid paper towels or toilet paper.
- If spurting persists with direct pressure, apply pressure to the artery between the heart and injury site.
- Maintain pressure until bleeding stops or help arrives.
- If bandage is saturated with blood, do not remove; apply additional bandages on top of the bandage.
- If unable to control bleeding with direct pressure and a tourniquet is available, follow the instructions contained in the tourniquet kit and apply tourniquet 2 to 3 inches above the bleeding site. Do not apply tourniquet over a joint.
- Write the time the tourniquet was applied on the tourniquet so emergency personnel know when the tourniquet was applied. Tourniquets can be in place for 2 hours before the risk of tissue damage.
- To control persistent bleeding after a tooth extraction or traumatic tooth loss, bite down on a moistened black tea bag for 20 minutes.

Additional Instructions

_____

_____

_____

Report the Following Problems to Your PCP/Clinic/ED
- Swelling/bleeding occurs >24 hours after bleeding is under control
- Signs of infection: increased pain, drainage, fever, swelling, pus, streaks, or redness

Seek Emergency Care Immediately If Any of the Following Occur
- Signs of shock:
  - lightheadedness
  - pale, cold, or moist skin
  - excessive thirst
  - rapid pulse

If the caller agrees with the advice given, document the call and encourage the caller to call back or see PCP if the problem worsens. If the caller does not agree with the advice given, reevaluate and advise the caller to follow up with PCP, Clinic, or ED.

Blood/Body Fluid Exposure

 Key Questions Name, Age, Onset, Cause, Source, Risk, Area Exposed, Immunization Status, Medications, History

 Other Protocols to Consider Bites, Animal/Human (76); Hepatitis (329); HIV Exposure (340); Piercing Problems (445); Tattoo Problems (604); Sexual Assault (539); Sexually Transmitted Disease (542).

Reminder: Document caller response to advice, home care instructions, and when to call back.

B

ASSESSMENT	ACTION

A. Are any of the following present?

- Contact with a person who is known to have HIV infection or hepatitis B, or is at high risk for infection, and any of the following have occurred:
  - unprotected sexual contact
  - open wounds (sores, cuts, scrapes), eyes, or mouth exposed to infected person's blood or body fluids
  - puncture with a contaminated needle

 YES "Seek medical care now to discuss options"

NO Go to B

B. Are any of the following present?

- Contact with a person whose HIV or hepatitis B status is unknown, and any of the following have occurred:
  - puncture with a contaminated needle
  - human bite
  - open wounds (sores, cuts, scrapes), eyes, or mouth exposed to infected person's blood or body fluids

YES "Seek medical care within 2 hours to discuss options"

NO Go to C

C. Are any of the following present?

- Contact with a person whose HIV or hepatitis B status is unknown, and any of the following have occurred:
  - unprotected sexual contact
  - suspected date rape
  - injury, and no tetanus immunization, immunization status unknown, or last tetanus immunization >5 years ago

 YES "Seek medical care within 24 hours to discuss options" and Follow **Home Care Instructions**

NO Follow **Home Care Instructions**

Home Care Instructions
Blood/Body Fluid Exposure

- If wound is present, wash with povidone-iodine (Betadine) if available or soap and water and watch for signs of infection: increased redness, pain, drainage, fever, warmth, or streaks.
- Rinse exposed eyes or mouth with running water for 5 minutes.
- Consult with PCP or Health Department (# _____) for:
  - HIV testing on self and contact person.
  - hepatitis B vaccine (if not previously vaccinated).
- Remember that casual contact cannot transmit disease.
- Check with PCP; tetanus booster may be needed in the event of a needlestick.

Additional Instructions

Report the Following Problems to Your PCP/Clinic/ED

- Known blood or body fluid exposure to person with HIV infection, hepatitis B, or STD
- Exposure to person who has high-risk factors for HIV or hepatitis infection, including intravenous drug user or multiple sexual partners

If the caller agrees with the advice given, document the call and encourage the caller to call back or see PCP if the problem worsens. If the caller does not agree with the advice given, reevaluate and advise the caller to follow up with PCP, Clinic, or ED.

Bone, Joint, and Tissue Injury

 Key Questions Name, Age, Onset, Cause, Location, Medications, Pain Scale, History

 Other Protocols to Consider Ankle Injury (31); Arthritis Problems (48); Back/Neck Injury (59); Bruising (109); Extremity Injury (222); Foot Problems (265); Hand/Wrist Problems (301); Hip Pain/Injury (334); Joint Pain/Swelling (390); Knee Pain/Swelling (393).

B

Reminder: Document caller response to advice, home care instructions, and when to call back.

ASSESSMENT	ACTION

A. Are any of the following present?

- Altered mental status
- Difficulty breathing
- Severe pain and inability to use extremity
- Bone protrudes through the skin

YES "Call ambulance"
or
"Seek emergency care now"

NO Go to B

B. Are any of the following present?

- Deformity
- Fingers or toes cold or blue compared with other fingers or toes
- Numbness, tingling, or weakness in arms, legs, fingers, or toes
- Severe pain
- Injury in infant younger than 6 months
- Facial injury with vision problems

YES "Seek emergency care now"

NO Go to C

C. Are any of the following present?

- Inability to move joint above or below the injured area
- Inability to use the part or bear weight
- Suspicious explanation for injury, especially in children and the elderly
- Jaw injury with difficulty opening jaw, increased pain with movement, or teeth do not line up properly

YES "Seek medical care within 2 to 4 hours"
and
"Support the injured part"

Follow **Home Care Instructions**

NO Go to D

D. Are any of the following present?

- Joint is painful or swollen, and movement is limited
- Swelling or bruising increased after 48 hours
- Pain, swelling, or discoloration occurred within 30 minutes of the injury

YES "Seek medical care within 24 hours if no improvement"
and
Follow **Home Care Instructions**

NO Follow **Home Care Instructions**

Home Care Instructions
Bone, Joint, and Tissue Injury

- Apply ice pack to the injured area to reduce swelling and pain for the first 24 to 48 hours. Then, alternate ice and heat. Do not apply ice directly to the skin; use a washcloth or other cloth barrier between ice and the skin.
- Elevate the affected part higher than the heart to help reduce swelling.
- Support the affected part with splints (pillows, magazines, cardboard) extending above and below the injury.
- Rest.
- Apply heat (moist hot packs or heating pack) after 48 hours. Do not sleep on a heating pad. Do not apply heating pad directly to the skin without a cloth barrier between the heating pad and the skin.
- Take your usual pain medication (aspirin, acetaminophen, or ibuprofen) for discomfort. Do not give aspirin to a child. Avoid aspirin-like products if age <20 years. Avoid acetaminophen if liver disease is present. Avoid ibuprofen if kidney disease or stomach problems exist or in the case of pregnancy. Follow the directions on the label.

Additional Instructions

Report the Following Problems to Your PCP/Clinic/ED

- Increasing pain
- No improvement in pain, swelling, or ability to walk or bear weight or use the limb after 48 hours

Seek Emergency Care Immediately If Any of the Following Occur

- Affected part turns cold or blue
- No pulse in affected part
- Numbness, tingling, or weakness in arms, legs, fingers, or toes

If the caller agrees with the advice given, document the call and encourage the caller to call back or see PCP if the problem worsens. If the caller does not agree with the advice given, reevaluate and advise the caller to follow up with PCP, Clinic, or ED.

Breastfeeding Problems

 Key Questions Name, Age, Onset, Problem, Frequency of Feedings, Medications, History

 Other Protocols to Consider Breast Problems (107); Crying, Excessive, in Infants (176); Newborn Problems (421); Postpartum Problems (461); Spitting Up Infant (570).

Reminder: Document caller response to advice, home care instructions, and when to call back.

ASSESSMENT	ACTION

A. Is the breastfeeding infant having any of the following problems?

- Respiratory distress
- Extreme lethargy
- Projectile vomiting
- Infant unresponsive, unable to awaken
- Temperature >100.4°F (38.0°C) in an infant <8 weeks of age

YES "Call ambulance"
or
"Seek emergency care now"

NO Go to B

B. Are any of the following present?

- Infant refuses to breastfeed because of intermittent lethargy, irritability, or fever
- Newborn jaundice (yellow skin) below the waist
- Signs of dehydration in an infant:
  - fewer than six wet diapers per day by age 5 days
  - fewer than three wet diapers per day after birth before day 5
  - sunken fontanel
  - dry mouth
  - more than three brick-dust urinations
- Infant with fewer than three yellow stools per day after day 5
- Pus-like drainage from the woman's nipple
- Woman has temperature >100°F (37.7°C), muscle aches, chills, fatigue, or headache

YES "Seek medical care within 2 to 4 hours"

NO Go to C

C. Are any of the following present?

- Mother's milk not in by day 5
- Swelling and soreness of breast that is unresponsive to home care measures
- Hard, red, warm area of breast
- Red streak on the breast tissue
- Swollen node on the same side as painful breast
- Unable to get infant to latch on for feeding
- Sudden searing, stabbing, or burning or radiating pain in breasts
- Infant seems consistently hungry after feeding
- Infant has not urinated in >8 hours or passed stool in >24 hours

YES "Seek medical care within 24 hours"

NO Go to D

B

D. Are any of the following present?

- Breasts are engorged (hardness, swelling, and tenderness)
- Nipples are cracked, red, or sore
- Infant has difficulty grasping nipple and maintaining vacuum while sucking
- Infant pulls away or pushes off breast and cries during feeding
- Insufficient milk supply for breastfeeding
- Painful breasts during weaning
- Uterine cramping and increased vaginal bleeding in new mother during breastfeeding

YES "Call back or call PCP for appointment if no improvement" and
Follow **Home Care Instructions**

NO Follow **Home Care Instructions**

Home Care Instructions
Breastfeeding Problems

Signs of Infection
- Apply moist hot packs to the affected area 10 to 15 minutes, 4 times a day.
- Express milk manually or pump to help prevent engorgement.
- Breastfeed frequently (every 1 to 3 hours, even on the affected side).
- Limit activity (encourage others to help with housework).
- Do not wean at this time.

Engorgement
- Apply warm water compress to breast or shower before feeding.
- Massage breast toward nipple.
- Manually express milk or use a breast pump immediately before a feeding to soften the area around the nipple/areola.
- Breastfeed on both sides at each feeding.
- Wear a supportive bra.
- Apply ice packs after breastfeeding (frozen vegetable bags covered in a lightweight towel can be used).

Sore, Cracked Nipples
- Establish rooting reflex by stroking infant's cheek and compress as much breast tissue as possible into the infant's mouth.
- Wait until the infant has a wide open mouth, like a yawn. The lips should be flanged.
- If only the nipple is in the infant's mouth, the nipple may become sore, bruised, cracked, or irritated.
- Break suction by putting a finger in the corner of the infant's mouth. Do not pull the nipple out of the infant's mouth without first breaking the suction.
- Clean the breast with plain water only. Do not use soap or antiseptic on the breast.
- A thin layer of lanolin or breast milk can be applied to the nipples after feedings. Allow nipples to air-dry briefly after each feeding.
- Rotate breastfeeding positions (cradle, football, side-lying).
- Start each feeding on the least sore side.

Infant Has Difficulty Grasping Breast, Pulls Away, Pushes Off
- Express breast milk before feeding if breast is too full. This also helps aid letdown.
- Encourage rooting reflex and wait until the infant's mouth is wide open.
- Compress and hold the breast tissue until the infant has a good latch and starts suckling for a minute.
- Massage breast while infant's swallowing is slowing down.
- Try different breastfeeding positions (cradle, football, side-lying).

Insufficient Milk Supply
- Remember that frequent breastfeeding stimulates milk supply.
- Try breastfeeding every 2 to 3 hours (minimum of eight breastfeedings per 24 hours).

- May need to awaken infant and offer breastfeeding.
- Offer both breasts at one feeding.
- Massage breast and use a warm water compress before breastfeeding.
- Encourage nutritive (active swallowing) feeding by stimulating the infant during feedings (rub back, tickle toes, touch under jaw).
- Remember that six wet diapers per 24 hours after day 5 is adequate output.
- Infant should have a minimum of three yellow stools per 24 hours from day 5 until the age of 6 to 8 weeks.
- Stooling decreases at 6 to 8 weeks.
- Sudden softening of breast at 6 to 8 weeks after delivery is normal because milk supply is adjusting and becoming efficient.
- Cluster feedings (every 1 to 1½ hours) occur often during growth spurts.
- Avoid emotional stress and anxiety and estrogen-containing birth control pills.
- Do not give solids before infant is 4 months old because solids reduce the infant's sucking and the mother's milk supply.
- Minimize use of pacifiers.
- Contact PCP or obstetrics/gynecology provider if taking estrogen-containing birth control pills.

Uterine Cramping and Increased Vaginal Bleeding
- Cramping is normal with breastfeeding in the early postpartum period.
- Call PCP if saturating one pad per hour (bright red bleeding).
- Breastfeeding helps the uterus return to normal state faster.

Exhaustion
- Remember that taking care of an infant is hard work.
- Try to nap while the infant naps.
- Take care of yourself by eating a well-balanced diet.
- Drink enough fluids to keep your urine light yellow.
- Take vitamins and iron supplements as directed by your PCP.
- Avoid drugs, smoking, and drinking alcohol and limit caffeine consumption.
- Postpartum depression may contribute to exhaustion. If depression lasts longer than 2 weeks, contact your PCP.
- If infant is feeding often at night, gently stimulate and awaken the infant every 2 to 3 hours during the day.

Painful Breasts During Weaning
- Wear a supportive bra.
- Avoid weaning too rapidly; lengthen weaning time if needed.
- Decrease one to two feedings (at same time each day) every 2 to 4 days.
- Wait until breasts become accustomed to the change before decreasing another feeding.
- Use ice packs to reduce swelling.
- Manually express small amounts of milk or use a breast pump until a little relief is felt.

B

Sleepy Infant

- Unwrap blankets and undress infant to change diaper.
- Massage infant's legs, back, and arms.
- Give infant a back rub by walking your fingers down his or her spine.
- Try infant "sit-ups" by holding the infant away from you and gently lift him or her toward your face.
- If newborn has not eaten in 6 hours, feed infant pumped breast milk or formula.

Additional Instructions

Report the Following Problems to Your PCP/Clinic/ED

- Condition persists or worsens
- Signs of infection develop
- Symptoms of infection persist >2 to 3 days or fever suddenly rises
- Signs of thrush (sudden breast pain)
- Infant shows signs of dehydration
- Infant refuses to breastfeed, has jaundice below the waist, or <3 yellow stools per day after day 5

Seek Emergency Care Immediately If the Following Occur

- Infant has respiratory distress, extreme lethargy, or projectile vomiting
- Temperature >100.4°F (38.0°C) in an infant <8 weeks of age

If the caller agrees with the advice given, document the call and encourage the caller to call back or see PCP if the problem worsens. If the caller does not agree with the advice given, reevaluate and advise the caller to follow up with PCP, Clinic, or ED.

Breast Problems

 Key Questions Name, Age, Onset, Cause, Medications, History (if breastfeeding, see Breastfeeding Problems [93]).

 Other Protocols to Consider Fever, Adult (250), Child (253); Laceration (395); Menstrual Problems (404); Piercing Problems (445); Pregnancy Problems (481); Tattoo Problems (604); Wound Healing and Infection (664).

> *Nurse Alert:* If new piercing or tattoo and signs of infection, irritation, or feeling ill go to Piercing Problems (445) or Tattoo Problems (604).

Reminder: Document caller response to advice, home care instructions, and when to call back.

ASSESSMENT	ACTION
A. Are any of the following present?	
• Chills or fever and headache during postpartum period • Recent trauma or piercing to breast and laceration or signs of infection • Muscle aches, fever, and painful red area on breast during postpartum period • Foul-smelling discharge from nipple • Severe pain • Puncture and leaking of breast implant • Recent breast surgery and chills, fever, worsening pain, redness, drainage, or swelling at the incision site	**YES** "Seek medical care within 2 to 4 hours" **NO** Go to B
B. Are any of the following present?	
• History of red, hot, lumpy breasts • Skin ulceration • Bloody discharge • Nipple drainage in nonpregnant woman • Sudden searing, stabbing, or burning pain in breasts • New tattoo and pain at wound site, chills, feeling ill, or headache	**YES** "Seek medical care within 24 hours" and Follow **Home Care Instructions** **NO** Go to C

B

C. Are any of the following present?

- Recent trauma to the breast and pain, swelling, or bruising
- Lumpy breasts and no other symptoms
- Lump is unrelated to premenstrual cycle
- Lump in a male
- Female's last breast examination >1 year ago
- Lumps appear 1 week before menstruation and disappear after menses
- Dimpling or change in nipple position
- Nipple soreness or curdlike drainage after taking antibiotics

YES "Call back or call PCP for appointment if no improvement" and
Follow **Home Care Instructions**

NO Follow **Home Care Instructions**

Home Care Instructions
Breast Problems

- Watch for signs of infection: fever; nipple or fissure discharge; red, hot, painful area; or red streaks. Apply moist hot packs to the affected area for 10 to 15 minutes, 4 times a day, until symptoms subside.
- If trauma is related, apply ice packs every 2 to 4 hours for the first 24 to 48 hours, then apply hot packs for 10 to 15 minutes, 4 times a day. Do not place ice or hot packs directly on the skin. Apply a cloth barrier between the ice pack or heat source.
- Keep nipples clean and dry.
- Avoid clothing that irritates nipples.
- For premenstrual swelling and tenderness, reduce intake of salty foods, caffeine, chocolate, and cola beverages.
- Follow PCP recommendations for regular self-breast checks and mammograms.

B

Additional Instructions

_____

_____

_____

Report the Following Problems to Your PCP/Clinic/ED

- Lump persists for 48 hours after a trauma
- Condition persists or worsens
- Signs of infection
- Bloody, green, brown, or yellow drainage
- Severe pain

If the caller agrees with the advice given, document the call and encourage the caller to call back or see PCP if the problem worsens. If the caller does not agree with the advice given, reevaluate and advise the caller to follow up with PCP, Clinic, or ED.

Breathing Problems

 Key Questions Name, Age, Onset, Cause, Medications, History

 Other Protocols to Consider Allergic Reaction (25); Asthma (52); Chest Pain (123); Chronic Obstructive Pulmonary Disease (COPD) (138); Choking (135); Common Cold Symptoms (146); Congestion (153); Congestive Heart Failure (CHF) (157); Cough (170); Foreign Body, Inhaled (271); Hyperventilation (350); Wheezing (657).

Nurse Alert: If known respiratory problems, prescribed inhalers, O_2, or peak flow meters (to measure how well air is moving out of the lungs). Assess baseline functioning, O_2 saturation level, and % oxygen delivery amount and method.

Peak flow values are divided into three zones:
Green: 80% of baseline or higher (mild attack)
Yellow: 50% to 80% of baseline (moderate attack)
Red: <50% of baseline (severe attack)

Reminder: Document caller response to advice, home care instructions, and when to call back.

ASSESSMENT	ACTION

A. Are any of the following present?

- Chest pain
- Blue lips or tongue
- Clammy skin
- Feeling of suffocation
- Frothy pink or copious white sputum
- Altered mental status
- Severe shortness of breath with sudden onset
- History of pulmonary embolus, blood clots, or lung collapse
- Severe wheezing and history of asthma not relieved with inhaler
- Inability to speak
- Drooling and inability to swallow
- Difficulty breathing after inhalation of smoke, flames, or fumes

YES "Call ambulance"

NO Go to B

B. Are any of the following present?

- Difficulty taking a deep breath because of severe pain
- Severe SOB, wheezing, or noisy breathing started within past 2 hours
- Recent trauma, surgery, or childbirth
- Inhalation of a foreign body
- Exposure to something that previously caused a significant reaction (sting, medication, plant, chemical, food, or animal)
- Speaking in short words
- Inability to breathe lying down or need to sit up to breathe
- Immunosuppressed, age >60, history of sickle cell anemia or diabetes, or bedridden and temperature >101°F (38.3°C)
- Peak flow rate <50% of baseline
- Adult with temperature >103°F (39.4°C)
- Progressively worsening shortness of breath
- Persistent wheezing after treatment
- Severe wheezing or cough and usual nebulizer or inhaler not available

YES "Seek emergency care now"

NO Go to C

C. Are any of the following present?

- Speaking in partial sentences
- Tight cough
- Mild audible wheezes at rest
- Pain increasing with breathing
- Upper respiratory infection and prior hospitalizations for same symptoms
- Inability to sleep >1 to 2 hours due to coughing or difficulty breathing
- History of diabetes or heart disease
- Peak flow rate 50% to 80% of baseline

YES "Seek medical care within 2 to 4 hours"

NO Go to D

D. Are any of the following present?

- Fever
- Productive cough with gray, green, or yellow sputum
- Peak flow rate >80% of baseline

YES "Seek medical care within 24 hours"

NO Go to E

E. Are any of the following present?

- Numbness or tingling in the fingers or face
- Recent exposure to a stressful event or situation
- Exposure to environmental irritants, allergies, or recent cold or flulike symptoms
- Nasal congestion
- Productive cough with clear sputum

YES "Call back or call PCP for appointment if no improvement" and Follow **Home Care Instructions**

NO Follow **Home Care Instructions**

Home Care Instructions
Breathing Problems

- Use routine prescriptions as directed.
- Rest or sleep with head elevated on a couple of pillows if lying flat increases breathing difficulty or a recliner.
- Increase fluid intake unless your physician has prescribed a fluid-restricted regimen.
- Avoid environmental irritants (smoke, smog, garden cuttings, chemicals, animals) and other irritants that seem to worsen your symptoms.
- If rapid breathing, tingling in the face or hands, and anxiety are present, breathe into a small paper bag held loosely around the mouth and nose for 5 minutes. The problem should resolve within that time period.
- Rest and relax as much as possible.
- If the problem is caused by excitement, heavy exertion (and resolved within a few minutes and there are no cardiac risk factors), or nasal congestion, there is no real cause for concern. Normal breathing should resume in a short period of time.
- Monitor peak flow rates.

Additional Instructions

_____

_____

_____

Report the Following Problems to Your PCP/Clinic/ED

- Condition worsens or no improvement in 2 days
- Temperature >101°F (38.3°C)
- Peak flow rate 50% to 80% of baseline

Seek Emergency Care Immediately or Call Ambulance If Any of the Following Occur

- Chest pain
- Blue lips or tongue, pale or gray face
- Clammy skin
- Feeling of suffocation
- Frothy pink or copious white sputum
- Decreased level of consciousness
- Inability to speak
- Drooling, unable to swallow saliva
- Peak flow rate <50% of baseline
- Persistent wheezing after treatment
- Severe wheezing or cough and usual nebulizer or inhaler not available

If the caller agrees with the advice given, document the call and encourage the caller to call back or see PCP if the problem worsens. If the caller does not agree with the advice given, reevaluate and advise the caller to follow up with PCP, Clinic, or ED.

Bruising

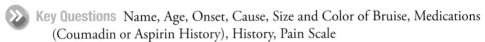

>> **Key Questions** Name, Age, Onset, Cause, Size and Color of Bruise, Medications (Coumadin or Aspirin History), History, Pain Scale

>> **Other Protocols to Consider** Bone, Joint, and Tissue Injury (95); Child Abuse (132); Domestic Abuse (202); Elder Abuse (216); Extremity Injury (222); Eye Injury (225); Falls (240); Hip Pain/Injury (334); Scrotal Problems (529); Swelling (597).

Reminder: Document caller response to advice, home care instructions, and when to call back.

ASSESSMENT	ACTION

A. Are any of the following present?

- Severe pain and bruising on the lower back, pelvis, chest, or abdomen
- Bruising caused by a blow to the eye and
  - severe bleeding in the colored part of the eye
  - reduced or double vision
  - difficulty moving eye in all directions
  - severe pain in the eye

YES "Seek emergency care now"

NO Go to B

B. Are any of the following present?

- Severe pain and bruising on extremities
- Severe swelling at the site
- Multiple bruises of unknown cause
- Suspected child abuse
- History of bleeding problems or use of blood thinners

YES "Seek medical care within 2 to 4 hours"

NO Go to C

109

C. Are any of the following present?

- Movement is limited
- Signs of infection: increased pain, swelling, redness, drainage, fever, heat, or red streaks extending from the area
- Frequent falls
- Recent abrupt cessation of drugs (OTC, prescription, recreational), alcohol, or caffeine

YES "Seek medical care within 24 hours"

NO Go to D

D. Are any of the following present?

- Slight swelling
- Slight discomfort

YES "Call back or call PCP for appointment if no improvement" and
Follow **Home Care Instructions**

NO Follow **Home Care Instructions**

Home Care Instructions
Bruising

- Rest involved area.
- Do not massage or rub area; this may increase bruising.
- Apply ice pack to the injured area to reduce swelling and pain for the first 24 to 48 hours. Do not apply ice directly to the skin; use a washcloth or other cloth barrier between ice and the skin.
- Elevate the affected part to help reduce swelling and bleeding.
- Apply warm moist packs for 20 minutes, 4 times a day, beginning 48 hours after injury.
- **If abuse is suspected**, offer resources for help. Important questions to ask:
  - Is the person in a safe environment right now?
  - Is the person alone?
  - Are there other family members at risk?
  - Has the person been abused in the past?
  - Where is the abuser right now?
  - Are there family or friends who can help?
  - Have the police been called, Adult Protective Services, or anyone else for help?
  - Are telephone numbers for Family Adult Shelters or family crisis lines desired?
    - Encourage the person to contact someone who has been supportive in the past.
    - Offer referral numbers for local resources, including social workers, crisis services, battered adult shelters, family services, and counseling services.
    - Encourage the person to notify Adult Protective Services and/or the police.
    - Provide reassurance and reinforce that no one deserves to be hit, abused, or assaulted and that the abuser is likely to hit again.

B

Additional Instructions

Report the Following Problems to Your PCP/Clinic/ED

- Severe pain
- Restricted movement
- Frequent bruising
- No improvement or condition worsens after 48 hours

If the caller agrees with the advice given, document the call and encourage the caller to call back or see PCP if the problem worsens. If the caller does not agree with the advice given, reevaluate and advise the caller to follow up with PCP, Clinic, or ED.

Burns, Chemical

>> **Key Questions** Name, Age, Onset, Cause, Name of Agent, Area Burned, First Aid Treatment, Tetanus Immunization Status, Medications, History

>> **Other Protocols to Consider** Burns, Electrical (115), Thermal (118); Eye Injury (225); Shock, Suspected (547); Skin Lesions: Lumps, Bumps, and Sores (556); Wound Healing and Infection (664).

Nurse Alert: Important to remove substance causing the burn as quickly as possible to stop the burning process and prevent exposing other areas of the body to the causative agent.

Reminder: Document caller response to advice, home care instructions, and when to call back.

ASSESSMENT	ACTION
A. Are any of the following present?	
• Difficulty breathing • Altered mental status • Chest pain or rapid or irregular heartbeat	**YES** "Call ambulance" and "Flush eye or skin" Follow **Home Care Instructions** **NO** Go to B
B. Are any of the following present?	
• Eye exposed to an acid such as battery acid or caustic substance (drain cleaner, lye) • Severe pain and the burned area is red, blistered, white, or charred • Burns larger than the size of a hand to the face, ears, genitals, neck, hands, feet, or over a major joint • Burn circles the neck or an extremity • Exposed to methamphetamine lab chemicals and symptomatic	**YES** "Seek emergency care now" **NO** Go to C

C. Are any of the following present?

- Persistent pain >20 minutes after following home care measures
- Persistent redness, discharge, or watering of eye
- Vision changes
- Colored part of the eye appears white or cloudy
- Signs of infection develop: increased redness, pain, swelling, drainage, or warmth
- Moderate-to-severe pain after home treatment
- Suspected abuse
- History of impaired peripheral circulation and burn on extremity
- History of diabetes

YES "Seek medical care within 2 to 4 hours"
and
Follow **Home Care Instructions**

NO Go to D

D. Are any of the following present?

- Tetanus immunization >5 years ago
- Multiple open blisters

YES "Seek medical care within 24 hours"
and
Follow **Home Care Instructions**

"Call back or call PCP for appointment if no improvement"
and
NO Follow **Home Care Instructions**

B

Home Care Instructions
Burns, Chemical

Eye
- Remove contact lens if present. Flush the eye for 15 to 20 minutes in a basin of water or under a running faucet. Position head under faucet so that water drains from inner eye to outer eye while holding lids open with fingers. Flush until pain subsides.
- After flushing, cover both eyes with a dressing or clean cloth and seek medical attention.
- Do not rub eyes.
- For capsaicin exposure (chili peppers, pepper spray), irrigate eye with carton of whole milk; will act like a detergent and remove the offending substance.

Skin
- Remove jewelry or shoes from burned limb before limb begins to swell. Remove clothing and flush the area with cool water for 20 minutes. Do not rub area. Cover with a dressing or clean cloth.
- Watch for signs of infection.
- Do not apply ointments, grease, butter, or pain-killing lotions.
- Take your usual pain medication (aspirin, acetaminophen, ibuprofen) for discomfort. Do not give aspirin to a child. Avoid aspirin-like products if age <20 years. Avoid acetaminophen if liver disease is present. Avoid ibuprofen if kidney disease or stomach problems exist or in the case of pregnancy. Follow the directions on the label.
- Do not puncture and drain blisters.
- For capsaicin exposure (chili peppers, pepper spray), irrigate eye with carton of whole milk; will act like a detergent and remove the offending substance.

Additional Instructions

Report the Following Problems to Your PCP/Clinic/ED
- Signs of infection
- Blisters break open
- Swelling
- No improvement in 48 hours or condition worsens
- Last tetanus immunization was >10 years ago

Seek Emergency Care Immediately If Any of the Following Occur
- Difficulty breathing
- Chest pain
- Rapid or irregular heartbeat

If the caller agrees with the advice given, document the call and encourage the caller to call back or see PCP if the problem worsens. If the caller does not agree with the advice given, reevaluate and advise the caller to follow up with PCP, Clinic, or ED.

Burns, Electrical

B

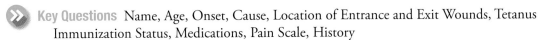 **Key Questions** Name, Age, Onset, Cause, Location of Entrance and Exit Wounds, Tetanus Immunization Status, Medications, Pain Scale, History

Other Protocols to Consider Altered Mental Status (28); Burns, Thermal (118); Electrical Injury (219); Seizure (531); Wound Healing and Infection (664).

Reminder: Document caller response to advice, home care instructions, and when to call back.

ASSESSMENT	ACTION

A. Are any of the following present?

- High-voltage shock
- Unconsciousness or no pulse or respirations
- Chest pain
- Rapid or irregular heart rate
- Difficulty breathing
- Burns above the neck
- Obvious entrance and exit wounds
- Burns caused by lightning

YES "Call ambulance"
and
"Start CPR or rescue breathing if no pulse or respirations"

NO Go to B

B. Are any of the following present?

- Burn caused by arc or flash
- Hair singed or missing but no burn to the skin
- Burn in mouth or lip, particularly in infant or toddler
- Burn circles the neck or an extremity
- Burn over a joint
- Amnesia or any period of unconsciousness
- Thrown from electrical source and difficulty breathing, chest or abdominal pain
- Numbness, tingling, or paralysis; vision, hearing, or speech problems
- Burn to head, face, neck, hands, feet, or genital area

YES "Seek emergency care now"

NO Go to C

C. Are any of the following present?

- Low-voltage small burn
- Pregnancy >20 weeks

 "Seek medical care immediately"

NO Go to D

D. Are any of the following present?

- No tetanus immunization, immunization status unknown, or last tetanus immunization >5 years ago
- Burns are not healing well
- Signs of infection: redness, streaks, swelling, or drainage
- No other symptoms, but person or parent concerned

YES "Seek medical care within 24 hours"

NO Follow **Home Care Instructions**

Home Care Instructions
Burns, Electrical

- Stop the burning process. Remove any clothing on fire and jewelry.
- Cool the burned area with moist, clean, cool cloths.
- Do not apply ointments, grease, butter, or pain-killing lotions.
- Keep area clean and cover with clean, dry, nonstick dressing.
- Watch for signs of infection.
- Take your usual pain medication. Do not give aspirin to a child. Avoid aspirin-like products if age <20 years. Avoid acetaminophen if liver disease is present. Avoid ibuprofen if kidney disease or stomach problems exist or in the case of pregnancy. Follow the directions on the label.
- Do not puncture or drain blisters.
- If electrical burn is caused by an appliance, do not use until repaired. Install GFCIs to ground outlets, especially in bathrooms, kitchens, and outside. If no GFCI outlets, use GFCI extension cord.

B

Additional Instructions

Report the Following Problems to Your PCP/Clinic/ED

- Burns are not healing well
- Signs of infection: redness, streaks, swelling, or drainage
- Muscle pain or weakness
- Post-lightning strike headache, ear pain, or memory loss
- Condition worsens or no improvement

Seek Emergency Care Immediately If Any of the Following Occur

- Seizure
- Difficulty breathing
- Chest pain
- Numbness, tingling, or paralysis; vision, hearing, or speech problems

If the caller agrees with the advice given, document the call and encourage the caller to call back or see PCP if the problem worsens. If the caller does not agree with the advice given, reevaluate and advise the caller to follow up with PCP, Clinic, or ED.

Burns, Thermal

 Key Questions Name, Age, Onset, Cause (see Burns, Chemical protocol (112) for chemical burns), Area of Burn, First Aid Treatment, Medications, History

 Other Protocols to Consider Breathing Problems (106); Burns, Electrical (115); Child Abuse (132); Domestic Abuse (202); Electric Injury (219); Foreign Body, Inhaled (271), Skin (278); Shock, Suspected (547); Sunburn (588); Wound Healing and Infection (664).

Nurse Alert: Estimate percentage of body affected. One percent of the body surface area is about the size of the palm of the hand. Instruct to remove jewelry, clothing, or other constricting clothing on the affected part.

Reminder: Document caller response to advice, home care instructions, and when to call back.

ASSESSMENT	ACTION

A. Are any of the following present?

- Extensive burn is white and painless
- Severe pain and extensive burn area is red and blistered
- Difficulty breathing
- Altered mental status
- Chest pain or rapid or irregular heartbeat
- Singed facial or nasal hairs
- Soot near nares
- Swelling at back of throat

YES "Call ambulance"

NO Go to B

B. Are any of the following present?

- Burn area charred
- Blistered or white painless burn area larger than the size of a hand
- Burn circles the neck or an extremity
- Smoke inhalation
- Burn over a joint
- >10% body surface burned
- Burn >1 inch square and located on the face, eyes, ears, neck, hands, feet, or genital area

YES "Seek emergency care now"

NO Go to C

C. Are any of the following present?

- Recent burn and increased redness, pain, swelling, red streaks, thick drainage, warmth, or fever
- History of diabetes
- Moderate-to-severe pain after home treatment and OTC medications

YES "Seek medical care within 2 to 4 hours"

NO Go to D

D. Are any of the following present?

- No tetanus immunization, immunization status unknown, or last tetanus immunization >5 years ago
- Pain for >48 hours
- Multiple open blisters

YES "Seek medical care within 24 hours" and Follow **Home Care Instructions**

NO Follow **Home Care Instructions**

B

Home Care Instructions
Burns, Thermal

- Apply cool packs to area until pain is relieved when cool packs are removed (may take several hours). May submerge in cool water. Do not apply ice directly to the burned area.
- Do not apply ointments, grease, butter, or pain-killing lotions.
- May apply milk of magnesia, aloe vera, or yogurt for soothing effect. Ask pharmacist for additional OTC products suggestions. Follow instructions on the label.
- Keep area clean and cover with clean, dry, nonstick dressing.
- Watch for signs of infection.
- Take your usual pain medication (aspirin, acetaminophen, or ibuprofen). Do not give aspirin to a child. Avoid aspirin-like products if age <20 years. Avoid acetaminophen if liver disease is present. Avoid ibuprofen if kidney disease or stomach problems exist or in the case of pregnancy. Follow the directions on the label.
- Use your usual antibiotic ointment (Mycitracin, Neosporin, Polysporin) after burn begins to heal to help prevent infection. Follow instructions on the label.
- Do not puncture and drain blisters.

Additional Instructions

Report the Following Problems to Your PCP/Clinic/ED

- Increased redness, pain, swelling, red streaks, pus or cloudy drainage, or fever
- Multiple blisters break open
- No improvement after 48 hours
- Tetanus immunization >10 years ago

Seek Emergency Care Immediately If Any of the Following Occur

- Significant decrease in urine
- Significant swelling
- Difficulty breathing
- Chest pain or rapid or irregular heartbeat

If the caller agrees with the advice given, document the call and encourage the caller to call back or see PCP if the problem worsens. If the caller does not agree with the advice given, reevaluate and advise the caller to follow up with PCP, Clinic, or ED.

Cast/Splint Problems

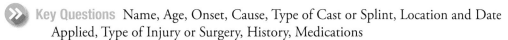 **Key Questions** Name, Age, Onset, Cause, Type of Cast or Splint, Location and Date Applied, Type of Injury or Surgery, History, Medications

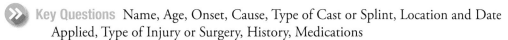 **Other Protocols to Consider** Extremity Injury (222); Itching (382); Leg Pain/Swelling (398); Postoperative Problems (457); Wound Healing and Infection (664).

Reminder: Document caller response to advice, home care instructions, and when to call back.

ASSESSMENT	ACTION
A. Are any of the following present?	
• Sudden onset of signs of poor circulation: fingers or toes cold, blue, or numb compared to other extremity • New onset of difficulty breathing	**YES** "Seek emergency care now" **NO** Go to B
B. Are any of the following present?	
• Severe pain, swelling, or tightness unrelieved by elevation or home care measures • Signs of infection: pain, swelling, drainage, warmth, or red streaks from the wound • Numbness or tingling in fingers or toes unrelieved by elevation or home care measures	**YES** "Seek medical care within 2 hours" **NO** Go to C
C. Are any of the following present?	
• Some relief in swelling, pain, or tightness with home care measures • Cracked or unstable cast/splint • New onset of inability to move fingers or toes	**YES** "Seek medical care within 24 hours" **NO** Go to D
D. Are any of the following present?	
• Wet cast • Itching or pain without swelling in fingers or toes • Persistent swelling or tightness that improves with home care measures • Cast feels too loose or too tight	**YES** "Call back or call PCP for appointment if no improvement" and Follow **Home Care Instructions** **NO** Follow **Home Care Instructions**

C

Home Care Instructions
Cast/Splint Problems

- If cast feels too tight, elevate the part higher than the heart.
- If splint feels too tight, loosen the bandage, elevate the part, and apply ice pack to the area for 20 minutes every 2 hours for the first 24 to 48 hours. Do not apply ice directly to the skin; use a washcloth or other cloth barrier between ice and the skin.
- If cast or splint is damaged, provide support with wide adhesive tape or elastic bandage, and see PCP the next day for repairs.
- If cast or splint is wet, dry with a towel and blow-dry on low setting as needed.
- If itching is present, apply a light dusting of talc powder or use blow-dryer set on cold setting. Do not stick anything in the cast. Scratched skin could become infected.

Additional Instructions

Report the Following Problems to Your PCP/Clinic/ED

- Cast or splint is unstable or damaged
- New onset of pain inside the cast
- No improvement or pain worsens
- Signs of infection

Seek Emergency Care Immediately If Any of the Following Occur

- Signs of circulation problems: fingers or toes become blue, cold, or numb
- Severe pain or swelling unrelieved by elevation or home care measures
- Difficulty breathing

If the caller agrees with the advice given, document the call and encourage the caller to call back or see PCP if the problem worsens. If the caller does not agree with the advice given, reevaluate and advise the caller to follow up with PCP, Clinic, or ED.

Chest Pain

>> **Key Questions** Name, Age, Onset, History of Myocardial Infarction, Coronary Artery Disease, Diabetes, Pulmonary Embolus, Deep Vein Thrombosis, Associated Symptoms, Medications, Pain Scale, History, Implanted Device in Chest

>> **Other Protocols to Consider** Anxiety (36); Breathing Problems (106); Common Cold Symptoms (146); Congestion (153); Congestive Heart Failure (157); Cough (170); Dizziness (199); Heartburn (316); Heart Rate Problems (320); Indigestion (368); Vomiting, Adult (642); Sweating, Excessive (594); Weakness (649).

Nurse Alert: There are many conditions that cause chest pain; some can be potentially life-threatening. Err on the side of caution when triaging callers with chest pain. Chest Pain: Causes and Characteristics Appendix S (712) is provided to help the nurse gain a better understanding of the many conditions causing chest pain. It is NOT to be used to try and diagnose a caller's condition.

Reminder: Document caller response to advice, home care instructions, and when to call back.

ASSESSMENT	ACTION

A. Are any of the following present?

- Continuous or intermittent pain, tightness, pressure, or discomfort accompanied by:
  - shortness of breath
  - dizziness or weakness
  - cool, moist skin
  - nausea or vomiting
  - pain in the neck, shoulders, jaw, back, or arms
  - blue or gray face, lips, earlobes, or fingernails
  - heart palpitations or fluttering
- Chest pain persists, unrelieved by rest, pain medication, antacids, or nitroglycerin every 5 minutes for three doses

 "Call ambulance" and "Chew one adult aspirin unless allergic to aspirin"

 Go to B

123

B. Are any of the following present?

- Change in chest pain pattern in known cardiac patient
- Pain not relieved by two nitroglycerin tablets
- Chest pain at rest or that awakens person
- Recent period of prolonged sitting (such as during traveling)
- Strong family history of heart disease, heart attack, stroke, or diabetes
- History of diabetes, heart disease, CHF (Congestive Heart Failure), or blood clotting problems
- Age >30 years and heavy smoker with high blood pressure, high cholesterol, or obesity
- Pain, swelling, warmth, or redness of leg
- Sudden onset of swollen ankles
- Coughing up blood
- Fever, cough, congestion, and shortness of breath
- Trauma, childbirth, or surgery in past month
- History of blood clotting problems
- Recreational street drug or prescription drug abuse within past 24 hours
- Age >35 years and heart palpitations or fluttering
- Repeated shocks and internal defibrillator in place

YES "Seek emergency care now"
"Do not drive yourself. If another driver is not available, call an ambulance."

NO Go to C

C. Are any of the following present?

- Localized area of painful blisters or rash
- Recent injury and pain increases with movement
- Chest pain with exertion that is relieved with rest
- Fracture <2 months previously

YES "Seek medical care within 24 hours"

NO Go to D

D. Are any of the following present?

- Pain occurs with deep breathing
- Pain occurs when pressure is applied to the area
- Intermittent mild chest discomfort with deep productive coughing

YES "Call back or call PCP for appointment if no improvement" and
Follow **Home Care Instructions**

NO Follow **Home Care Instructions**

Home Care Instructions
Chest Pain

- For heartburn or GERD (Gastroesophageal Reflux Disease):
  - Take your usual antacid (Maalox, Mylanta, Riopan, Tums, Pepcid, Prilosec, or other antacid) for indigestion and follow instructions on the label.
  - Liquids provide faster relief than tablets.
  - Consult with PCP if taking other medications.
  - Do not give Pepto-Bismol to a child.
  - Avoid eating 2 to 3 hours before bedtime.
- Take your usual pain medication (aspirin, acetaminophen, or ibuprofen). Do not give aspirin to a child. Avoid aspirin-like products if age <20 years. Avoid acetaminophen if liver disease is present. Avoid ibuprofen if kidney disease or stomach problems exist or in the case of pregnancy. Follow the directions on the label.
- Take nitroglycerin as directed by PCP if pain is typical anginal chest pain; if no relief after 3 to 5 minutes, take aspirin and another nitroglycerin dose and have someone drive you to the ED or call an ambulance. Do not take aspirin if you are currently on anticoagulant therapy.
- If pain is related to an injury that occurred 24 hours ago or longer and pain increases with movement, apply heat to the area for 20 minutes, 4 times a day.
- For a cough:
  - Drink 6 to 8 glasses of water daily (if no fluid restrictions prescribed).
  - Breathe steam from a shower or tea kettle with towel held over the head for 10 to 15 minutes to loosen phlegm. Do not place face too close to the steam from the tea kettle in order to prevent the face and eyes from burning.
  - Elevate head of bed to reduce coughing at night.
  - Drink warm lemonade, apple cider, or tea to help soothe cough.
  - Avoid irritants such as smoking, smog, and chemicals.
  - Turn down the heat, open the windows, or go out into cooler air to help suppress cough.
  - Take cough suppressants (ask your pharmacist for product suggestions) if cough is interfering with activity, causing chest pain or vomiting, or interrupting sleep at night. Follow instructions on the label. Do not use if age <1 year.
  - If congested, avoid milk products.
  - Take OTC medications as needed, being sure to follow instructions on the label: for a wet cough, use a decongestant; for a dry cough, use an expectorant during the day and suppressant at night; for an allergy, use an antihistamine or decongestant. Ask your pharmacist for product suggestions.

C

Additional Instructions

Report the Following Problems to Your PCP/Clinic/ED

- No improvement or condition worsens
- Localized area of painful blisters or rash

Seek Emergency Care Immediately If Any of the Following Occur

- Continuous or intermittent pain, tightness, pressure, or discomfort accompanied by
  - shortness of breath
  - dizziness
  - cool, moist skin
  - nausea or vomiting
  - pain in the neck, shoulders, jaw, teeth, back, or arms
  - blue or gray face, lips, earlobes, or fingernails
  - heart palpitations or fluttering
- No relief from repeated nitroglycerin every 5 minutes for two doses
- Repeated shocks with internal defibrillator in place
- Severe pain

If the caller agrees with the advice given, document the call and encourage the caller to call back or see PCP if the problem worsens. If the caller does not agree with the advice given, reevaluate and advise the caller to follow up with PCP, Clinic, or ED.

Chest Trauma

 Key Questions Name, Age, Onset, Cause, Medications, Pain Scale, History

 Other Protocols to Consider Bleeding, Severe (90); Breathing Problems (106); Chest Pain (123); Cough (170); Shock, Suspected (547); Weakness (649).

Reminder: Document caller response to advice, home care instructions, and when to call back.

ASSESSMENT	ACTION

A. Recent injury to the chest or trunk and are any of the following present?

- Severe shortness of breath
- Altered mental status
- Lips or face is blue, very pale, or gray
- Air bubbles in chest wound with inspiration
- Severe pain in chest wall or over breastbone
- Foreign object impaled in chest wall
- Difficulty breathing, pain, and chest moves in with inspiration and out with expiration

 "Call ambulance" and Follow **Emergency Home Care Instructions**

 Go to B

B. Are any of the following present?

- Increasing pain with movement or breathing
- Increasing shortness of breath
- Coughing up blood or pink frothy sputum

YES "Seek emergency care now"

NO Go to C

C. Are any of the following present?

- Persistent pain >48 hours
- Fever
- Green, yellow, or brown sputum >48 hours
- Light-headedness develops after 24 hours

 "Seek medical care within 24 hours"

NO Follow **Home Care Instructions**

Home Care Instructions
Chest Trauma

Emergency Instructions

- For sucking chest wound, cover wound with plastic wrap or layers of tape to prevent the movement of air into the wound. Seal in place when patient is exhaling.
- Do not remove objects impaled in chest.
- Take your usual pain medication (aspirin, acetaminophen, or ibuprofen). Do not give aspirin to a child. Avoid aspirin-like products if age <20 years. Avoid acetaminophen if liver disease is present. Avoid ibuprofen if kidney disease or stomach problems exist or in the case of pregnancy. Follow the directions on the label.
- Support painful ribs with a pillow if movement increases pain.

Additional Instructions

 Report the Following Problems to Your PCP/Clinic/ED

- Increased difficulty breathing, fever, pain, or light-headedness
- Green, yellow, or brown sputum

 Seek Emergency Care Immediately If Any of the Following Occur

- Altered mental status
- Sudden severe pain or shortness of breath
- Cool, clammy, pale skin
- Coughing up blood or pink frothy sputum

If the caller agrees with the advice given, document the call and encourage the caller to call back or see PCP if the problem worsens. If the caller does not agree with the advice given, reevaluate and advise the caller to follow up with PCP, Clinic, or ED.

Chickenpox

Key Questions Name, Age, Onset, Known Exposure to Chickenpox, Date of Exposure, Pregnancy Status, Immunization Status, Description of the Lesions and Location, History, Medications

Other Protocols to Consider Breathing Problems (106); Communicable Diseases Table, Appendix M (696); Cough (170); Fever, Adult (250), Child (253); Immunization Reactions (358); Itching (382); Rash, Adult (500), Child (505); Shingles, Suspected or Exposure (544).

Nurse Alert:

- Use this protocol if known or suspected exposure to chickenpox and stages of lesions have progressed from small red bumps to blisters, then brown dry scabs on several parts of the body.

- Communicable Disease Table, Appendix M (684) is provided to help the nurse gain a better understanding of many communicable diseases, the mode of disease transmission, incubation period, and contagious period. It is NOT to be used to try and diagnose a caller's condition.

Reminder: Document caller response to advice, home care instructions, and when to call back.

ASSESSMENT	ACTION

A. Are any of the following present?

- Difficulty in awakening
- Confusion or delirium
- Difficulty breathing

YES "Call ambulance"
or
"Seek emergency care now"

NO Go to B

B. Are any of the following present?

- Severe headache
- Fast breathing
- Stiff neck
- Red, painful area of skin or red streaks
- Severe pain or swelling of the face
- Child age <1 month and lesions present
- Fever >104.9°F (40.5°C)
- Current/recent steroid treatment or immunocompromised

YES "Seek medical care within 2 hours"

NO Go to C

C

C. Are any of the following present?

- Cough or fever unresponsive to home care measures
- Vomiting >3 to 4 times
- Dry brown scab changes to soft and golden or drains pus
- Fever for >4 days
- Severe itching unresponsive to home care measures
- No history of chickenpox or immunization and pregnant
- Secondary case within the household
- No history of chickenpox or immunization and exposure <5 days
- Infant's mother had chickenpox <5 days before or <2 days after delivery

YES "Seek medical care within 24 hours"

NO Go to D

D. Are any of the following present?

- Fever and general tiredness
- Rash with red spots progressing to blisters
- Swollen and tender lymph nodes

YES "Call back or call PCP for appointment if no improvement" and
Follow **Home Care Instructions**

NO Follow **Home Care Instructions**

Home Care Instructions
Chickenpox

- Increase fluid intake.
- Take cool baths every 3 to 4 hours and take your usual medication (acetaminophen) for fever. Follow instructions on the label. Do not take aspirin.
- To control itching, try OTC preparations (Benadryl [oral], Caladryl, Cortaid, Cortizone [topical]) and follow instructions on the label, or take an oatmeal bath (Aveeno).
- Infected person should stay home until all lesions are dry.
- Avoid contact with pregnant women.
- Remember that
  - new eruptions will occur for 5 to 6 days
  - the contagious period is usually 7 days
  - symptoms occur 10 to 14 days after exposure

C

Additional Instructions

_____

_____

_____

Report the Following Problems to Your PCP/Clinic/ED

- Signs of infection: increased redness, pain, drainage, pus, red streaks
- Itching interferes with sleep
- Persistent fever >4 days
- Cough or difficulty breathing

Seek Emergency Care Immediately If Any of the Following Occur

- Stiff neck or severe headache
- Confusion or altered mental status
- Difficulty breathing

If the caller agrees with the advice given, document the call and encourage the caller to call back or see PCP if the problem worsens. If the caller does not agree with the advice given, reevaluate and advise the caller to follow up with PCP, Clinic, or ED.

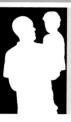

Child Abuse

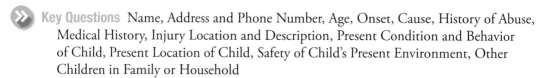

Key Questions Name, Address and Phone Number, Age, Onset, Cause, History of Abuse, Medical History, Injury Location and Description, Present Condition and Behavior of Child, Present Location of Child, Safety of Child's Present Environment, Other Children in Family or Household

Other Protocols to Consider Bone, Joint, and Tissue Injury (95); Bruising (109); Burns, Chemical (112), Electrical (115), Thermal (118); Domestic Abuse (202); Extremity Injury (222); Sexual Assault (539).

Reminder: Document caller response to advice, home care instructions, and when to call back.

ASSESSMENT	ACTION

A. Are any of the following present?

- Abuse occurring at time of call
- Severe injuries
- Unresponsive

YES "Call ambulance"
or
"Seek emergency care now and call police"

NO Go to B

B. Are any of the following present?

- Bruises in various stages of healing or in unusual areas, yellow bruises >18 hours
- Burns (such as from cigarettes or hot water)
- Extremities swollen, tender, or deformed
- Suspected fractures or dislocations
- Multiple abrasions
- Bite, buckle, or slap marks on face or body
- Parent wants to place child in a receiving home temporarily because of crisis or fear of abusing the child
- Caller suspects injured child is victim of abuse
- Caller or another person has thoughts about hurting the child

YES "Seek medical care within 2 to 4 hours"

NO Go to C

132

C. Are any of the following present?

- Suspected child abuse but no physical signs or symptoms present
- Request to discuss suspected abuse with a health-care professional

YES "Seek medical care within 24 hours"

NO Follow **Home Care Instructions**

C

Home Care Instructions
Child Abuse

- Keep in mind that a safe environment must be provided for the child.
- Refer parent or caregiver to local resources: child protective services; social services; county or state health department; area housing shelters; local police; Child Abuse Registry Hotline; family services; counseling services; or crisis hotline.
- Follow state-mandated laws for reporting alleged abuse or neglect.
- Place a follow-up call to parent or caregiver within 1 hour.
- If caller is advised to call child protective services, place a follow-up call to the caller within 1 hour; make sure the call to child protective services was made.

Referral Telephone Numbers

_____

_____

_____

Additional Instructions

_____

_____

_____

Report the Following Problem to Your PCP/Clinic/ED
- Child has been abused or abuse is suspected

If the caller agrees with the advice given, document the call and encourage the caller to call back or see PCP if the problem worsens. If the caller does not agree with the advice given, reevaluate and advise the caller to follow up with PCP, Clinic, or ED.

Choking

 Key Questions Name, Age, Onset, Cause, Pain Scale, History

 Other Protocols to Consider Breathing Problems (106); Cough (170); Foreign Body, Swallowing of (280); Sore Throat (564); Swallowing Difficulty (591); Weakness (649).

> *Nurse Alert:* If actively choking and unable to speak, cough, or breathe, instruct caller to call Emergency Medical Services (EMS) or 911. Dispatchers are specially trained in giving emergency procedure instructions over the phone while the ambulance is on the way. If caller is unable to call 911, make the call for them.

Reminder: Document caller response to advice, home care instructions, and when to call back.

ASSESSMENT	ACTION
A. Is the following present?	
• Person is conscious and unable to speak, cough, or breathe	**YES** "Call EMS/911 for emergency choking procedures"
	NO Go to B
B. Is the following present?	
• Person is unconscious and not breathing	**YES** "Call ambulance and begin CPR"
	NO Go to C
C. Are any of the following present?	
• Difficulty breathing • Blue lips or face	**YES** "Call ambulance"
	NO Go to D

C

D. Are any of the following present?

- Foreign body aspirated into lungs
- Coughing up blood or severe pain after dislodging foreign body from throat
- Unable to remove foreign object from throat and no other symptoms

 "Seek emergency care now"

NO Go to E

E. Are any of the following present?

- Able to speak and cough
- No difficulty breathing
- Frequent episodes of choking on saliva, foods, or fluids

YES "Call back or call PCP for appointment if no improvement" and
Follow **Home Care Instructions**

NO Follow **Home Care Instructions**

Home Care Instructions
Choking

- For frequent choking, eat slowly, taking smaller bites.
- If there is a sensation that a fish bone is stuck in the throat, try washing down the bone with bread and milk.

Additional Instructions

Report the Following Problems to Your PCP/Clinic/ED

- Fish bone in throat and persistent scratchy throat >2 hours
- Signs of infection: persistent sore throat, fever, drainage
- Difficulty swallowing
- No improvement or condition worsens

Seek Emergency Care Immediately If Any of the Following Occur

- Difficulty breathing
- Unable to swallow saliva or fluids
- Coughing up blood or severe pain after dislodging foreign body from the throat

If the caller agrees with the advice given, document the call and encourage the caller to call back or see PCP if the problem worsens. If the caller does not agree with the advice given, reevaluate and advise the caller to follow up with PCP, Clinic, or ED.

Chronic Obstructive Pulmonary Disease (COPD)

 Key Questions Name, Age, Onset, Prior COPD History, Severity, Peak Flow Measurement (if used), Prior Treatment, Medications, Prior History, Suspected or Known Triggers

 Other Protocols to Consider Ankle Problems (33); Asthma (52); Breathing Problems (106); Chest Pain (123); Choking (135); Congestion (153); Fever (250); Fatigue (244); Leg Pain/Swelling (398); Swelling (597); Weakness (649); Wheezing (657).

> *Nurse Alert:* Use this protocol only if previously diagnosed with COPD. The person with COPD often adapts to the symptoms of severe tiredness and shortness of breath and/or coughing with activity, which may be mistaken for the normal aging process, or a persistent cough common in long-term smokers. Poorly controlled COPD can lead to a heart attack or pulmonary hypertension (high blood pressure in the arteries that go from the heart to the lungs). Peak flow meters may be useful in measuring how well air is moving out of the lungs and help to gauge the severity of an attack in persons with worsening or severe COPD. Peak flow values are divided into three zones, and a plan must have already been developed with the PCP for treatment of the COPD based on symptoms and peak flow readings:
> Green: 80% of normal baseline or higher (mild attack)
> Yellow: 50% to 80% of normal baseline (moderate attack)
> Red: <50% of normal baseline (severe attack)

Reminder: Document caller response to advice, home care instructions, and when to call back.

ASSESSMENT	ACTION

A. Are any of the following present?

- Persistent wheezing after a treatment
- Difficulty breathing or shortness of breath
- Pain or tightness in the chest
- Inability to breathe lying down; must sit up to breathe
- Dusky or blue lips, tongue, or face
- Sudden onset of wheezing after medication, exposure to known allergen, or other triggers
- Weakness, listlessness, restlessness, or extreme tiredness
- Speaking in partial, 2- to 3-word sentences
- Peak flow rate <50% of normal baseline
- Severe wheezing or cough, and nebulizer or inhaler not available

YES "Seek emergency care now." "If breathing difficulty is severe, call ambulance"

NO Go to B

B. Are any of the following present?

- Vomiting and inability to retain medication
- Upper respiratory infection symptoms and history of:
  - steroid treatment
  - prior hospitalization for same symptoms
  - intubations
- Peak flow rate 50% to 80% of normal baseline and no improvement after using nebulizer or inhaler
- Nebulizer or inhaler used every 4 hours or less

| YES | "Seek medical care within 2 to 4 hours" |
| NO | Go to C |

C. Are any of the following present?

- Fever >100.5°F (38.1°C)
- Cough unresponsive to medication
- Minimal or temporary relief of COPD symptoms with current medications
- Chronic cough with mucous that is clear, white, yellow, or green
- Swelling in the feet, ankles, or legs
- Headaches in the morning (caused by decreased breathing during sleep, less oxygen leading to an increase in carbon dioxide)
- Peak flow rate >50% to 80% of normal baseline

| YES | "Seek medical care within 24 hours" |
| NO | Follow **Home Care Instructions** |

C

Home Care Instructions
Chronic Obstructive Pulmonary Disease (COPD)

- Quit smoking and encourage smokers in the home to smoke outside.
- Avoid known triggers, second-hand smoke, smoky or dusty areas, or pollution.
- Follow a COPD "action plan" or "management plan" developed with the PCP for use of peak flow meter if indicated, medication, and inhalers to best control COPD.
- Treat symptoms early to decrease severity of COPD. Use preventive medication as prescribed by the PCP.
- Increase fluid intake, unless on a daily fluid restriction; drink 8 to 10 glasses of water and clear liquids daily to keep the mucous thinned and easier to cough up.
- Pace activities of daily living. Slow down if activity causes increased difficulty breathing.
- Exercise regularly to help improve the lung's strength and endurance; discuss pulmonary rehabilitation with the PCP if needed to help increase ability for increased activity.
- Eat a healthy diet each day; take nutritional supplements as advised by the PCP.
- Follow-up regularly with the PCP.
- Join a COPD support group for tips on managing the disease.

Additional Instructions

Report the Following Problems to Your PCP/Clinic/ED

- No improvement after medication
- Difficulty breathing
- Prescribed treatment plan is unclear
- Peak flow rate 50% to 80% of normal baseline
- Nebulizer or inhaler used every 4 hours or less

Seek Emergency Care Immediately If Any of the Following Occur

- Breathing difficulty worsens
- Face, tongue, or lips become dusky or blue
- Pain or tightness in the chest
- Weakness, listlessness, restless
- Peak flow rate <50% of normal baseline

If the caller agrees with the advice given, document the call and encourage the caller to call back or see PCP if the problem worsens. If the caller does not agree with the advice given, reevaluate and advise the caller to follow up with PCP, Clinic, or ED.

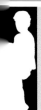

Circumcision Care

 Key Questions Name, Age, Date of Circumcision, Onset, History

 Other Protocols to Consider Genital Problems, Male (294); Wound Healing and Infection (664).

Reminder: Document caller response to advice, home care instructions, and when to call back.

ASSESSMENT	ACTION
A. Are any of the following present?	
• Difficulty controlling persistent bleeding at circumcision site • Head of penis dark blue or black	**YES** "Seek emergency care now" **NO** Go to B
B. Are any of the following present?	
• Few drops or no urine in >8 hours • Age <12 weeks and fever >100.4°F (38.0°C) • New onset of blisters • Red streaks extending down penis shaft	**YES** "Seek medical care within 2 to 4 hours" **NO** Go to C
C. Are any of the following present?	
• Swelling • Discharge or drainage from the site • Plastic ring remains in place >14 days • Plastic ring shifted to shaft of penis	**YES** "Seek medical care within 24 hours" **NO** Go to D
D. Is the following present?	
• Redness at circumcision site	**YES** "Call back or call PCP for appointment if no improvement" and Follow **Home Care Instructions** **NO** Follow **Home Care Instructions**

C

Home Care Instructions
Circumcision Care

- Apply petroleum jelly to the head of the penis every time the diaper is changed to help prevent the scab from sticking to the diaper for the first 4 days.
- Wash the penis gently with warm water and pat dry with a soft towel twice a day and when soiled. Fasten the diaper loosely to prevent friction and bleeding.
- Do not use baby wipes or alcohol to clean the circumcision site.
- Use your normal antibiotic ointments (bacitracin or Neosporin) if the circumcision is red. Follow the instructions on the label.
- The plastic ring will fall off naturally in 7 to 14 days. Do not pull the ring off even if it is loose and barely connected.

Additional Instructions

Report the Following Problems to Your PCP/Clinic/ED

- Bleeding from circumcision site
- Red streaks extending down penis shaft
- Head of penis dark blue or black
- Few drops or no urine in >8 hours
- Age <12 weeks and fever >100.4°F (38.0°C)
- New onset of blisters

If the caller agrees with the advice given, document the call and encourage the caller to call back or see PCP if the problem worsens. If the caller does not agree with the advice given, reevaluate and advise the caller to follow up with PCP, Clinic, or ED.

Cold Exposure Problems

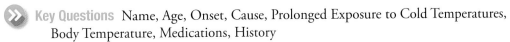

>> **Key Questions** Name, Age, Onset, Cause, Prolonged Exposure to Cold Temperatures, Body Temperature, Medications, History

>> **Other Protocols to Consider** Altered Mental Status (28); Breathing Problems (106); Confusion (150); Dizziness (199); Fainting (237); Frostbite (284); Hypotension (352).

Nurse Alert:

- The risk of serious cold injury, especially hypothermia, is higher in people who are young, elderly, lacking in insulating body fat, abusing drugs or alcohol, smoking, suffering from cardiac disease, fatigued, or malnourished. Hypothermia can be a sign of sepsis in neonates and the elderly.

- Use Frostbite protocol (279) if there has been prolonged exposure to freezing conditions and skin changes are present.

Reminder: Document caller response to advice, home care instructions, and when to call back.

ASSESSMENT	ACTION

A. Prolonged exposure to the cold (indoors or outdoors) and are any of the following present?

- Altered mental status or loss of consciousness
- Persistent rigid muscles
- Persistent purple fingers, toes, and nail beds
- Stumbling, poor coordination
- Impaired judgment, confusion, incoherence
- Difficulty breathing
- Temperature: <94°F (34.4°C) oral; <95°F (35°C) rectal
- Infant with bright red and cold skin
- Persistent numbness in hands or feet

 YES "Call ambulance" or "Seek emergency care now" and Follow **Home Care Instructions**

 NO Go to B

143

B. Prolonged exposure to the cold and are any of the following present?

- Infant, elderly, disabled, or immunosuppressed person
- Persistent shivering after warming
- Cold pale skin after exposure and unresponsive to home care measures
- Faintness
- Unable to raise body temperature to normal after 4 hours of home care

 YES "Seek medical care within 2 to 4 hours"
and
Follow **Home Care Instructions**

NO   Go to C

C. Prolonged exposure to the cold and are any of the following present?

- Cold skin
- Shivering
- Wet
- Able to talk and drink fluids

YES "Call back or call PCP for appointment if no improvement"
and
Follow **Home Care Instructions**

NO   Follow **Home Care Instructions**

Home Care Instructions
Cold Exposure Problems

- Warm the body slowly starting with the person's trunk first and then the hands and feet.
- Warm chest, neck, and groin by wrapping in blankets or skin-to-skin contact under loose blankets.
- Remove from the cold exposure and avoid reexposure, if possible.
- Do not walk on frozen feet.
- If severe exposure is <24 hours, rewarm affected part in warm water for 10 to 30 minutes or apply warm wet packs. Avoid dry heat. Stop rewarming when part is warm, red, and pliable. Do not submerge the person in warm water or a warm bath. Warming the person too quickly can cause heart problems.
- Do not place frozen part in the snow.
- Remove wet clothing and change into warm, dry clothing.
- Warm with own body and/or blankets or a sleeping bag.
- Drink warm fluids if alert and oriented.
- Eat high-energy food, such as candy, fruit, and health bars.
- Do not drink alcoholic beverages or caffeine.
- Do not massage frozen areas.
- Do not put cold-exposed person in front of a fireplace.
- Once the temperature returns to normal, keep the person wrapped in a warm blanket, including the head and neck.

Additional Instructions

Report the Following Problems to Your PCP/Clinic/ED
- Body temperature does not return to normal after 4 hours of warming
- Symptoms persist or worsen

If the caller agrees with the advice given, document the call and encourage the caller to call back or see PCP if the problem worsens. If the caller does not agree with the advice given, reevaluate and advise the caller to follow up with PCP, Clinic, or ED.

Common Cold Symptoms

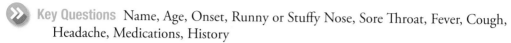 **Key Questions** Name, Age, Onset, Runny or Stuffy Nose, Sore Throat, Fever, Cough, Headache, Medications, History

Other Protocols to Consider Asthma (52); Avian Influenza (Bird Flu) Exposure (55); Breathing Problems (106); Chest Pain (123); Congestion (153); Cough (170); Earache (206); Fever, Adult (250), Child (253); Hay Fever Problems (305); Severe Acute Respiratory Syndrome (SARS) (536); Sore Throat (564); Swine Flu (H1N1 Virus) Exposure (600); West Nile Virus (653); Wheezing (657).

Reminder: Document caller response to advice, home care instructions, and when to call back.

ASSESSMENT	ACTION

A. Is there difficulty breathing for reasons other than nasal congestion?

YES	Go to Breathing Problems protocol (101)
NO	Go to B

B. Is chest pain present unrelated to deep breathing or coughing?

YES	Go to Chest Pain protocol (118)
NO	Go to C

C. Are any of the following present?

- Signs of dehydration:
  - decreased urine
  - sunken eyes
  - pinched skin does not spring back
  - excessive thirst or dry mouth
- crying without tears
- Fever and neck pain bending head forward
- Altered mental status, change in behavior or responsiveness
- Immunosuppressed, age >60 years, history of diabetes or sickle cell anemia, or bedbound with temperature >101°F (38.3°C)
- Infant < 3 months with temperature >100.4°F (38.0°C)
- Child with temperature >105°F (40.6°C)
- Adult with temperature >103°F (39.4°C)
- Fever and child appears very ill
- Change in child's breathing pattern: labored, noisy, wheezing, or chest retractions >30 minutes

YES "Seek emergency care now"

NO Go to D

D. Are any of the following present?

- Sore throat or fever >2 days
- Wheezing and age <4 years
- Persistent wheezing unrelieved by home care measures
- Ear pain or drainage
- Sinus pain >24 hours
- Fever and history of asthma, cancer, chronic obstructive pulmonary disease, CHF, diabetes, heart disease, or renal disease
- Honey-colored crusts in nostril or ear canal or around the mouth
- Fever and age >65 years
- Green, brown, or yellow sputum or nasal discharge >7 days and condition worsening

YES "Seek medical care within 24 hours"

NO Go to E

E. Are any of the following present?

- Green, brown, or yellow sputum or nasal discharge <7 days
- Blood streaks in sputum
- History of asthma, cancer, chronic obstructive pulmonary disease, CHF, diabetes, heart disease, or renal disease
- Yellow eye drainage

YES "Call back or call PCP for appointment if no improvement" and Follow **Home Care Instructions**

NO Follow **Home Care Instructions**

Home Care Instructions
Common Cold Symptoms

- Do not give cold or cough medications to a child <6 years old.
- Take pain reliever of choice for fever and discomfort. Do not give aspirin to a child. Avoid aspirin-like products if age <20 years. Avoid acetaminophen if liver disease is present. Avoid ibuprofen if kidney disease or stomach problems exist or in the case of pregnancy. Follow the directions on the label.
- Rest.
- Drink 6 to 8 glasses of liquids daily, especially warm liquids, such as tea with lemon and honey. Do not give honey to a child <1 year old.
- Take decongestant of choice for congestion (unless there is a history of hypertension or the child is <6 years old).
- Take expectorant of choice for cough. For child >1 year of age, give ½ tsp lemon juice.
- Suction secretions from infant's nose with soft rubber suction bulb.
- Use saline nose drops as needed for nasal congestion. (For homemade saline nasal drops, add ¼ tsp regular salt to ½ cup warm water.) Place three drops in each nostril and wait 1 minute, then attempt to blow nose or suction with a soft rubber suction bulb.
- Apply petroleum jelly to nasal opening to protect from irritation.
- Use a vaporizer or humidifier to keep air moist, especially at night, and change the water daily.
- If the throat is sore, gargle several times a day with warm water. Use frozen cough drops or hard candy, or sip warm chicken broth for additional relief if age >4 years.
- Use water to rinse red eyes and wipe with moistened cotton balls. Discard cotton ball after use in each eye.
- Clear nose of child before breast- or bottle-feeding.
- Remember that colds are very contagious and have an incubation period of 2 to 5 days. Use good hygiene, wash hands, dispose of used tissues, and cover mouth when sneezing or coughing.
- Avoid smoking and exposure to second-hand smoke.

Additional Instructions

_____

_____

_____

 Report the Following Problems to Your PCP/Clinic/ED

- Persistent fever >3 days or temperature of 105°F (40.6°C)
- Nasal discharge >10 days
- Persistent earache, sinus pain, or yellow eye drainage
- Formation of honey-colored crusts under nostrils
- Productive cough or fever
- Condition persists or worsens

 Seek Emergency Care Immediately If Any of the Following Occur

- Difficulty breathing for reasons other than nasal congestion
- Severe chest pain

If the caller agrees with the advice given, document the call and encourage the caller to call back or see PCP if the problem worsens. If the caller does not agree with the advice given, reevaluate and advise the caller to follow up with PCP, Clinic, or ED.

C

Confusion

 Key Questions Name, Age, Onset, Cause, Medications, History, Pain Scale

 Other Protocols to Consider Alcohol Problems (21); Altered Mental Status (28); Fever, Adult (250), Child (253); Headache (308); Mental Health Challenges in Telephone Triage (App V 720); Seizure (531); Seizure, Febrile (533); Substance Abuse, Use, or Exposure (5).

Nurse Alert: Signs of confusion may include irritability; less responsive to voice or touch; drowsiness; combative, uncooperative, nonsensical verbalizing; sudden change in behavior, thinking process, or ability to communicate; auditory (voices, buzzing, clicks), sensory (bug crawling), or visual hallucinations.

- In the elderly, confusion may be one of the first indicators of a UTI, dehydration, or a stroke.
- In a child, confusion may be one of the first indicators of rapidly progressing meningitis or a head injury after trauma.

Reminder: Document caller response to advice, home care instructions, and when to call back.

ASSESSMENT	ACTION

A. Are any of the following present?

- History of recent head trauma
- Exposure to chemicals or drug ingestion
- Diabetes
- History of stroke, high blood pressure, or cardiac disease
- Disorientation to name, date, place, or situation
- Fruity breath
- Flushing or dry skin
- Severe vomiting
- Temperature >102°F (38.9°C)
- Stiff neck, severe headache, rigidity
- Sudden weakness on one side of body
- Facial drooping on one side with smile
- Difficulty speaking
- Sudden change in vision
- Pale, diaphoretic, and light-headed or weak
- Ill child and sudden change in behavior; combative, uncooperative, nonsensical verbalizing

YES "Call ambulance"
or
"Seek emergency care now"

NO Go to B

B. Are any of the following present?

- New onset of hallucinations or paranoia
- History of drug or alcohol abuse
- Temperature >101°F (38.3°C) in a child, the elderly, or immunosuppressed
- Seizure disorder

YES "Seek medical care within 2 hours"

NO Go to C

C. Are any of the following present?

- Currently taking medications known to cause confusion
- Recently taking a new medication
- Temperature >101°F (38.3°C)
- History of dementia or chronic brain syndrome and change in mental status
- Recent abrupt cessation of drugs (OTC or prescription), alcohol, or caffeine

YES "Seek medical care within 24 hours"

NO Go to D

D. Is the following present?

- History of dementia or chronic brain syndrome and no change in status

YES "Call back or call PCP for appointment if no improvement" and Follow **Home Care Instructions**

NO Follow **Home Care Instructions**

C

Home Care Instructions
Confusion

- If taking medications that can cause delirium (antihistamines, belladonna, alkaloids), discontinue use and call back or call PCP if no improvement within 1 hour.
- Keep person comfortable in a well-lighted room in familiar surroundings and with someone in attendance.
- Give usual medication for fever (such as acetaminophen). Give cool baths to reduce fever. Do not give aspirin to a child. Avoid aspirin-like products if age <20 years. Avoid acetaminophen if liver disease is present. Avoid ibuprofen if kidney disease or stomach problems exist or in the case of pregnancy. Follow the directions on the label.

Additional Instructions

Report the Following Problems to Your PCP/Clinic/ED

- Persistent confusion >1 hour
- Persistent confusion after fever is controlled
- Other symptoms are present after delirium clears

Seek Emergency Care Immediately If Any of the Following Occur

- Severe headache or stiff neck or rigidity
- Sudden weakness on one side of body
- Difficulty speaking
- Pale, diaphoretic, and light-headed or weak
- Hallucination, paranoia, or suicidal threat or attempt
- Ill child and sudden change in behavior
- Severe vomiting
- Fruity breath
- Flushing or dry skin

If the caller agrees with the advice given, document the call and encourage the caller to call back or see PCP if the problem worsens. If the caller does not agree with the advice given, reevaluate and advise the caller to follow up with PCP, Clinic, or ED.

Congestion

 Key Questions Name, Age, Onset, Prior Treatment, Medications, History

 Other Protocols to Consider Asthma (52); Breathing Problems (106); Chest Pain (123); Common Cold Symptoms (146); Congestive Heart Failure (157); Cough (170); Earache, Drainage (206); Fever, Adult (250), Child (253); Hay Fever Problems (305); Influenza (372); Severe Acute Respiratory Syndrome (SARS) (536); Sore Throat (564); Swine Flu (H1N1 Virus) Exposure (600); Wheezing (657).

Reminder: Document caller response to advice, home care instructions, and when to call back.

ASSESSMENT	ACTION
A. Is there difficulty breathing for reasons other than nasal congestion?	
	YES Go to Breathing Problems protocol (101)
	NO Go to B
B. Is chest pain present?	
	YES Go to Chest Pain protocol (118)
	NO Go to C
C. Is wheezing present?	
	YES Wheezing protocol (652)
	NO Go to D

D. Are any of the following present?

- Fever >101°F (38.3°C) and age >60 years, bedridden, or weakened immune system
- Fever >100.4°F (38.0°C) and age <3 months
- Adult with fever >103°F (39.4°C)
- Child or elderly person appears very ill
- Young child with signs of dehydration:
  - sunken eyes or fontanel
  - pinched skin that does not spring back
  - infant cries without tears
- Child with severe pain, swelling, or redness of the upper part of the face

YES "Seek emergency care now"

NO Go to E

E. Are any of the following present?

- Several signs of dehydration:
  - infrequent urination
  - dark yellow urine
  - sunken eyes
  - pinched skin that does not spring back
  - excessive thirst
  - dry mouth or mucous membranes
- Severe pain, swelling, or redness of the upper part of the face

YES "Seek medical care within 2 to 4 hours"

NO Go to F

F. Are any of the following present?

- Sore throat or fever >2 days
- Persistent fever >100.4°F (38.0°C) >3 days
- Weakness and listlessness
- Wheezing in a child younger than 4 years
- Ear pain or drainage
- History of asthma, cancer, chronic obstructive pulmonary disease, CHF, diabetes, heart disease, renal disease, or weakened immune system
- Adult with green, brown, or yellow sputum or nasal discharge >72 hours
- Child with green, brown, or yellow sputum or nasal discharge >7 days and condition worsening
- Persistent pain >24 hours after home care

YES "Seek medical care within 24 hours"

NO Go to G

G. Are any of the following present?

- Blood streaks in sputum
- Green, brown, or yellow sputum or nasal discharge <72 hours
- Persistent sinus congestion >7 days after home care

YES "Call back or call PCP for appointment if no improvement" and Follow **Home Care Instructions**

NO Follow **Home Care Instructions**

Home Care Instructions
Congestion

- Do not give cold or cough medications to a child <6 years old.
- Take your usual pain reliever (acetaminophen, ibuprofen) for fever and discomfort. Do not give aspirin to a child. Avoid aspirin-like products if age <20 years. Avoid acetaminophen if liver disease is present. Avoid ibuprofen if kidney disease or stomach problems exist or in the case of pregnancy. Follow the directions on the label.
- Rest and drink 6 to 8 glasses of water a day. Warm liquids, such as tea with lemon and honey, are also soothing. Do not give honey to a child <1 year old.
- Take OTC decongestants (ask the pharmacist for product suggestions) for congestion. Follow the instructions on the label. (Many decongestants are contraindicated if there is a history of hypertension, asthma, heart disease, glaucoma, or enlarged prostate.) Try a vaporizer, a humidifier, or a hot steamy shower and saline nose drops first; if no relief occurs, try decongestants.
- For sinus pain, inhale the vapor of peppermint tea. Peppermint has anti-inflammatory compounds and pain relievers like menthol that relax constricted sinuses.
- Take an expectorant (ask your pharmacist for product suggestions) for cough. Follow the instructions on the label.
- Try antihistamine if congestion is due to allergy.
- Use saline nose drops as needed for nasal congestion. (For homemade saline nasal drops, add ¼ tsp of regular salt to ½ cup of warm water.) Blow each nostril separately.
- Use a vaporizer or humidifier to keep the air moist, especially at night, and change the water daily.
- If the throat is sore, gargle several times a day with warm water. Use frozen cough drops for additional relief.
- Remember that infants <3 months old often have congestion and wheezing. Use saline nose drops and a humidifier to reduce congestion. Suction secretions from the infant's nose with a soft rubber suction bulb.
- Apply petroleum jelly to the nasal opening to protect it from irritation.
- Clear the child's nose before breast- or bottle-feeding.
- Remember, colds are contagious; use good hygiene, wash hands, and dispose of used tissues. Cover the mouth with a tissue or inside the elbow sleeve when sneezing or coughing.
- Avoid smoking or exposure to second-hand smoke.

C

Additional Instructions

Report the Following Problems to Your PCP/Clinic/ED

- Persistent temperature >101°F (38.3°C) and age >4 months
- Sore throat >2 days
- Green or yellow sputum
- Persistent earache, sinus pain, or yellow eye drainage
- Chest pain
- Severe pain, swelling, or redness of the upper part of the face
- Difficulty breathing
- Fever >100.4°F (38.0°C) and age <3 months

Seek Emergency Care Immediately If Any of the Following Occur

- Chest pain unrelated to coughing or deep breathing
- Difficulty breathing for reasons other than congestion
- Young child with sign of dehydration

If the caller agrees with the advice given, document the call and encourage the caller to call back or see PCP if the problem worsens. If the caller does not agree with the advice given, reevaluate and advise the caller to follow up with PCP, Clinic, or ED.

Congestive Heart Failure

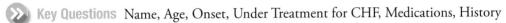 **Key Questions** Name, Age, Onset, Under Treatment for CHF, Medications, History

Other Protocols to Consider Ankle Problems (33); Breathing Problems (106); Chest Pain (123); Cough (170); Dizziness (199); Fatigue (244); Leg Pain/Swelling (398); Swelling (597); Weakness (649); Wheezing (657).

Nurse Alert: Use this protocol only if previously diagnosed with CHF and currently under treatment for CHF. Shortness of breath is the most common complaint with CHF. Person may have altered mental status or increased anxiety.

C

Reminder: Document caller response to advice, home care instructions, and when to call back.

ASSESSMENT	ACTION

A. Are any of the following present?

- Sudden onset of severe difficulty breathing
- Chest pain or pressure
- Altered mental status
- Dusky or blue lips, tongue, or fingernails
- Pale or gray face
- Unable to speak >2- to 3-word sentences due to shortness of breath
- Extreme exhaustion
- Coughing up frothy pink or copious white sputum
- Feeling of suffocation

YES "Call ambulance"
or
"Seek emergency care now"

NO Go to B

B. Are any of the following present?

- Sweating
- Increased anxiety
- Gradual increase in shortness of breath when lying flat or with activity
- Shortness of breath with exertion
- Speaking in partial sentences
- Upper respiratory infection with fever and cough
- Sudden weight gain 3 to 4 lb in 1 to 4 days
- Sudden increased swelling in legs, feet, or abdomen

YES "Seek medical care immediately"

NO Go to C

C. Are any of the following present?

- Difficulty sleeping
- Increased ankle swelling
- Increasing fatigue or weakness
- Frequent dry hacking cough
- Weight gain >3 lb in 1 day
- Increased wheezing

YES "Seek medical care within 24 hours"

NO Go to D

D. Are any of the following present?

- Congestion, sneezing, cough, and no fever
- Caregiver or person concerned and no other symptoms
- Intermittent ankle swelling

YES "Call back or call PCP for appointment if no improvement" and Follow **Home Care Instructions**

NO Follow **Home Care Instructions**

Home Care Instructions
Congestive Heart Failure

- Take medications as prescribed.
- Keep appointments with PCP and laboratory testing.
- Weigh daily before breakfast and after toileting. Keep a record and take it to appointments.
- Follow low-salt diet as instructed by health-care provider.
- Pace activities. Slow down if activity causes increased difficulty breathing.
- Avoid alcohol and smoking.

Additional Instructions

Report the Following Problems to Your PCP/Clinic/ED

- Increased difficulty breathing, wheezing, coughing, or fatigue
- Difficulty sleeping due to breathing problems or increased urination
- >3 lb weight gain in any 1 day
- Worsening ankle swelling
- Condition worsens or no improvement

Seek Emergency Care If Any of the Following Occur

- Sudden onset of severe difficulty breathing
- Chest pain or pressure
- Altered mental status
- Dusky or blue lips, tongue, face, or fingernails
- Inability to speak
- Extreme exhaustion
- Coughing up frothy pink or copious amounts of white sputum
- Feeling of suffocation

If the caller agrees with the advice given, document the call and encourage the caller to call back or see PCP if the problem worsens. If the caller does not agree with the advice given, reevaluate and advise the caller to follow up with PCP, Clinic, or ED.

Constipation

 Key Questions Name, Age, Onset, Last Bowel Movement, Medications, History, Pain Scale

 Other Protocols to Consider Abdominal Pain, Adult (9), Child (13); Abdominal Swelling (16); Diarrhea, Adult (192), Child (195); Foreign Body, Rectum (280); Hemorrhoids (327); Postoperative Problems (457); Vomiting, Adult (642), Child (645); Rectal Bleeding (510); Rectal Problems (513).

Reminder: Document caller response to advice, home care instructions, and when to call back.

ASSESSMENT	ACTION

A. Is the following present?

- Severe abdominal pain, swelling, distension, or vomiting

YES "Seek emergency care now"

NO Go to B

B. Are any of the following present?

- Persistent vomiting and progressive abdominal swelling
- Severe pain or cramping
- Vomiting brown, yellow, or green bitter-tasting emesis
- Significant rectal bleeding with no history of hemorrhoids or bleeding with constipation
- Infant <1 month, breastfeeding, and signs of dehydration

YES "Seek medical care within 2 to 4 hours"

NO Go to C

C. Are any of the following present?

- No bowel movement in 5 to 7 days and constipation unresponsive to home care measures
- Recent surgery, injury, or childbirth and no relief with home care measures
- History of diverticulitis and fever
- Infant has no stool for >6 to 10 days
- Child/infant crying, bloating, passing hard stools, and not responding to home care measures
- Fever for 24 to 48 hours, cause unknown
- Infant younger than 2 months had first stool after 24 hours and is now constipated

YES "Seek medical care within 24 hours"

NO Go to D

D. Are any of the following present?

- Dry hard stools
- Pain with bowel movements
- Recent change in stools or bowel habits
- Chronic constipation
- Small, frequently occurring liquid or hard stools
- Intermittent constipation
- Recent decrease in activity or bed rest
- Taking narcotic pain medications with codeine or other medications that increase constipation
- Blood on tissue or surface of stool

YES "Call back or call PCP for appointment if no improvement" and
Follow **Home Care Instructions**

NO Follow **Home Care Instructions**

C

Home Care Instructions
Constipation

- Make sure diet is adequate in volume (quantity), bulk (high fiber), and fluids (6 to 8 [8 ounce] glasses a day, unless on a restricted fluid diet). Add prunes or prune juice, fresh fruits, beans, and whole grains to the diet.
- Avoid constipating foods (dairy, rice, bananas, white bread, and processed foods).
- Drink a hot beverage each morning, such as coffee, tea, or hot water with lemon.
- Establish a regular time for privacy and elimination each day.
- Increase exercise as tolerated.
- Adults may try OTC bulk-forming laxatives (Metamucil, Miralax, glycerin suppositories, MOM) or an enema if other measures are unsuccessful. Follow instructions on the label. Ask pharmacist for other product suggestions.
- Infants:
  - For infants >1 month, if the infant is drinking juice, give prune or apricot juice mixed with water to help relieve constipation. Do not give enemas or laxatives.
  - For infants >2 months, give fruit juice (1 ounce per month of age, twice a day).
  - For infants >4 months, add baby foods high in fiber such as prunes, peaches, pears, or sweet potatoes.
- Children: Increase fruit juice and decrease milk to 1 pint a day. Increase high-fiber foods, such as bran cereals, oatmeal, bran muffins, or popcorn (if child >4 years). Avoid laxatives and enemas.
- May use stool softeners such as Citrucel, Metamucil, Colace, or mineral oil. (½ to 1 tbsp per day is usually sufficient. However, read directions on container label before administering.)
- For rectal pain due to constipation, sit in a warm bath for 20 minutes.
- For painful and bleeding hemorrhoids, sit in a warm tub of water after each bowel movement. Try OTC medications for hemorrhoids.
- Avoid a delay in toileting when the urge for a bowel movement is present.

Additional Instructions

Report the Following Problems to Your PCP/Clinic/ED
- Condition persists or worsens
- Fever, vomiting, and pain
- Home care measures are ineffective

Seek Emergency Care Immediately If Any of the Following Occur
- Severe abdominal pain, swelling, or vomiting

If the caller agrees with the advice given, document the call and encourage the caller to call back or see PCP if the problem worsens. If the caller does not agree with the advice given, reevaluate and advise the caller to follow up with PCP, Clinic, or ED.

Contact Lens Problems

 Key Questions Name, Age, Onset, Cause, Type of Contact, Pain Scale, Medications

 Other Protocols to Consider Eye Injury (225); Eye Problems (228); Foreign Body, Eye (269); Vision Problems (639).

Reminder: Document caller response to advice, home care instructions, and when to call back.

ASSESSMENT	ACTION

A. Are any of the following present?

- Sudden loss of vision
- Severe pain
- Penetrating injury (such as hard lens embedded in the surface of the eye)
- Severe pain after insertion of lenses that were not properly cleaned and rinsed before insertion

YES "Seek emergency care now"

NO Go to B

B. Are any of the following present?

- Hard lens broken in eye
- Persistent pain that is unresponsive to home care
- Blurred or changed vision

YES "Seek medical care within 2 to 4 hours"

NO Go to C

C. Are any of the following present?

- Pus-like drainage from eye
- No improvement or condition worsens after home care treatment
- Inability to remove contact lens
- Persistent sensation of a foreign body in the eye
- Severe sensitivity to light

YES "Seek medical care within 12 hours"

NO Go to D

D. Are any of the following present?

- Discomfort
- Eyes red or swollen and no change in vision
- Scratchy sensation
- Frequent tearing

YES "Call back or call PCP for appointment if no improvement" and Follow **Home Care Instructions**

NO Follow **Home Care Instructions**

Home Care Instructions
Contact Lens Problems

- Wash hands thoroughly before any eye care.
- To remove hard contact lens:
  - Penlight or magnification is helpful.
  - Eyelid may need to be turned inside out.
  - Place several drops of saline in eye.
  - Move lens with gentle pressure through the eyelid.
- To remove soft contact lens:
  - Place several drops of saline in the eye.
  - Gently move lens to white part of the eye.
  - Grasp lens with thumb and forefinger and remove.
- Gently irrigate affected eye with saline or water for 10 to 20 minutes.
- Rest eyes in a darkened room. Apply cold compresses or ice packs to eyes to reduce swelling.
- Take your usual pain medication (aspirin, acetaminophen, or ibuprofen) to relieve discomfort. Do not give aspirin to a child. Avoid aspirin-like products if age <20 years. Avoid acetaminophen if liver disease is present. Avoid ibuprofen if kidney disease or stomach problems exist or in the case of pregnancy. Follow the directions on the label.
- Begin wearing lenses for limited periods of time 1 week after the problem is resolved or as directed by provider.
- For eye drainage, apply warm compresses to eyes for 10 minutes several times a day. Use separate towels and wash cloths for other family members. Do not wear contact lenses when eye drainage is present. Wash hands frequently.
- Avoid rubbing or scratching eyes.
- Check contact lens for tears or irregularities.
- Sterilize contact lenses thoroughly before reinserting them after infection resolves.

Additional Instructions

Report the Following Problems to Your PCP/Clinic/ED

- Persistent redness or irritation to eyes
- Pus-like drainage or frequent tearing
- Light sensitivity
- No improvement or condition worsens
- Inability to remove lens

Seek Emergency Care Immediately If Any of the Following Occur

- Sudden loss of vision
- Severe pain to one or both eyes

If the caller agrees with the advice given, document the call and encourage the caller to call back or see PCP if the problem worsens. If the caller does not agree with the advice given, reevaluate and advise the caller to follow up with PCP, Clinic, or ED.

Contraception, Emergency (EC)

 Key Questions Name, Age, Onset (number of hours since last unprotected intercourse), Cause, Medications, Birth Control History, Other Symptoms

 Other Protocols to Consider Blood/Body Fluid Exposure (93); Domestic Abuse (202); Foreign Body, Rectum (276), Vagina (282); Sexual Assault (539); Sexually Transmitted Disease (STD); Vaginal Bleeding (633); Vaginal Discharge/Pain/Itching (636).

Reminder: Document caller response to advice, home care instructions, and when to call back.

ASSESSMENT	ACTION

A. Is the following present?

- Recently taken emergency contraception pills and signs of allergic reaction (difficulty breathing or swallowing, sudden throat or tongue swelling, inability to speak, or chest pain)

 "Go to Allergic Reaction protocol (26)"

 Go to B

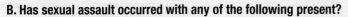

B. Has sexual assault occurred with any of the following present?

- Vaginal or anal tears or bleeding
- Request for sexual assault examination and evidence collection
- Victim is a minor

 "Seek emergency care now" and "Do not shower or change clothes to allow for evidence collection"

 Go to C

C. Are any of the following present?

- Sexual assault or forced sex occurred and medical examination without collection of evidence has been requested
- Unprotected intercourse occurred <120 hours (5 days) and person requests protection from sexually transmitted disease and pregnancy
- Copper IUD as EC has been requested; unprotected intercourse has occurred within past 5 days

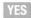 "Seek medical care within 24 hours"

 Go to D

D. Are any of the following present?

- Questions or concerns about EC
- Unprotected sex >120 hours and person has concerns about pregnancy
- EC pills taken and concerns about side effects exist; or person has nausea/vomiting, abdominal pain, dizziness, fatigue, headache, menstrual changes, or breast tenderness

YES "Call back or call PCP for appointment if no improvement" and
Follow **Home Care Instructions**

NO Follow **Home Care Instructions**

C

Home Care Instructions
Contraception, Emergency (EC)

- Provide reassurance and general information:
  - EC pills are for emergencies and should not be used for ongoing contraception.
  - EC pills do not protect against sexually transmitted diseases.
  - EC pills are most effective in the first 72 hours but can be taken up to 120 hours after unprotected sex. (The EC product "Next Choice" is taken within 72 hours [telephone 866-9WATSON]. "Plan B" is taken within 120 hours. [1-888-not-2-late or 1-668-2-5283].)
  - EC can be obtained without a prescription from select pharmacies if age is ≥16 years (some states may vary in age restrictions). If age ≤16 years, a prescription is required. Check with your pharmacy for any age requirements.
  - Additional information about EC can be located at http://ec.princeton.edu or at the hotline 1-888-not-2-late (1-668-2-5283).
  - If pregnancy is a concern, advise a urine pregnancy test be taken. Urine pregnancy tests can be purchased at most drug stores and many markets with pharmacy products.
- To prevent nausea and vomiting, Dramamine II or Benadryl may be taken 1 hour before the first EC dose.
- Provide reassurance; nausea usually passes in a short period of time.
- If vomiting occurs within 1 hour of taking EC pills, repeat the dose along with an antinausea medication.
- If side effects such as nausea/vomiting, abdominal pain, dizziness, fatigue, or breast tenderness persist >24 hours after taking EC pills, contact the PCP.
- After taking EC pills within 120 hours and having had no menses within 21 days, take a urine pregnancy test. If positive, follow up with the PCP. If negative, wait another 7 days. If no menses occur, take another urine pregnancy test and follow up with the PCP with results.

Additional Instructions

Report the Following Problems to Your PCP/Clinic/ED

- Persistent nausea/vomiting, abdominal pain, dizziness, fatigue, or breast tenderness >24 hours
- Pelvic pain with or without fever
- Concerns about pregnancy or sexually transmitted disease
- Vaginal drainage

Seek Emergency Care Immediately If Any of the Following Occur After Taking EC Pills

- Signs of allergic reaction; difficulty breathing, sudden throat or tongue swelling, rash, or hives
- Skin or lips turn gray, blue, or pale
- Sudden onset of profuse sweating
- Decrease in level of consciousness

If the caller agrees with the advice given, document the call and encourage the caller to call back or see PCP if the problem worsens. If the caller does not agree with the advice given, reevaluate and advise the caller to follow up with PCP, Clinic, or ED.

C

Cough

 Key Questions Name, Age, Onset, Prior Treatment, Related Symptoms, Medications, History

 Other Protocols to Consider Asthma (52); Breathing Problems (106); Chest Pain (123); Choking (135); Common Cold Symptoms (146); Congestion (153); Congestive Heart Failure (157); Foreign Body, Inhaled (271); Influenza (372); Pertussis (441); Severe Acute Respiratory Syndrome (SARS) (536); Sore Throat (564); Wheezing (657).

Reminder: Document caller response to advice, home care instructions, and when to call back.

ASSESSMENT	ACTION

A. Is coughing caused by choking on a foreign body, food, or vomit?

YES	Go to Choking protocol (130)
NO	Go to B

B. For reasons other than nasal congestion, is the following present?

- Sudden shortness of breath, rapid breathing, or wheezing

YES	Go to Breathing Problems protocol (101)
NO	Go to C

C. Is chest pain present?

YES	Go to Chest Pain protocol (118)
NO	Go to D

D. Are any of the following present?

- Blue lips or tongue
- Feeling of suffocation
- Frothy pink sputum
- Difficulty breathing and inability to speak
- Difficulty breathing after smoke, flame, or fume inhalation
- Sudden onset after exposure to something that previously caused a significant reaction (sting, medication, plant, chemical, food, or animal)

 YES "Call ambulance"
or
"Seek emergency care now"

NO Go to E

E. Are any of the following present?

- Cough is unrelated to cold symptoms and person has a history of
  - chest trauma >48 hours
  - blood clots or recent long sedentary period
  - recent surgery
  - recent childbirth
  - recent heart attack
  - asthma and unresponsiveness to home care measures or medication
- Coughing up blood
- Child younger than 6 months with rapid breathing and persistent cough
- Child appears very ill
- Change in child's breathing pattern: labored, noisy, wheezing, or chest retractions >30 minutes

 YES "Seek medical care within 2 hours"

NO Go to F

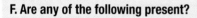

F. Are any of the following present?

- Persistent fever >72 hours that is unresponsive to fever-reducing measures
- Green or brown sputum >72 hours
- Child has a "barking" cough that is unrelieved by exposure to cool air, humidifier, or steam

YES "Seek medical care within 24 hours"

NO Go to G

G. Are any of the following present?

- Cough caused by exercise
- Persistent or worsening cough during a period of several weeks or months
- Intermittent mild chest discomfort with deep productive coughing
- Child with temperature >101°F (38.3°C) for >24 hours
- Cough with weight loss

YES "Call back or call PCP for appointment if no improvement"
and
Follow **Home Care Instructions**

NO Follow **Home Care Instructions**

Home Care Instructions
Cough

- Drink 6 to 8 glasses of water daily.
- Warm mist may help improve conditions. Breathe through a warm wet washcloth placed over the mouth and nose or sit in a steam-filled bathroom for 20 to 30 minutes.
- Elevate head of bed to reduce coughing at night.
- For children younger than 1 year, give ½ tsp lemon mixed with ½ tsp corn syrup to soothe cough.
- Give older children and adults ½ tsp lemon mixed with ½ tsp honey or corn syrup. (DO NOT give honey to a child <1 year.)
- Drink warm lemonade, apple cider, or tea to help soothe cough.
- Avoid irritants such as smoking, smog, and chemicals.
- Turn down the heat, open the windows, or go out into cooler air to help suppress cough.
- Take cough suppressants (ask your pharmacist for product suggestions) if cough is interfering with activity, causing chest pain or vomiting, or interrupting sleep at night. Do not give cough suppressants to a child <1 year. Follow instructions on the label.
- If congested, avoid milk products.
- Take OTC medications as needed, being sure to follow instructions on the label: for a wet cough, use a decongestant; for a dry cough, use an expectorant during the day and suppressant at night; for an allergy, use an antihistamine or decongestant. Ask your pharmacist for product suggestions.

Additional Instructions

Report the Following Problems to Your PCP/Clinic/ED

- No improvement or condition worsens
- Fever for >72 hours
- Green, brown, or gray sputum develops and lasts >72 hours
- Coughing up blood (more than streaks or flecks)

Seek Emergency Care Immediately If Any of the Following Occur

- Blue lips or tongue
- Feeling of suffocation
- Frothy pink sputum
- Difficulty breathing and inability to speak

If the caller agrees with the advice given, document the call and encourage the caller to call back or see PCP if the problem worsens. If the caller does not agree with the advice given, reevaluate and advise the caller to follow up with PCP, Clinic, or ED.

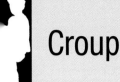

Croup

 Key Questions Name, Age, Onset, Description of Cough, Prior Treatment, Medications, Associated Symptoms, History

 Other Protocols to Consider Breathing Problems (106); Congestion (153); Cough (170); Fever, Adult (250), Child (253); Influenza (372); Pertussis (441); Sore Throat (564).

Reminder: Document caller response to advice, home care instructions, and when to call back.

ASSESSMENT	ACTION

C

A. Are any of the following present?

- Drooling, difficulty swallowing, and child looks ill
- Lips blue or dusky
- Severe difficulty breathing
- Chest caves in when breathing

YES "Call ambulance"

NO Go to B

B. Are any of the following present?

- Crowing sound when breathing in that does not clear after 20 minutes of steam, or more than three episodes during the last 24 hours
- Child appears very ill

YES "Seek emergency care now"

NO Go to C

C. Are any of the following present?

- History of pneumonia or other lung problems
- History of asthma and no improvement after home breathing treatment and usual bronchodilator

YES "Seek medical care within 2 hours"

NO Go to D

D. Are any of the following present?

- Condition worsens when lying down
- Condition interferes with sleep
- Temperature >104°F (40°C)

YES "Seek medical care within 24 hours"

NO Go to E

E. Are any of the following present?

- Barking cough >5 days
- Cough worse at night
- Barking cough heard during daytime hours

YES "Call back or call PCP for appointment if no improvement" and
Follow **Home Care Instructions**

NO Follow **Home Care Instructions**

Home Care Instructions
Croup

- Warm mist may help improve condition: breathe through a warm wet washcloth placed over the mouth and nose or sit in a steam-filled bathroom for 20 to 30 minutes.
- Continuous cool mist may help. Use a cool-mist humidifier or go out into the cool night air.
- Drink warm clear fluids to soothe cough.
- Use usual medication for fever (children's Motrin, ibuprofen, children's Tylenol, acetaminophen). Do not give aspirin to a child. Avoid aspirin-like products if age <20 years. Avoid acetaminophen if liver disease is present. Avoid ibuprofen if kidney disease or stomach problems exist or in the case of pregnancy. Follow the directions on the label.

C

Additional Instructions

Report the Following Problems to Your PCP/Clinic/ED
- No improvement or condition worsens
- Difficulty breathing
- Temperature >104°F (40°C)
- Condition persists in child with asthma after home breathing treatment

Seek Emergency Care Immediately If Any of the Following Occur
- Drooling, difficulty swallowing, and child looks ill
- Lips turn blue or dusky
- Severe difficulty breathing
- Child appears very ill
- Chest caves in with breathing
- Crowing sound that does not clear after 20 minutes of home care measures or more than three episodes in a 24-hour period

If the caller agrees with the advice given, document the call and encourage the caller to call back or see PCP if the problem worsens. If the caller does not agree with the advice given, reevaluate and advise the caller to follow up with PCP, Clinic, or ED.

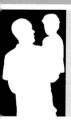

Crying, Excessive, in Infants

 Key Questions Name, Age, Onset, Cause, Medications, History

 Other Protocols to Consider Breastfeeding Problems (98); Earache, Drainage (206); Sore Throat (564); Teething (608).

Reminder: Document caller response to advice, home care instructions, and when to call back.

ASSESSMENT	ACTION

A. Are any of the following present?

- Respiratory distress
- Extreme lethargy
- Exhausted parent expressing fear that he or she may hurt the infant
- Temperature >100.4°F in infant younger than 12 weeks

YES "Call ambulance"
or
"Seek emergency care now"

NO Go to B

B. Are any of the following present?

- Projectile vomiting
- Constant crying >2 hours and unresponsive to home care measures
- Intermittent lethargy or irritability
- Temperature >104°F in infant older than 12 weeks

YES "Seek medical care within 2 hours"

NO Go to C

C. Are any of the following present?

- New onset of crying
- Infant appears sick to parent
- Crying accompanied by fever, vomiting, or pulling on ears
- Fussiness >48 hours
- Inability to sleep at night without feeding
- Crying when infant tries to sleep

YES "Seek medical care within 24 hours"

NO Go to D

D. Are any of the following present?

- Mother breastfeeding and has unrestricted diet
- Crying mostly at night from 6 pm to midnight in infant younger than 12 weeks
- Recent immunizations with fever
- Temperature >101°F (38.3°C)
- Teething with red gums and infant is 4 to 8 months old

YES "Call back or call PCP for appointment if no improvement" and
Follow **Home Care Instructions**

NO Follow **Home Care Instructions**

C

Home Care Instructions
Crying, Excessive, in Infants

- When infant begins to cry, check immediate needs for food, diaper changing, holding, or fever.
- Do not feed infant every time he/she cries; try to comfort for 15 to 20 minutes. If crying persists, lay down the infant for 15 to 20 minutes and repeat the process. Look for other causes: pulling on ears, diarrhea, eyelash in eye, or hair around finger, toe, or penis. Hold, comfort, and burp the infant. Periods of irritability are normal.
- If crying mainly at evening or night, infant may have colic pain. Rhythmic soothing activities such as rocking, swinging, or cradling often help. Apply a blanket or towel warmed in the dryer to infant's stomach; give a warm bath, provide a pacifier, and play recordings of monotonous sounds. Keep infant from sleeping >3 hours between daytime feedings to help increase nighttime sleep. A car ride in the car seat and sounds of vacuum cleaner, dishwasher, dryer, or washing machine may help soothe infant.
- If breastfeeding, avoid excessive caffeine and smoking. Breastfeed on demand, rather than on a rigid schedule.
- Acetaminophen may be given for pain or fever. Do not give aspirin to an infant or to a child. Avoid aspirin-like products if age <20 years. Avoid acetaminophen if liver disease is present. Avoid ibuprofen if kidney disease or stomach problems exist or in the case of pregnancy. Follow the directions on the label.
- If the infant is teething, provide a cold teething ring, frozen ice wrapped in a cloth, frozen banana, or frozen bagel (as appropriate for age) for the infant to chew. Avoid teething gels with benzocaine because they may numb the throat and cause choking or a drug reaction.
- Ibuprofen may be helpful in infants older than 6 months. Follow the instructions on the label.
- If taking cough or cold medications, discontinue them.

Additional Instructions

Report the Following Problems to Your PCP/Clinic/ED

- Crying becomes severe, constant, and/or interferes with infant's sleep >2 hours
- Any new signs or symptoms
- Crying does not resolve after 2 days
- Parent/caregiver becomes exhausted

Seek Emergency Care Immediately If Any of the Following Occur

- Respiratory distress
- Extreme lethargy
- Exhausted parent expresses fear that he or she may hurt the infant

If the caller agrees with the advice given, document the call and encourage the caller to call back or see PCP if the problem worsens. If the caller does not agree with the advice given, reevaluate and advise the caller to follow up with PCP, Clinic, or ED.

C

Dehydration

 Key Questions Name, Age, Onset, Cause, Medications, History, Caller or Triager Concerned about Possible Dehydration Symptoms

 Other Protocols to Consider Diabetes Problems (187); Diarrhea, Adult (192), Child (195); Fever, Adult (250), Child (253); Heat-Exposure Problems (323); Vomiting, Adult (642), Child (645); Sweating, Excessive (594).

Nurse Alert: Dehydration can quickly become a serious emergency requiring prompt medical attention. Persistent or frequent bouts of dehydration can lead to urinary tract infections, kidney stones, and kidney failure. Common causes include inadequate fluid intake, diarrhea, excessive sweating, diseases like diabetes and dementia, and medications like diuretics.

- Signs of moderate or severe dehydration
  - infrequent urination (urinate <1 time in >12 hours)
  - very dark yellow or amber urine
  - excessive thirst
  - very dry mouth, lips, and eyes
  - cries without tears
  - dizziness interferes with standing or walking
  - rapid or faint heartbeat
- Signs of mild dehydration
  - infrequent urination (urinate <3 to 4 times in >24 hours)
  - dark yellow urine
  - excessive thirst
  - weakness or unusual fatigue
  - dry mouth, tongue, thick saliva

Reminder: Document caller response to advice, home care instructions, and when to call back.

ASSESSMENT	ACTION

A. Are several of the following present?

- Altered mental status: listlessness, unusual irritability, confusion, delirium, or difficulty arousing
- Severe headache, stiff neck, or pain bending head forward
- Vomiting bright red blood or dark coffee grounds–like emesis
- Bloody or black stools
- Severe abdominal or chest pain
- Difficulty breathing
- Fever >103°F (39.4°C) without urination in >12 hours
- Hard or fast breathing, or child or the elderly appears very ill
- Signs of dehydration in a child or the elderly:
  - infrequent urination (<1 void in >12 hours)
  - dark yellow urine
  - sunken eyes or fontanel
  - pinched skin does not spring back
  - excessive thirst
  - dry mouth or mucous membranes
  - infant cries without tears

YES "Seek emergency care now"

NO Go to B

B. Are several of the following present?

- Child and no urine in 4 to 6 hours
- Signs of dehydration in an adult:
  - infrequent urination (<1 void in >12 hours)
  - dark yellow urine
  - sunken eyes or fontanel
  - pinched skin does not spring back
  - excessive thirst
  - dry mouth or mucous membranes
- Persistent vomiting, diarrhea, or fever >24 hours
- Diabetes and persistent vomiting, diarrhea, or fever
- Age >60 years, bedridden, or weakened immune system
- Dizziness, light-headedness, unsteady walking or standing

YES "Seek medical care within 2 to 4 hours"

NO Go to C

C. Are any of the following present?

- Dizzy when rising to a sitting or standing position
- Feeling faint
- Decreased urine production

YES "Seek medical care within 24 hours" "Call back or call PCP for appointment if no improvement" and

NO Follow **Home Care Instructions**

Home Care Instructions
Dehydration

- Cool down if dehydration is due to heat exposure. Remove excess clothing, apply damp towels, or spray mist the skin. If no air-conditioning, place person near fans or in the shade if outside.
- Do not eat or drink anything for 20 minutes after the last emesis. Then take small sips of fluids.
- Increase fluid intake as tolerated. Start with clear liquids, such as sports drinks, weak tea, ginger ale, clear broth, gelatin, flavored ice in very small amounts (1 ounce every 10 to 15 minutes).
- In infants younger than 1 year:
  - Introduce 1 tsp Lytren, Pedialyte, Infalyte, Rehydrate, Resol, Ricelyte, or KAO-Lectrolyte every 5 minutes and increase as tolerated.
  - Formula-fed infant needs more fluid, supplement with extra Pedialyte.
  - If breastfeeding, offer breast milk for 4 to 5 minutes every 30 to 60 minutes and offer electrolyte solution between breastfeeds, 1 tsp every 5 to 15 minutes. It is usually not necessary to discontinue breastfeeding.
- In children:
  - A child should have nothing to eat or drink for 30 minutes after last emesis.
  - Drink 1 tbsp every 5 minutes for 4 hours (fruit juice diluted with water, weak tea with sugar, clear broth, gelatin, flavored ice, sport drink diluted 50:50 with water).
  - Avoid milk and any dairy products for 12 to 24 hours after vomiting subsides.
  - Slowly introduce bland foods as tolerated (rice, potatoes, soda crackers, pretzels, dry toast, applesauce, bananas) after 8 hours without vomiting.

Additional Instructions

Report the Following Problems to Your PCP/Clinic/ED

- High fever, weakness, or abdominal pain >2 hours
- No improvement in 24 hours or condition worsens
- Persistent signs of dehydration in an adult
- Dizziness, light-headedness, unsteady walking or standing

Seek Emergency Care Immediately If Any of the Following Occur

- Altered mental status
- Vomiting blood or dark coffee grounds–like emesis
- Black or bloody stools
- Severe headache, stiff neck, or pain bending head forward
- Difficulty breathing
- Fever >103°F (39.4°C)
- Persistent signs of dehydration in the elderly or child

If the caller agrees with the advice given, document the call and encourage the caller to call back or see PCP if the problem worsens. If the caller does not agree with the advice given, reevaluate and advise the caller to follow up with PCP, Clinic, or ED.

D

Depression

Key Questions Name, Age, Onset, Trigger, Recent Related Event, Prior Suicide Attempts and Date of Last Attempt, History, Medications

Other Protocols to Consider Alcohol Problems (21); Altered Mental Status (28); Anxiety (36); Appetite Loss, Adult (39), Child (42); Domestic Abuse (202); Elder Abuse (216); Fatigue (244); Mental Health Challenges in Telephone Triage (App V, 720); Substance Abuse, Use, or Exposure (5); Suicide Attempt, Threat (585).

Nurse Alert: Obtain as much history as possible with potentially high-risk individuals: elderly with multiple somatic complaints, recent loss of a partner or major life-changing event, history of prior suicide attempts, severe eating disorders, substance abuse, inability to perform daily living activities.

Reminder: Document caller response to advice, home care instructions, and when to call back.

ASSESSMENT	ACTION

A. Are any of the following present?

- Suicidal thoughts with a plan and means to carry out the plan
- Intent to harm others
- Suicidal thoughts and injured self
- Overdose
- Altered mental status: confusion, delusional, psychotic

YES "Call ambulance" or "Seek emergency care now"

NO Go to B

B. Are any of the following present?

- Suicidal thoughts without a plan or means to carry out the plan
- New onset of delusional ideas
- Past inpatient admission for depression
- Adolescent acting out, provocative or risk-taking behavior
- New onset and recent change or addition of new medication

YES "Seek medical care within 2 to 4 hours"
Call Crisis #_____

NO Go to C

C. Are any of the following present?

- Previous suicide attempts
- Depression interfering with ability to work or function
- Loss of appetite and eating poorly
- Abrupt cessation of drugs (OTC or Rx), alcohol, or caffeine
- Drug or alcohol abuse

YES "Seek medical care within 24 hours"

NO Go to D

D. Are several of the following present?

- Difficulty concentrating
- Difficulty sleeping
- Reduced interest in sexual activity or impotency
- Irregular or absent menstruation
- No interest in activity
- Change in interpersonal relationships
- Increased use/abuse of alcohol or drugs
- Pregnant or recent childbirth
- Recent major life change
- History of depression

YES "Call back or call PCP for appointment if no improvement" and
Follow **Home Care Instructions**

NO Follow **Home Care Instructions**

D

Home Care Instructions
Depression

- If currently in counseling, call counselor for an appointment.
- Call local crisis intervention _____
  - Community counseling services _____
  - Family services _____
  - Drug and alcohol services _____
  - AA _____
- Contact friends or family for support.
- Increase exercise and enjoyable activities.
- Eat a balanced diet, drink plenty of fluids, and rest as needed.
- Alcohol or other recreational drugs can worsen depression. If heavy use of drugs or alcohol, contact counselor or PCP for help to reduce consumption.

Additional Instructions

_____

_____

_____

Report the Following Problems to Your PCP/Clinic/ED
- Suicidal thoughts without a plan or means to carry out the plan
- Depression interferes with daily activities
- Persistent inability to sleep

Seek Emergency Care Immediately If Any of the Following Occur
- Suicidal thoughts and a plan and means to carry out the plan
- Injury to self or others
- Altered mental status: confusion, delusional, psychotic

If the caller agrees with the advice given, document the call and encourage the caller to call back or see PCP if the problem worsens. If the caller does not agree with the advice given, reevaluate and advise the caller to follow up with PCP, Clinic, or ED.

Diabetes Problems

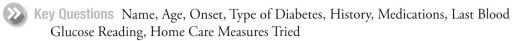 **Key Questions** Name, Age, Onset, Type of Diabetes, History, Medications, Last Blood Glucose Reading, Home Care Measures Tried

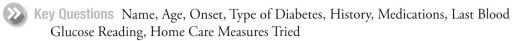 **Other Protocols to Consider** Altered Mental Status (28); Confusion (150); Diarrhea, Adult (192), Child (195); Fainting (237); Fever, Adult (250), Child (253); Vomiting, Adult (642), Child (645); Wound Healing and Infection (664).

Nurse Alert: Use this protocol only if previously diagnosed with diabetes.

Reminder: Document caller response to advice, home care instructions, and when to call back.

ASSESSMENT	ACTION
A. Are any of the following present?	
• Gradual onset of high blood glucose symptoms and	**YES** "Seek emergency care now"
• decreased level of consciousness or confusion, excessive thirst, dry mouth, frequent urination, or dry flushed skin	or "Call ambulance"
• deep and rapid breathing	**NO** Go to B
• breath smells fruity	
• weakness, fatigue, or drowsiness	
• High glucose and ketones in urine	
• After taking insulin or oral diabetic medications:	
• weakness, pale moist skin, shallow breathing, blurred or double vision, profuse sweating, light-headedness or dizziness, headache, confusion, or irritability and no improvement 15 minutes after eating something containing fast-acting sugar	
• Seizure	
• Severe dehydration	
• Insulin overdose	
• Persistent diarrhea and rapid or labored breathing	

D

B. Are any of the following present?

- High glucose level, some ketones in urine, and person is alert
- Open or infected wound unresponsive to home care measures
- Persistent vomiting for >12 hours and unable to keep down medication
- Blood glucose >300 in children or >400 in adults
- Abdominal pain
- Blood glucose <80 and unresponsive to usual methods to raise blood glucose level
- Temperature >100.4°F (38.0°C)

YES "Seek medical care within 2 to 4 hours"

NO Go to C

C. Are any of the following present?

- Progressive fatigue
- Upper respiratory infection with fever and productive cough
- Painful urination, back pain, or cloudy or bloody urine
- Poor compliance with insulin or oral medication and feels ill

YES "Seek medical care within 24 hours"

NO Go to D

D. Are any of the following present?

- Taking insulin or oral hypoglycemic agents, and blood glucose is 200 to 300
- Vomiting or diarrhea, no fever, and diabetes under control
- Requests dietary guidance and blood glucose control
- Beginning signs of insulin reaction and responsive to sugar intake (improved glucose level)
- Requests blood glucose medication refill
- Slow-healing wound

YES "Call back or call PCP for appointment if no improvement" and Follow **Home Care Instructions**

NO Follow **Home Care Instructions**

Home Care Instructions
Diabetes Problems

- When first signs of insulin reaction occur, immediately drink orange juice or cola, or suck on a hard candy or a sugar cube, but only if the person is conscious.
- Person with diabetes should continue taking insulin when ill, unless he/she is not able to eat. Regularly check blood or urine for glucose and acetone during illness.
- Exercise regularly.
- Pay special attention to the feet. Avoid cuts, sores, blisters, ill-fitting shoes, or going barefoot. Promptly treat injuries to the feet.
- Take medications as directed by physician.
- Drink extra water or noncaffeinated, nonsugared drinks to prevent dehydration. If low blood glucose is a frequent problem, keep quick-sugar foods with you at all times. Examples are table sugar, fruit juice or regular soda pop, fat-free milk, honey or corn syrup, jam, raisins, gumdrops, Life Savers candy, hard candy, glucose tablets, and glucose gel. Expect the blood glucose to rise in 15 to 20 minutes.

Additional Instructions

D

Report the Following Problems to Your PCP/Clinic/ED

- Signs of infection: increased swelling, pain, redness, drainage, or warmth
- No improvement or condition worsens
- Persistent vomiting for >12 hours and unable to keep down medication
- Blood glucose >300 in children and >500 in adults

Seek Emergency Care Immediately If Any of the Following Occur

- Person with diabetes becomes unconscious; call ambulance
- Signs of high blood glucose: decreased level of consciousness or confusion, excessive thirst, dry mouth, frequent urination, or dry flushed skin
- Signs of insulin reaction with no improvement 15 minutes after eating something with sugar
- Persistent diarrhea and rapid or labored breathing
- Severe dehydration

If the caller agrees with the advice given, document the call and encourage the caller to call back or see PCP if the problem worsens. If the caller does not agree with the advice given, reevaluate and advise the caller to follow up with PCP, Clinic, or ED.

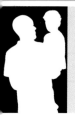

Diaper Rash

 Key Questions Name, Age, Onset, History, Medications, Description of the Rash

 Other Protocols to Consider Bedbug Exposure or Concerns (67); Bed-Wetting (70); Diarrhea, Child (195), Adult (192); Skin Lesions: Lumps, Bumps, and Sores (556).

Reminder: Document caller response to advice, home care instructions, and when to call back.

ASSESSMENT	ACTION

A. Are any of the following present?

- Large painful blisters or open sores
- Pus, boils, pimples, or crusting
- Bleeding
- Discomfort that interferes with sleep
- Rash that spreads beyond the diaper area
- Solid bright red rash
- Sore or scab on end of penis
- Unexplained temperature of >100.4°F (38°C)

YES "Seek medical care within 24 hours"

NO Go to B

B. Are any of the following present?

- Rash >3 days
- Red or weeping rash in groin and diaper area

YES "Call back or call PCP for appointment if no improvement" and Follow **Home Care Instructions**

NO Follow **Home Care Instructions**

Home Care Instructions
Diaper Rash

- Air-dry skin as much as possible—at least 1 hour a day.
- Change diapers frequently. Check each hour for wetness or soiling.
- Clean area with warm water at every diaper change. Wash with a mild soap once a day and allow to dry.
- Once skin is dry, apply a protective barrier, for example, OTC A and D Ointment, Desitin, or zinc oxide. The barrier helps to protect the skin, especially if diarrhea is present.
- Apply diaper loosely. Pin diaper front and back to T-shirt and leave sides of diaper open.
- If using cloth diapers, avoid plastic pants until rash is gone.
- Place undiapered infant on blanket next to a window in the sunlight to help heal the rash. Check infant frequently to ensure heat does not burn the skin.
- At night, use disposable diapers that keep wetness inside the diaper, away from the skin.
- Avoid diaper wipes.
- If red rash involves skin creases or has lasted >3 days, apply OTC Lotrimin to involved area.

D

Additional Instructions

Report the Following Problems to Your PCP/Clinic/ED

- Rash turns bright red or raw
- Blisters, pus, pimples, or crusting
- Persistent rash >3 days that is unresponsive to home care measures
- Rash worsens
- Unexplained fever

If the caller agrees with the advice given, document the call and encourage the caller to call back or see PCP if the problem worsens. If the caller does not agree with the advice given, reevaluate and advise the caller to follow up with PCP, Clinic, or ED.

Diarrhea, Adult

 Key Questions Name, Age, Onset, Medications, History, Associated Symptoms

 Other Protocols to Consider Abdominal Pain, Adult (9); Abdominal Swelling (16); Constipation (160); Dehydration (180); Diabetes Problems (187); Hemorrhoids (327); Rectal Bleeding (510); Stools, Abnormal (573); Vomiting, Adult (642); Weakness (649).

Nurse Alert: Diarrhea is not generally of serious concern as it is the body's way of getting rid of toxins in the digestive tract. It can be caused by the bacteria in spoiled food, laxatives, too much fiber, medications like antibiotics, chemotherapy, anxiety, or intolerance to certain foods like dairy products. If diarrhea is chronic or severe, it may be caused by more serious conditions such as colon cancer, infection, diabetes, severe constipation, or other medical problems that require prompt medical attention. Be on the alert for signs of dehydration, a common side effect of diarrhea.

Reminder: Document caller response to advice, home care instructions, and when to call back.

ASSESSMENT	ACTION

A. Are any of the following present?

- Diarrhea and severe weakness, lethargy, or faintness
- Severe abdominal pain, swelling, and fever
- Diabetic and rapid or labored breathing

YES "Seek emergency care now"

NO Go to B

B. Are any of the following present?

- Severe abdominal pain
- Grossly bloody stool
- Signs of dehydration:
  - decreased urination
  - sunken eyes
  - loose dry skin
  - excessive thirst, dry mouth
  - dry mucous membranes
- Dizziness upon standing
- Persistent vomiting and diarrhea

YES "Seek medical care within 2 to 4 hours"

NO Go to C

C. Are any of the following present?

- Diarrhea every 30 to 60 minutes for >6 hours
- Diarrhea for >5 days
- Mucus, pus, yellow, green, or frothy stool >2 days
- Persistent fever
- New onset of loss of bowel control
- No improvement with home care measures

YES "Seek medical care within 24 hours"

NO Go to D

D. Are any of the following present?

- Recent change in diet
- Other family members have diarrhea
- Recent travel to a foreign country
- Recent antibiotics in past 2 months
- New prescription
- Tube feedings

YES "Call back or call PCP for appointment if no improvement" and
Follow **Home Care Instructions**

NO Follow **Home Care Instructions**

D

Home Care Instructions
Diarrhea, Adult

- Take clear liquid diet first 12 to 24 hours (sips of water, flat soda, clear broth, gelatin [not red], flavored ice).
- During the next 12 hours, progress to eating soup (avoiding cream soups), dry toast, soda crackers, white rice, pretzels, bananas, applesauce, and potatoes.
- Progress to a regular diet after soft-formed stools occur.
- Avoid dairy products, citrus juices, raw fruits and vegetables, and fried or spicy foods for 2 to 5 days after diarrhea subsides.
- After 6 hours of diarrhea and cramping, or if pain persists, OTC antidiarrheal medications (Imodium, Kaopectate, Pepto-Bismol) can be used. Follow instructions on the label.
- Acetaminophen can be given for fever. Do not give aspirin to a child. Avoid aspirin-like products if age <20 years. Avoid acetaminophen if liver disease is present. Avoid ibuprofen if kidney disease or stomach problems exist or in the case of pregnancy. Follow the directions on the label.

Additional Instructions

Report the Following Problems to Your PCP/Clinic/ED

- No improvement or diarrhea worsens after 48 hours of home care measures
- Yellow, frothy, bloody, or green stool occurs more than one time
- Signs of dehydration
- Fever, weakness, or lethargy
- Persistent vomiting
- Person with insulin-dependent diabetes changes diet plan

Seek Emergency Care Immediately If Any of the Following Occur

- Person has diabetes and rapid or labored breathing
- Severe abdominal pain, swelling, and fever

If the caller agrees with the advice given, document the call and encourage the caller to call back or see PCP if the problem worsens. If the caller does not agree with the advice given, reevaluate and advise the caller to follow up with PCP, Clinic, or ED.

Diarrhea, Child

 Key Questions Name, Age, Onset, Frequency, Medications, History, Associated Symptoms

 Other Protocols to Consider Abdominal Pain, Child (13); Abdominal Swelling (16); Altered Mental Status (28); Confusion (150); Constipation (160); Dehydration (180); Fever, Child (253); Rectal Bleeding (510); Stools, Abnormal (573); Vomiting, Child (645).

Nurse Alert: Diarrhea is not generally of serious concern as it is the body's way of getting rid of toxins in the digestive tract. It can be caused by the bacteria in spoiled food, laxatives, too much fiber, medications like antibiotics, chemotherapy, anxiety, or intolerance to certain foods like dairy products. If diarrhea is chronic or severe, it may be caused by more serious conditions such as colon cancer, infection, diabetes, severe constipation, or other medical problems that require prompt medical attention. Be on the alert for signs of dehydration, a common side effect of diarrhea.

Reminder: Document caller response to advice, home care instructions, and when to call back.

D

ASSESSMENT	ACTION

A. Are any of the following present?

- Diarrhea and severe weakness, lethargy, listlessness, or faintness
- Vomiting with right-sided abdominal pain
- Infant younger than 3 months with diarrhea and temperature >100.4°F (38°C)
- Cold and gray skin
- Grossly bloody stool
- Breathing fast and hard
- Severe pain, drawing knees to chest with cramping

YES "Seek emergency care now"

NO Go to B

B. Are any of the following present?

- Signs of dehydration:
  - decreased urination
  - no urine for >4 to 6 hours in child younger than 1 year
  - no urine for >12 hours in child older than 1 year
- Temperature >104°F (40°C), age >3 months, and unresponsive to fever-reducing measures
  - crying without tears
  - sunken eyes or fontanels
  - excessive thirst, dry mouth
- Listlessness
- Persistent vomiting and diarrhea
- Diarrhea every hour for >8 hours
- Blood in stool

YES "Seek medical care within 2 to 4 hours"

NO Go to C

C. Are any of the following present?

- >3 diarrhea stools in 24 hours in a child younger than 1 month
- Diarrhea for >3 days or diarrhea while receiving antibiotic therapy
- Pus or mucus in stool
- No improvement with home care measures
- Temperature >103°F (39.4°C) or temperature >101°F (38.3°C) for > 48 hours
- Fever unresponsive to fever-reducing measures

YES "Seek medical care within 24 hours"

NO Go to D

D. Are any of the following present?

- Chronic diarrhea
- Recent change in diet
- Other family members or pets have diarrhea
- Recent travel to a foreign country
- New prescription
- Recent contact with a snake, lizard, or turtle

YES "Call back or call PCP for appointment if no improvement" and Follow **Home Care Instructions**

NO Follow **Home Care Instructions**

Home Care Instructions
Diarrhea, Child

Breastfeeding Infants ≤1 Year Old
- Continue to feed every 2 hours and offer rehydration fluids (Pedialyte, Infalyte, Rehydralyte) between feedings. Stools usually follow feeding. Diarrhea is a sudden increase in the frequency of stools with loose consistency.
- Do NOT give Jell-O water mixtures or sports drinks as these do not contain enough sodium, and the sugar content can make diarrhea worse.

Formula-Fed Infants ≤1 Year Old
- Give Pedialyte, Infalyte, or Rehydralyte for the first 4 to 6 hours only. Each hour, give at least 2 tsp for every pound your child weighs. Then resume full-strength formula, but give more often than usual. If diarrhea is severe, use a soy formula or soy with added rice (AR) until diarrhea has been gone for 3 days, or switch to soy or lactose-free formula if diarrhea lasts longer than 3 days.
- Do NOT give Jell-O water mixtures or sports drinks as these do not contain enough sodium, and the sugar content can make diarrhea worse.

All Infants ≥4 Months and ≤12 Months
- Offer solids, such as infant cereal (especially rice), strained applesauce, carrots, bananas, mashed potatoes, or other high-fiber foods. These starchy foods are more easily digested when your child has diarrhea.
- Avoid all fruit juices, as these will make diarrhea worse.
- If your child refuses the solids, offer extra formula rather than water.

Children ≥1 Year Old
- Fluids: Avoid juices and increase water and other fluids that are caffeine-free. Eat or drink less milk and milk products for 2 to 3 days. If solids are being taken well, milk products can still be used and should be well tolerated.
- Maintain regular diet if tolerated well.
- Avoid foods that would normally cause loose stools in your child, such as spicy sauces or beans.

Additional Home Care Advice
- Acetaminophen can be given for fever. Do not give aspirin to a child. Avoid aspirin-like products if age <20 years. Avoid acetaminophen if liver disease is present. Avoid ibuprofen if kidney disease or stomach problems exist or in the case of pregnancy. Follow the directions on the label.
- Diarrhea often is very contagious. Wash hands with soap and water after using the toilet or changing a diaper.
- If diaper rash or redness occurs in the anus, wash with running water, dry, and apply petroleum jelly or other barrier ointment to protect the area, particularly at night and during naps.

D

Additional Instructions

_____

_____

_____

Report the Following Problems to Your PCP/Clinic/ED

- No improvement or diarrhea worsens after 48 hours of home care measures
- Yellow, frothy, bloody, or green stool occurs more than once
- Signs of dehydration: decreased urination, dry mouth, no tears
- Fever, weakness, or lethargy
- Watery diarrhea and vomiting clear fluid >3 times

Seek Emergency Care Immediately If Any of the Following Occur

- Rapid or labored breathing
- Severe abdominal pain, swelling, and fever
- Infant <2 months and fever >100.4°F (38.0°C)
- Gross bloody stools
- Cold and gray skin
- Severe listlessness or fainting

If the caller agrees with the advice given, document the call and encourage the caller to call back or see PCP if the problem worsens. If the caller does not agree with the advice given, reevaluate and advise the caller to follow up with PCP, Clinic, or ED.

Dizziness

 Key Questions Name, Age, Onset, History, Medications

 Other Protocols to Consider Breathing Problems (106); Chest Pain (123); Confusion (150); Dehydration (180); Earache and Drainage (206); Fainting (237); Falls (240); Headache (308); Heart Rate Problems (320); Heat-Exposure Problems (323); Hypertension (347); Hyperventilation (350); Neurologic Symptoms (418); Rectal Bleeding (510); Stroke Suspected (576); Substance Abuse, Use, and Exposure (582); Weakness (649).

> *Nurse Alert:* Dizziness can be a minor symptom caused by inadequate fluid or food intake, heat or sun exposure, or standing up too quickly. It may also be an indication of a serious condition related to an infectious process, cardiovascular, respiratory, gastrointestinal, or neurologic disorder. Dizziness may be described as light-headedness, feeling faint, fuzzy, woozy, or a sensation of motion by the person or the environment such as spinning or whirling.

D

Reminder: Document caller response to advice, home care instructions, and when to call back.

ASSESSMENT	ACTION
A. Is chest pain present?	
	YES Go to Chest Pain protocol (118)
	NO Go to B
B. In addition to the dizziness, are any of the following present?	
• Sudden onset of weakness or numbness in the face, arms, or legs on one side of the body • Difficulty speaking or walking, confusion, facial droop • Fainting spells or loss of consciousness • Heart rate <50 or >130 bpm or irregular heart rhythm • Persistent severe headache or change in vision • Fever, pale skin, and weakness	**YES** "Seek emergency care now" **NO** Go to C

C. Are any of the following present?

- History of recent trauma or blow to the head <48 hours ago
- Recent history of severe vomiting, diarrhea, or bleeding and dizziness and pulse increase when sitting or standing
- History of diabetes

YES "Seek medical care within 2 to 4 hours"

NO Go to D

D. Are any of the following present?

- Earache, ringing in the ears, or loss of hearing
- Fever unresponsive to fever-reducing measures
- Persistent light-headedness >3 days
- Recent abrupt cessation of drugs (OTC or prescription), alcohol, or caffeine

YES "Seek medical care within 24 hours"

NO Go to E

E. Are any of the following present?

- Dizziness interferes with activities
- History of dieting, and dizziness does not improve after eating
- Dizziness occurs after taking a new medication
- Increase in stress
- Dizziness occurs during or after drinking alcohol
- Dizziness occurs when moving the head

YES "Call back or call PCP for appointment if no improvement" and Follow **Home Care Instructions**

NO Follow **Home Care Instructions**

Home Care Instructions
Dizziness

- During the dizzy spell, reach out and touch something, then lie flat or sit with head down on your lap and take deep breaths for a few minutes.
- If dizziness is accompanied by anxiety, rapid breathing, and numbness in the face or fingers, breathe into a paper bag for 5 to 10 minutes, making sure the mouth and nose are covered by the bag.
- Sit up or stand up slowly. Avoid sudden changes in posture.
- If diagnosed with labyrinthitis, consider having someone else provide transportation. Dizziness can take up to 4 weeks to resolve after starting treatment.
- In the case of persistent dizziness, avoid noisy environments.
- Limit intake of caffeinated beverages and alcohol.
- If dehydrated, drink plenty of water or sports drinks.
- Use a night light.
- Consider OTC motion sickness medications (Benadryl, Bonine) if dizziness is related to motion, and follow the instructions on the label.
- If dizziness is caused by Ménière disease, reinforce the importance of restricting salt intake.
- When feeling a "dizzy attack" coming on, stop moving for a few minutes. Reach out and lightly touch something solid and firm, then sit down and stay still.

D

Additional Instructions

Report the Following Problems to Your PCP/Clinic/ED

- Problem persists >1 week or worsens
- Persistent vomiting and dizziness

Seek Emergency Care Immediately If Any of the Following Occur

- Chest pain
- Decrease in level of consciousness
- Weakness or difficulty speaking
- Heart rate <50 or >130 bpm or irregular heart rhythm

If the caller agrees with the advice given, document the call and encourage the caller to call back or see PCP if the problem worsens. If the caller does not agree with the advice given, reevaluate and advise the caller to follow up with PCP, Clinic, or ED.

Domestic Abuse

 Key Questions Name, Age, Drug or Alcohol Issues or Concerns, Onset, Cause, History of Abuse, Medications, Other Family Members in the Home, History

 Other Protocols to Consider Alcohol Problems (21); Bites, Animal/Human (76); Bone, Joint, and Tissue Injury (95); Bruising (109); Burns, Chemical (112); Burns, Thermal (118); Child Abuse (132); Elder Abuse (216); Extremity Injury (222); Sexual Assault (539); Substance Abuse, Use, and Exposure (582).

Reminder: Document caller response to advice, home care instructions, and when to call back.

ASSESSMENT	ACTION

A. Are any of the following present?

- Person is being abused and/or threatened at time of call
- Victim is seriously injured or unresponsive
- Excessive bleeding
- Difficulty breathing

YES "Call ambulance" or "Seek emergency care now and call police"

NO Go to B

B. Are any of the following present?

- Bruises, including hand print or fingerprint
- Cigarette, scalding water, friction, or chemical burns
- Extremity swollen, tender, or deformed
- Suspected fracture or dislocation
- Other injuries or lacerations from blows
- Human bites or scratches
- Weapon used during the assault
- Pregnancy
- Victim does not feel safe
- Children are threatened or assaulted

YES "Seek medical care within 2 to 4 hours"

NO Go to C

C. Are any of the following present?

- Abuse occurred >2 days ago and injuries are not severe
- Caller requesting help or referral

YES "Seek medical care within 24 hours" and Ask questions in **Home Care Instructions**

NO Follow **Home Care Instructions**

Home Care Instructions
Domestic Abuse

- Important questions to ask:
  - Are you in a safe environment right now?
  - Are you alone?
  - Do you have children at risk?
  - Have you been abused in the past?
  - Where is the abuser right now?
  - Do you have family or friends who can help you?
  - Have you called the police, Adult Protective Services, or anyone else for help?
  - Do you need the telephone numbers for Family Adult Shelters or family crisis lines?
- Encourage caller to contact someone who has been supportive in the past.
- Offer referral numbers for local resources, including social workers, crisis services, battered adult shelters, family services, and counseling services.
- Encourage caller to notify Adult Protective Services and/or the police.
- Provide reassurance and reinforce that no one deserves to be hit, abused, or assaulted and that the abuser is likely to hit again.
- Follow up the call in 1 hour.
- Instruct caller to apply ice pack to injury to reduce swelling and discomfort for 20 minutes, 4 times a day for 24 to 48 hours.

D

Additional Instructions

Report the Following Problem to Your PCP/Clinic/ED

- Persistent or worsening pain or swelling

Seek Emergency Care Immediately If Any of the Following Occur

- Serious injury
- Excessive bleeding
- Difficulty breathing
- Chest pain as a result of the abuse
- Caller does not feel safe

If the caller agrees with the advice given, document the call and encourage the caller to call back or see PCP if the problem worsens. If the caller does not agree with the advice given, reevaluate and advise the caller to follow up with PCP, Clinic, or ED.

Drowning (Near Drowning)

 Key Questions Name, Age, Onset, Cause, History, Water Source and Temperature (if known)

 Other Protocols to Consider Altered Mental Status (28); Back/Neck Injury (59); Breathing Problems (106); Choking (135).

Reminder: Document caller response to advice, home care instructions, and when to call back.

ASSESSMENT	ACTION

A. Victim experienced near drowning, and are any of the following present?

- Unresponsiveness
- Suspected injury
- Vomiting
- Respiratory distress
- Difficulty breathing
- Lips or face blue

YES "Call ambulance"
and
YES Follow **Home Care Instructions**

NO Go to B

B. Did a near drowning occur?

- Victim was submerged under water but is now breathing and responsive

"Seek medical care within 2 to 4 hours"
and
Follow **Home Care Instructions**

NO Follow **Home Care Instructions**

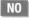

Home Care Instructions
Drowning (Near Drowning)

- For suspected neck injury, do not move victim unless absolutely necessary. Support the head and neck and allow to float in water. If necessary to move, support head and neck and torso as one unit.
- If vomiting occurs, turn victim to side and clear mouth.
- Do not press on abdomen, or vomiting may occur.
- Keep victim warm.

Additional Instructions

Report the Following Problem to Your PCP/Clinic/ED

- No improvement or condition worsens

If the caller agrees with the advice given, document the call and encourage the caller to call back or see PCP if the problem worsens. If the caller does not agree with the advice given, reevaluate and advise the caller to follow up with PCP, Clinic, or ED.

Earache, Drainage

 Key Questions Name, Age, Onset, Medications, Pain Scale

 Other Protocols to Consider Common Cold Symptoms (146); Crying, Excessive, in Infants (176); Ear Injury, Foreign Body (209); Fever, Adult (250), Child (253); Hearing Loss (314); Piercing Problems (445); Sore Throat (564).

Reminder: Document caller response to advice, home care instructions, and when to call back.

ASSESSMENT	ACTION

A. Is the following present?

- Earache, stiff neck, and fever

YES "Seek emergency care now"

NO Go to B

B. Are any of the following present?

- Swelling, pain, and redness on one side of the face
- Traumatic blow to the ear followed by severe pain, loss of hearing, bruising behind the ear, bleeding in the ear canal, or significant swelling
- Severe pain unresponsive to pain medication
- History of diabetes or immunosuppression
- Ear deviated outward
- Tenderness of bone behind ear

YES "Seek medical care within 2 to 4 hours"

NO Go to C

C. Are any of the following present?

- Sudden hearing loss and pain, ear drainage, or dizziness
- Bloody or clear drainage (different from usual ear wax)
- Swelling, pain, warmth, drainage, or fever
- Increased pain when moving or touching the ear
- Blisters or sores
- Fever, congestion, or sore throat
- Light-headedness

YES "Seek medical care within 24 hours"

NO Go to D

D. Are any of the following present?

- Unable to remove wax plug with medication and pain or decreased hearing
- Sunburned ears
- Pain after exposure to cold
- Muffled hearing but no pain
- Pain after swimming or exposure to water
- Itching
- Sudden pain with cracking or popping noise, decreased hearing and congestion
- Ringing in the ears
- Taking antibiotics for ear infection >3 days and earache persists

YES "Call back or call PCP for appointment if no improvement" and
Follow **Home Care Instructions**

NO Follow **Home Care Instructions**

E

Home Care Instructions
Earache, Drainage

- Do not instill liquid drops in the ear if pain is related to an injury or a ruptured eardrum is suspected (sudden pain, hearing loss, bleeding or discharge, ringing in the ears, dizziness).
- Apply cool compresses to sunburned ears or ice packs to swollen area caused by a blow to the ear.
- To remove excessive ear wax, use Debrox (carbamide peroxide) as directed for as long as 3 days or use two drops of mineral oil in the affected ear twice a day for 2 days.
- Apply warm compresses for ear pain for 15 to 20 minutes, 4 times a day, until resolved or while waiting for appointment. Fill a sock half full with rice. Knot the end. Microwave the sock until warm and apply against the ear. Check temperature against inner wrist before applying to the ear.
- Avoid swimming until ear pain and drainage subside.
- Swimmer's ear prevention: Mix equal parts of white vinegar and rubbing alcohol. Instill five drops of the mixture in each ear before and after swimming.
- Relieve ear congestion by frequent swallowing, chewing gum, and swallowing with the nose pinched closed.
- Avoid air travel when an earache or congestion is present. If travel is unavoidable, take a decongestant before flying, and chew gum during takeoff and landing.
- Take acetaminophen for earache or fever. Do not give aspirin to a child. Avoid aspirin-like products if age <20 years. Avoid acetaminophen if liver disease is present. Avoid ibuprofen if kidney disease or stomach problems exist or in the case of pregnancy. Follow the directions on the label.

Additional Instructions

Report the Following Problems to Your PCP/Clinic/ED

- No improvement in 3 days or condition worsens
- Persistent fever unresponsive to fever-reducing measures
- Vomiting, diarrhea, fatigue, lethargy, or stiff neck
- Fever or swelling

Seek Emergency Care Immediately If the Following Occur

- Earache, stiff neck, fever

If the caller agrees with the advice given, document the call and encourage the caller to call back or see PCP if the problem worsens. If the caller does not agree with the advice given, reevaluate and advise the caller to follow up with PCP, Clinic, or ED.

Ear Injury, Foreign Body

 Key Questions Name, Age, Onset, Cause, Medications, History, Pain Scale

Other Protocols to Consider Earache, Drainage (206); Head Injury (311); Hearing Loss (314); Piercing Problems (445).

Reminder: Document caller response to advice, home care instructions, and when to call back.

ASSESSMENT	ACTION
A. After an injury to the ear, are any of the following present?	
<ul><li>Loss of coordination</li><li>Facial paralysis or drooping</li><li>Whirling vertigo</li></ul>	**YES** "Seek emergency care now" **NO** Go to B
B. Are any of the following present?	
<ul><li>Hearing loss</li><li>Ear canal bleeding</li><li>Dizziness</li><li>Recent blow to head and clear or bloody ear canal drainage</li><li>Unable to remove foreign body or embedded piercing</li><li>Severe pain</li><li>Persistent ringing in ear</li><li>Lacerated earlobe</li><li>Insect in ear canal</li><li>Severe swelling of ear lobe</li><li>Persistent bleeding >30 minutes</li></ul>	**YES** "Seek medical care within 2 to 4 hours" **NO** Go to C
C. Are any of the following present?	
<ul><li>Persistent pain >48 hours</li><li>Earache after a blast of air, noise, or a blow to the head</li><li>External ear red and swollen</li><li>Recent use of Q-tips</li><li>Minor laceration and tetanus immunization >10 years</li><li>No improvement after 3 days of home care</li></ul>	**YES** "Seek medical care within 24 hours" **NO** "Call back or call PCP for appointment if no improvement" and Follow **Home Care Instructions**

E

Home Care Instructions
Ear Injury, Foreign Body

- Apply ice pack to ear for 20 minutes, 4 times a day, for the first 24 to 48 hours after injury. Do not apply ice directly to the skin; use a washcloth or other cloth barrier between ice and the skin.
- Point the ear toward the light and pull up on the ear to encourage an insect to crawl out of the ear toward the light.
- Do not try to remove foreign object if unable to remove by pointing ear down toward the ground and gently shaking the head while pulling up on the ear.
- Take your usual pain medication (aspirin, acetaminophen, or ibuprofen) for discomfort. Do not give aspirin to a child. Avoid aspirin-like products if age <20 years. Avoid acetaminophen if liver disease is present. Avoid ibuprofen if kidney disease or stomach problems exist or in the case of pregnancy. Follow the directions on the label.
- Watch for signs of infection: increased pain, drainage, fever, redness, or warmth.

Additional Instructions

Report the Following Problems to Your PCP/Clinic/ED

- Signs of infection: increased pain, drainage, fever, redness, or warmth
- Persistent pain >48 hours
- Dizziness
- Persistent ear canal drainage
- No improvement or condition worsens

Seek Emergency Care Immediately If Any of the Following Occur

- Loss of coordination
- Facial paralysis or drooping
- Whirling vertigo

If the caller agrees with the advice given, document the call and encourage the caller to call back or see PCP if the problem worsens. If the caller does not agree with the advice given, reevaluate and advise the caller to follow up with PCP, Clinic, or ED.

Ear Ringing

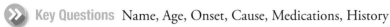

>> **Key Questions** Name, Age, Onset, Cause, Medications, History

>> **Other Protocols to Consider** Congestion (153); Dizziness (199); Earache, Drainage (206); Ear Injury, Foreign Body (209); Hearing Loss (314).

Reminder: Document caller response to advice, home care instructions, and when to call back.

ASSESSMENT	ACTION

A. Is the following present?

- Overdose or frequent ingestion of aspirin or aspirin products

YES "Seek emergency care now"

NO Go to B

B. Are any of the following present?

- Foreign body in the ear
- Severe ear pain unresponsive to home care measures

YES "Seek medical care within 2 to 4 hours"

NO Go to C

C. Are any of the following present?

- Recent ingestion of aspirin or medications containing aspirin, quinine, or streptomycin
- History of recent head injury or recent ear surgery
- Dizziness or vertigo
- Nausea or vomiting
- Persistent ear pain
- Ear drainage
- Persistent hearing loss

YES "Seek medical care within 24 hours"

NO Go to D

D. Are any of the following present?

- Upper respiratory infection
- Congestion associated with allergies
- Feeling of fullness in one or both ears
- Excessive wax buildup
- History of Ménière disease with similar symptoms

YES "Call back or call PCP for appointment if no improvement" and Follow **Home Care Instructions**

NO Follow **Home Care Instructions**

E

Home Care Instructions
Ear Ringing

- Take decongestants to relieve ear congestion. Follow instructions on the label. Ask your pharmacist for product suggestions.
- If taking medications containing aspirin, quinine, or streptomycin, stop taking and notify PCP.
- Do not poke at wax or try to remove with fingers or cotton swabs. These measures worsen the problem.
- Decrease use of salt, caffeine, and alcohol if history of Ménière disease is present.

Additional Instructions

Report the Following Problems to Your PCP/Clinic/ED

- Significant hearing loss or dizziness
- Ear pain or drainage
- Persistent vomiting, increased ringing, headache

If the caller agrees with the advice given, document the call and encourage the caller to call back or see PCP if the problem worsens. If the caller does not agree with the advice given, reevaluate and advise the caller to follow up with PCP, Clinic, or ED.

Ebola: Known or Suspected Exposure

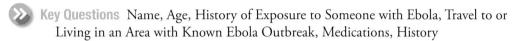 **Key Questions** Name, Age, History of Exposure to Someone with Ebola, Travel to or Living in an Area with Known Ebola Outbreak, Medications, History

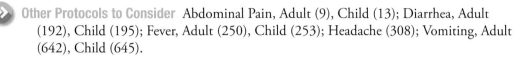 **Other Protocols to Consider** Abdominal Pain, Adult (9), Child (13); Diarrhea, Adult (192), Child (195); Fever, Adult (250), Child (253); Headache (308); Vomiting, Adult (642), Child (645).

> *Nurse Alert:* Use this protocol if
>
> - Diagnosed with Ebola
> - Known or suspected exposure to someone infected with Ebola
> - Caller or member of household has traveled to or lived in West Africa or an area with known Ebola outbreak within past 21 days
> - No known exposure but has questions about Ebola infection
> - It is important to stay current with potential changes in managing Ebola exposure. Regularly check the CDC website for updated outbreak information: www.cdc.gov/vhf/ebola, and add pertinent changes to this protocol per CDC guidelines.
> - See Home Care Instructions for additional information.
> - Emergency departments are better equipped to handle infected patients with use of protective clothing and the ability to prevent the exposure to other patients and staff. Some areas have designated facilities to handle patients with Ebola infection.
> - Incubation period is 2 to 21 days, usually 8 to 10 days, and thought to be contagious only after symptoms begin.

Reminder: Document caller response to advice, home care instructions, and when to call back.

E

ASSESSMENT	ACTION

A. Exposure to person with Ebola within past 21 days and are any of the following present?

- Unresponsive or altered mental status
- Severe difficulty breathing
- Fever >100.4°F (38.0°C), severe headache, muscle aches, abdominal pain, vomiting, diarrhea, unexplained or abnormal bleeding

 YES
"Call ambulance"
or
"Go to Emergency Department now"
and
"Notify 911 dispatchers and health-care workers of potential exposure to Ebola so they can be prepared with appropriate personal protective equipment"
"Do not use a taxi or public transportation"

 NO   Go to B

B. Exposure to person with Ebola within past 21 days and are any of the following present?

- No symptoms such as fever >100.4°F (38.0°C), severe headache, muscle aches, abdominal pain, vomiting, diarrhea, unexplained or abnormal bleeding

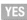 **YES**
"Notify PCP and Local Public Health Department within 24 hours of exposure"
and
Follow **Home Care Instructions**

 NO   Go to C

C. No known exposure to Ebola within past 21 days but has questions or has viral symptoms.

- No known exposure but has symptoms such as fever >100.4°F (38.0°C), severe headache, muscle aches, abdominal pain, vomiting, diarrhea, unexplained or abnormal bleeding and has concerns about Ebola infection

 YES
Follow
Home Care Instructions

Home Care Instructions
Ebola: Known or Suspected Exposure

- If going to the ED or calling 911, alert providers ahead of time so they can be prepared for arrival with appropriate protective equipment and a place for isolation. Do not use public transportation.
- If exposure to someone with Ebola within past 21 days, avoid public contact until you have remained symptom-free for 21 days since exposure.
- Caregivers or others nearby should avoid contact with infected person's body fluids, including blood, vomit, stool, semen, saliva, urine, sweat.
- Provide reassurance that the mode of transmission of Ebola is through body fluid exposure and is not airborne. As an added protective measure, if Ebola infected person is coughing or sneezing, maintain a distance of 6 feet to avoid contact with expelled saliva. Wash hands frequently.
- Monitor temperature twice a day, morning and night, and report fever or other new symptoms to PCP and health department.
- Notify health department of exposure even if no symptoms so they can assist with monitoring.
- If no exposure but has symptoms such as fever >100.4°F (38.0°C), severe headache, muscle aches, abdominal pain, vomiting, diarrhea, unexplained or abnormal bleeding. Triage using other protocols to consider. Use the protocol for the symptom that is most bothersome.

E

Additional Instructions

_____

_____

_____

Report the Following Problems to Your PCP/Clinic/ED
- No improvement or condition worsens

Seek Emergency Care Immediately If Any of the Following Occur
- Severe difficulty breathing
- Altered mental status
- Suspected exposure within 21 days and develops fever >100.4°F (38.0°C), severe headache, muscle aches, abdominal pain, vomiting, diarrhea, unexplained or abnormal bleeding

If the caller agrees with the advice given, document the call and encourage the caller to call back or see PCP if the problem worsens. If the caller does not agree with the advice given, reevaluate and advise the caller to follow up with PCP, Clinic, or ED.

Elder Abuse

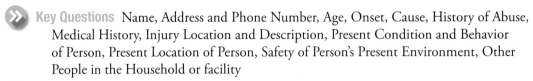

>> **Key Questions** Name, Address and Phone Number, Age, Onset, Cause, History of Abuse, Medical History, Injury Location and Description, Present Condition and Behavior of Person, Present Location of Person, Safety of Person's Present Environment, Other People in the Household or facility

>> **Other Protocols to Consider** Bone, Joint, and Tissue Injury (95); Bruising (109); Burns, Chemical (112), Electrical (115), Thermal (118); Domestic Abuse (202); Extremity Injury (222); Sexual Assault (539).

Nurse Alert: The National Center on Elder Abuse identifies three primary categories of abuse of elderly people >60 years of age: domestic (occurs in the home of the elderly or caregiver), institutional (occurs in a facility that is responsible for caring for the elderly), self-neglect (behavior is harmful to self). Elder abuse may be physical, verbal, psychological, or financial through intentional acts or lack of action. The most common risk factors for abuse are social isolation, depression, decision-making impairment, disability requiring assistance with daily activities, financial dependence by the caregiver, and aggressive behavior.

Reminder: Document caller response to advice, home care instructions, and when to call back.

ASSESSMENT	ACTION

A. Are any of the following present?

- Abuse occurring at time of call
- Severe injuries
- Unresponsive

YES "Call ambulance"
or
"Seek emergency care now and call police"

NO Go to B

B. Are any of the following present?

- Bruises in various stages of healing or in unusual areas, yellow bruises >18 hours
- Burns (such as from cigarettes or hot water)
- Extremities swollen, tender, or deformed
- Suspected fractures or dislocations
- Multiple abrasions
- Bite, buckle, or slap marks on face or body
- Caregiver wants to place person in a foster home temporarily because of crisis or fear of abusing the person
- Suspects injured person is victim of abuse
- Caregiver or another person has thoughts about hurting the person

YES "Seek medical care within 2 to 4 hours"

NO Go to C

C. Are any of the following present?

- Suspected abuse but no physical signs or symptoms present
- Significant sudden weight loss
- Unexplainable bruising
- Sudden fear of family or caregiver
- Request to discuss suspected abuse with a health-care professional

YES "Seek medical care within 24 hours"

NO Follow **Home Care Instructions**

E

Home Care Instructions
Elder Abuse

- Keep in mind that a safe environment must be provided for the person.
- In persons with advanced dementia or certain types of Alzheimer disease, abuse may be difficult to detect if there are delusions of persecution and aggression. Observe for changes in behavior from their baseline. Is the person more withdrawn, malnourished, acting differently, and with bed sores, unkempt, unexplained wounds or scars?
- Keep in mind that people who take blood thinning medications often bruise easily. Question when and how the bruise came about. Look for other areas of bruising.
- If you suspect or see signs of abuse, talk with the person in private to find out what's going on and takes steps to report it and stop it from happening again.
- For additional information, contact: The National Center on Elder Abuse (1-855-500-3537); ncea-info@aoa.hhs.gov; https://ncea.acl.gov
- Refer person or caregiver to local resources: adult protective services; social services; county or state health department; area housing shelters; local police; Elder Abuse Registry Hotline; family services; counseling services; or crisis hotline.
- Follow state-mandated laws for reporting alleged abuse or neglect.
- Place a follow-up call to person or caregiver within 1 hour.
- If caller is advised to call adult protective services (APS), place a follow-up call to the caller within 1 hour; make sure the call to APS was made. Call APS the next day to make sure a report was made. They will say yes or no but will not provide details.

Referral Telephone Numbers

Additional Instructions

Report the Following Problem to Your PCP/Clinic/ED

- Person has been abused or abuse is suspected.

If the caller agrees with the advice given, document the call and encourage the caller to call back or see PCP if the problem worsens. If the caller does not agree with the advice given, reevaluate and advise the caller to follow up with PCP, Clinic, or ED.

Electric Injury

Key Questions Name, Age, Onset, Cause, Medications, Location of Entrance Wound and Exit Wound, Tetanus Immunization Status, History

Other Protocols to Consider Altered Mental Status (28); Breathing Problems (106); Burns, Electrical (115); Heart Rate Problems (320); Seizure (531).

Reminder: Document caller response to advice, home care instructions, and when to call back.

ASSESSMENT	ACTION

A. Is the victim still engaged with the source of electricity?

YES	Instruct caller how to safely remove the victim from the electric source and call ambulance. Follow **Home Care Instructions**
NO	Go to B

B. After exposure to an electric shock, are any of the following present?

- Unconscious or altered mental status
- No pulse or respirations
- Rapid or irregular heart rate
- Difficulty breathing
- Burns above the neck
- Seizures
- High-voltage shock
- Obvious entrance and exit wounds

YES	"Call ambulance, and start CPR or rescue breathing if no pulse or respirations"
NO	Go to C

C. Are any of the following present?

- Numbness, tingling, paralysis
- Vision, hearing, or speech problems
- Burn to head, face, neck, hands, feet, or genital area
- Pale, sweaty, and light-headed or weak
- Thrown from electrical source and difficulty breathing, chest or abdominal pain
- Pain or deformity in hand or foot

YES	"Seek emergency care now"
NO	Go to D

E

D. Are any of the following present?

- Muscle pain
- Headache
- Irritability
- Fatigue
- 220-W voltage or greater

YES "Seek medical care within 2 to 4 hours"

NO Follow **Home Care Instructions**

Home Care Instructions
Electric Injury

- Remove victim from electrical source:
  - If possible, turn off the electrical current at the breaker box.
  - Do not touch a person who is connected to an electrical source.
  - Try to break the contact between the person and the source using a dry nonmetal object, such as a broom handle.
  - Use the nonmetal object to push the electrical source away from the victim.
- If the victim is in a car near a downed power line, advise the victim to stay in the car until help arrives.
- Do not go near a victim electrocuted by a high-voltage current until the power is turned off.
- Once the victim is removed from the source, check for breathing and a pulse. Begin CPR or rescue breathing if indicated. If the caller does not know CPR, provide instruction, or call emergency dispatcher for instruction.
- Keep the victim warm.
- Observe for entrance and exit wounds.

Additional Instructions

Report the Following Problems to Your PCP/Clinic/ED

- When electrical current passes through the body, internal damage can occur. Victims of electrical shock should seek medical care and evaluation.
- Signs of infection: increased redness, pain, swelling, drainage, red streaks, or fever
- Bloody or very cloudy urine

Call Ambulance Immediately If Any of the Following Occur

- Altered mental status
- Seizures
- Palpitations
- Pale, sweaty, and light-headed or weak

If the caller agrees with the advice given, document the call and encourage the caller to call back or see PCP if the problem worsens. If the caller does not agree with the advice given, reevaluate and advise the caller to follow up with PCP, Clinic, or ED.

Extremity Injury

 Key Questions Name, Age, Onset, Cause of Injury, Medications, History, Pain Scale

 Other Protocols to Consider Ankle Injury (31); Arm or Hand Problems (45); Finger and Toe Problems (257); Hand/Wrist Problems (301); Hip Pain/Injury (334); Joint Pain/ Swelling (390); Knee Pain/Swelling (393).

Reminder: Document caller response to advice, home care instructions, and when to call back.

ASSESSMENT	ACTION

A. Are any of the following present?

- Altered mental status
- Difficulty breathing
- Severe pain in the hip or thigh and unable to ambulate
- Bone protrudes through the skin

YES "Call ambulance"
or
"Seek emergency care now"

NO Go to B

B. Are any of the following present?

- Affected limb is deformed
- Fingers or toes of the affected limb are cold, blue, and numb

YES "Seek emergency care now"

NO Go to C

C. Are any of the following present?

- Severe pain with movement or weight bearing
- Difficulty moving the joint nearest the injury

YES "Seek medical care within 2 to 4 hours"
and
Follow **Home Care Instructions**

NO Go to D

D. Did any of the following occur within 30 minutes of the injury?

- Pain
- Swelling
- Discoloration

 "Seek medical care within 24 hours" and
Follow **Home Care Instructions**

 Go to E

E. Did pain, swelling, or discoloration occur within 24 to 48 hours?

YES   Follow **Home Care Instructions**

NO   Follow **Home Care Instructions**

E

Home Care Instructions
Extremity Injury

- Apply ice pack to the injured area to reduce swelling and pain for the first 24 to 48 hours. After that, alternate ice and heat. Do not apply ice directly to the skin; use a washcloth or other cloth barrier between ice and the skin.
- Elevate the affected part higher than the heart to help reduce swelling.
- For severe injuries, before going to the hospital, splint the affected limb (pillows, cardboard, or magazines can be used) above and below the injury.
- Cover open wounds with a sterile dressing.
- Take your usual medication for discomfort. Do not give aspirin to a child. Avoid aspirin-like products if age <20 years. Avoid acetaminophen if liver disease is present. Avoid ibuprofen if kidney disease or stomach problems exist or in the case of pregnancy. Follow the directions on the label.

Additional Instructions

Report the Following Problem to Your PCP/Clinic/ED

- No improvement in pain, swelling, or ability to use extremity after ice and elevation

Seek Emergency Care Immediately If Any of the Following Occur

- Extremity becomes cold, blue, and numb
- No pulse in affected extremity
- Difficulty breathing

If the caller agrees with the advice given, document the call and encourage the caller to call back or see PCP if the problem worsens. If the caller does not agree with the advice given, reevaluate and advise the caller to follow up with PCP, Clinic, or ED.

Eye Injury

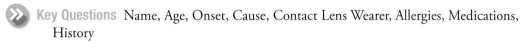

>> **Key Questions** Name, Age, Onset, Cause, Contact Lens Wearer, Allergies, Medications, History

>> **Other Protocols to Consider** Burns, Chemical (112); Eye Problems (228); Foreign Body, Eye (269); Head Injury (311); Piercing Problems (445); Vision Problems (639).

Reminder: Document caller response to advice, home care instructions, and when to call back.

ASSESSMENT	ACTION

A. Are any of the following present?

- Laceration or penetrating injury to the eye or eyelid
- Blow to the eye and sudden loss of vision
- Bulging eyeball
- Clear jellylike discharge from injured eye
- Blunt trauma to the eye
- Pupils of unequal size
- Blood in the colored part of the eye
- Persistent severe pain
- Exposure to acid such as battery acid or caustic substance (drain cleaner, lye)

YES "Seek emergency care now" and for chemical exposure, flush eye with cold running water and Follow **Home Care Instructions**

NO Go to B

B. Are any of the following present?

- Swelling, pain, and tearing >30 minutes
- Exposure to a strong light, such as a welder's arc or sun lamp
- Injury caused by hot water, chemical, pepper spray, or foreign body and pain persists after home care treatment or white part of eye becomes cloudy
- Persistent blurred or double vision

YES "Seek medical care within 2 hours" and for chemical exposure, flush eye with cold water and Follow **Home Care Instructions**

NO Go to C

E

C. Are any of the following present?

- Discomfort or irritation persists 24 hours after the injury or removal of a foreign body
- Signs of infection develop after an injury: pain, swelling, redness, drainage, or fever

YES "Seek medical care within 24 hours"

NO Go to D

D. Are any of the following present?

- Area surrounding the eye is black and blue
- Blood on white part of the eye for >3 days

YES "Call back or call PCP for appointment if no improvement" and
Follow **Home Care Instructions**

NO Follow **Home Care Instructions**

Home Care Instructions
Eye Injury

- Chemicals in the eye: Immediately flush eye with cold running water for 20 to 30 minutes. Tilt head under running water with injured eye down. While holding eyelids apart, allow water to run across the inner eye to the outer part of the eye.
- For capsaicin exposure (chili peppers, pepper spray) irrigate eye with carton of whole milk. It will act like a detergent and remove the offending substance.
- Do not rub eye.
- Apply ice pack or cool compresses to reduce swelling for the first 24 hours. Do not apply ice directly to the skin; use a washcloth or other cloth barrier between ice and the skin.
- Take acetaminophen for discomfort. Do not give aspirin to a child. Avoid aspirin-like products if age <20 years. Avoid acetaminophen if liver disease is present. Avoid ibuprofen if kidney disease or stomach problems exist or in the case of pregnancy. Follow the directions on the label.

Additional Instructions

Report the Following Problems to Your PCP/Clinic/ED

- Increased pain, swelling, drainage, or fever
- Changes in vision
- No improvement in pain after 48 hours
- Bruising around the eye or bleeding persists >2 weeks
- White part of eye becomes cloudy

Seek Emergency Care Immediately If Any of the Following Occur

- Any bleeding or jellylike discharge from the eye
- Sudden change in vision
- Persistent severe pain

If the caller agrees with the advice given, document the call and encourage the caller to call back or see PCP if the problem worsens. If the caller does not agree with the advice given, reevaluate and advise the caller to follow up with PCP, Clinic, or ED.

Eye Problems

 Key Questions Name, Age, Onset, Cause, Medications, History

 Other Protocols to Consider Neurologic Symptoms (418); Stye (580); Vision Problem (639). If injury or foreign body, see Eye Injury (225) or Foreign Body, Eye (269); Stroke Suspected (576).

Reminder: Document caller response to advice, home care instructions, and when to call back.

ASSESSMENT	ACTION

A. Are any of the following present?

- Sudden or severe pain
- Sudden vision loss or blurred or double vision
- Sudden onset of pupils of unequal size
- Curtain over field of vision
- Sudden increase in floaters
- Flashes of light
- Halos or rainbows around light
- Blood in the colored part of the eye
- Redness and unable to open eye or keep it open
- Fever, light sensitivity, bilateral swelling, and redness

YES "Seek emergency care now"

NO Go to B

B. Are any of the following present?

- Pain, redness, watering, eye drainage, and wears contact lenses
- Fever and swollen red eyelids
- Pain increases with pressure to the eye or eye movement
- Lesion on the eyeball or corner of the eye
- Eye swollen shut

YES "Seek medical care within 2 to 4 hours"

NO Go to C

C. Are any of the following present?

- Persistent pain unresponsive to home care measures
- Persistent itching, redness, burning, and drainage
- Persistent pain after removing contact lenses and irrigating eyes
- Swollen neck, lymph nodes, and redness around the entire eye
- Stye returns or bleeds
- Stye located on bottom eyelid near the nose is unresponsive to home care
- Eye pain or drainage and fever >100.5°F
- Excessive persistent tearing of eye

YES "Seek medical care within 24 hours"

NO Go to D

D. Are any of the following present?

- Blood in the white part of the eye >3 days
- History of eye pain late in the day
- History of wearing contact lenses too long or improper cleaning
- Tear duct area swollen and painful
- Small red, swollen, tender area on upper or lower lid
- Exposure to smoke, fumes, smog, pool water, known allergens, or sun lamp
- Eyes dry and itching
- Eyes crusted closed in the morning

YES "Call back or call PCP for appointment if no improvement" and
Follow **Home Care Instructions**

NO Follow **Home Care Instructions**

E

Home Care Instructions
Eye Problems

- If drainage is present, encourage family members to use separate towels and washcloths. Eye infections are highly contagious.
- Avoid rubbing or touching eyes.
- Clean crusting or discharge with cotton ball moistened in warm water. Discard cotton ball after use. Do not use same cotton ball for both eyes. Wash your hands after cleaning.
- Apply warm compresses to eyes for 15 to 20 minutes, 4 times a day.
- Wash hands frequently.
- Instill saline drops in dry itchy eyes.
- Avoid wearing contact lenses for several days until the problem is resolved.
- For styes: See Home Care Instructions in Stye protocol (580).

Additional Instructions

Report the Following Problems to Your PCP/Clinic/ED
- Condition persists or worsens after 48 hours
- Yellow or green discharge
- Fever
- Sores
- Red and swollen eyelids

Seek Emergency Care Immediately If Any of the Following Occur
- Severe pain
- Sudden loss of vision or blurred or double vision
- Sudden onset of unequal pupil size
- Blood in colored part of the eye
- Redness and unable to open eye or keep it open
- Fever, light sensitivity, bilateral swelling, and redness

If the caller agrees with the advice given, document the call and encourage the caller to call back or see PCP if the problem worsens. If the caller does not agree with the advice given, reevaluate and advise the caller to follow up with PCP, Clinic, or ED.

Facial Problems

 Key Questions Name, Age, Onset, Cause, Medications, History, Pain Scale

 Other Protocols to Consider Congestion (153); Facial Skin Problems (234); Mouth Problems (407); Numbness and Tingling (431); Piercing Problems (445); Rash, Adult (500), Child (505); Sinus Problems (554); Stroke Suspected (576); Tattoo Problems (604); Toothache (613).

Reminder: Document caller response to advice, home care instructions, and when to call back.

ASSESSMENT	ACTION

A. Are any of the following present?

- Sudden loss of vision
- Severe pain on one side of face, over eye, blurred vision, and red eye
- Adult with shoulder, chest, neck, or arm pain
- History of glaucoma
- Sudden onset of facial drooping on one side

YES "Seek emergency care now"

NO Go to B

B. Are any of the following present?

- Sudden severe pain interferes with activity
- Facial paralysis
- Pain, swelling, redness, warmth, drainage, or fever

YES "Seek medical care within 2 to 4 hours"

NO Go to C

C. Are any of the following present?

- Increased pain in afternoon or when bending over
- Green, brown, or yellow nasal discharge
- Pain along ridge between nose and lower eyelid
- Temperature >101°F (38.3°C)
- Persistent swelling
- Facial rash, blisters, or lesions

YES "Seek medical care within 24 hours"

NO Go to D

F

D. Are any of the following present?

- Recent red, blistered facial rash
- Pain, swelling, or bruising after blow to the face
- History of recent cold
- Pain follows ingestion of ice-cold foods or fluids
- Nose and eye drainage

YES "Call back or call PCP for appointment if no improvement" and
Follow **Home Care Instructions**

NO Follow **Home Care Instructions**

Home Care Instructions
Facial Problems

- Alternate cold and warm compresses to forehead and cheeks 1 minute each for 10 minutes, 4 times a day. A sock filled with rice and heated in the microwave works well.
- Increase fluid intake.
- Apply ice pack to face injury for 10 to 20 minutes, 4 times a day for first 24 hours to help reduce swelling. Do not place ice directly on the skin, use a washcloth or other cloth barrier between the ice and the skin.
- Sit in a steamy bathroom for 20 minutes several times a day to promote sinus drainage.
- Take OTC decongestants as needed for congestion and follow instructions on the label. Ask your pharmacist for product suggestions.
- Take usual pain medication (aspirin, acetaminophen, ibuprofen) for discomfort and fever. Do not give aspirin to a child. Avoid aspirin-like products if age <20 years. Avoid acetaminophen if liver disease is present. Avoid ibuprofen if kidney disease or stomach problems exist or in the case of pregnancy. Follow the directions on the label.

Additional Instructions

Report the Following Problems to Your PCP/Clinic/ED

- Persistent pain or condition worsens
- Temperature >101°F (38.3°C)
- Signs of infection: pain, swelling, redness, warmth, drainage, or red streaks
- Persistent nasal discharge
- Change in vision, hearing, smell, or taste

Seek Emergency Care Immediately If Any of the Following Occur

- Sudden loss of vision
- Severe pain on one side of face, over eye, blurred vision, and red eye
- Adult with shoulder, chest, neck, or arm pain
- Sudden facial drooping on one side of the face

F

If the caller agrees with the advice given, document the call and encourage the caller to call back or see PCP if the problem worsens. If the caller does not agree with the advice given, reevaluate and advise the caller to follow up with PCP, Clinic, or ED.

Facial Skin Problems

 Key Questions Name, Age, Onset, Medications, History

 Other Protocols to Consider Facial Problems (231); Mouth Problems (407);
Rash, Adult (500), Child (505); Shingles: Suspected or Exposure (544);
Skin Lesions: Lumps, Bumps, and Sores (556).

Reminder: Document caller response to advice, home care instructions, and when to call back.

ASSESSMENT	ACTION
A. Are any of the following present?	
• Sudden onset of facial drooping • Severe facial swelling • Rapidly spreading red or purple rash that develops into blisters on mucous membranes (lips, mouth, eyes, genitals) • Peeling or shedding large amount of skin • Unexplained widespread pain	**YES** "Seek emergency care now" **NO** Go to B
B. Are any of the following present?	
• Signs of infection: swelling, redness, pain, warmth, temperature >100°F (37.8°C), drainage, or red streaks • Large, open, draining lesions	**YES** "Seek medical care within 2 to 4 hours" **NO** Go to C
C. Are any of the following present?	
• Crusty, tender lesions around nostrils or lips • Blisters on one side of face preceded by pain and burning 1 to 2 days before rash appearance • Persistent flat or slightly raised lesions with irregular borders • Recent rapid change in color, size, or shape of mole	**YES** "Seek medical care within 24 hours" **NO** Go to D

D. Are any of the following present?

- Itching rash interferes with sleep
- Persistent acne unresponsive to OTC and home care measures
- Flushed face
- Blister, or red, rough, or painful area around mouth
- Swollen, tender lump under skin
- Sudden appearance of mole or painless lump
- Persistent sore >3 weeks

YES "Call back or call PCP for appointment if no improvement" and
Follow **Home Care Instructions**

NO Follow **Home Care Instructions**

F

Home Care Instructions
Facial Skin Problems

- Wash with mild soap (OTC products, i.e., Aveeno, Basis, Cetaphil, Dove, Neutrogena) and rinse well.
- For signs of infection, apply hot moist packs to area for 20 minutes, 4 to 6 times a day.
- Do not break open or squeeze lesions.
- Keep scalp hair off face.
- Apply lip protectant (Blistex) or analgesic (Campho-Phenique) to sores around mouth to reduce discomfort. Keep sores moist with petroleum jelly–based product. Follow instructions on the label. Ask your pharmacist for suggestions for other OTC products.

Additional Instructions

Report the Following Problems to Your PCP/Clinic/ED

- Persistent sores around mouth >14 days
- No improvement or condition worsens
- Signs of infection
- Severe pain or itching interferes with activity

Seek Emergency Care If Any of the Following Occur

- Sudden onset of facial drooping or numbness
- Severe facial swelling
- Rapidly spreading red or purple rash that develops into blisters on mucous membranes (lips, mouth, eyes, genitals)
- Peeling or shedding large amount of skin
- Unexplained widespread pain

If the caller agrees with the advice given, document the call and encourage the caller to call back or see PCP if the problem worsens. If the caller does not agree with the advice given, reevaluate and advise the caller to follow up with PCP, Clinic, or ED.

Fainting

 Key Questions Name, Age, Onset, Cause, Additional Injuries, Medications, History

 Other Protocols to Consider Alcohol Problems (21); Confusion (150); Diabetes Problems (187); Dizziness (199); Heart Rate Problems (320); Heat-Exposure Problems (323); Pregnancy Problems (481); Stroke Suspected (576); Weakness (649).

Reminder: Document caller response to advice, home care instructions, and when to call back.

ASSESSMENT	ACTION

A. Is the person still unconscious or has slow, irregular, or noisy breathing?

YES	"Call ambulance"
NO	Go to B

B. Is chest, jaw, neck, shoulder, or arm pain present?

YES	Go to Chest Pain protocol (118)
NO	Go to C

C. Are any of the following present?

- Loss of consciousness >1 to 2 minutes
- Loss of movement in arms or legs, confusion, difficulty speaking, numbness or tingling, or blurred vision
- History of recent head injury
- History of heart problems or diabetes
- Irregular or rapid heartbeat
- Severe headache
- Severe back or abdominal pain
- Recent bloody or black tarry stools
- Shortness of breath

YES	"Call ambulance" or "Seek emergency care now"
NO	Go to D

F

237

D. Are any of the following present?

- Signs of dehydration:
  - infrequent urination
  - dark yellow urine
  - sunken eyes
  - poor skin elasticity
  - excessive thirst
  - dry mouth or mucous membranes
- Continued light-headedness or dizziness

YES "Seek medical care within 2 to 4 hours"

NO Go to E

E. Are any of the following present?

- Person is older than 50 years and faintness occurs after turning head or looking up
- Pregnancy or LMP >6 weeks ago

YES "Seek medical care within 24 hours"

NO Go to F

F. In addition to light-headedness, are any of the following present?

- Several hours of exposure to the sun or a hot environment
- Prolonged period of time since eating
- Feeling faint after suddenly standing from a lying, sitting, or bending position
- Recent onset of an emotional event
- Feeling faint after strenuous exercise
- Faintness after prolonged standing in one spot
- New blood pressure medication
- Faintness occurred after a period of rapid breathing and numbness in hands, toes, or face

YES "Call back or call PCP for appointment if no improvement" and
Follow **Home Care Instructions**

NO Follow **Home Care Instructions**

Home Care Instructions
Fainting

- For faintness, raise legs higher than the head or sit and lower head between the knees until sensation passes.
- If there has been prolonged exposure to heat, sip cool fluids and apply cold compresses to cool the body.
- Avoid sudden posture changes: slowly stand from a lying, sitting, or bending position.
- If the person has diabetes, check blood sugar and take appropriate action. For low blood sugar, drink a glass of orange juice, cola, or milk.
- Eat frequent small protein snacks. Eat a well-balanced, sensible, weight-reduction diet if overweight.
- Avoid prolonged standing in one position. Shift weight from foot to foot. Walk around if possible.

Additional Instructions

Report the Following Problems to Your PCP/Clinic/ED

- Frequent episodes of light-headedness
- New blood pressure medication and faintness persists
- Condition persists or worsens
- New-onset, bloody or black tarry stools
- Possibility of pregnancy

F

Seek Emergency Care Immediately If Any of the Following Occur

- Chest, jaw, neck, shoulder, or arm pain
- Severe headache
- Severe back or abdominal pain
- Fainting recurs
- Shortness of breath

If the caller agrees with the advice given, document the call and encourage the caller to call back or see PCP if the problem worsens. If the caller does not agree with the advice given, reevaluate and advise the caller to follow up with PCP, Clinic, or ED.

Falls

 Key Questions Name, Age, Onset, Cause, Distance of Fall, Medications, History

 Other Protocols to Consider Alcohol Problems (21); Altered Mental Status (28); Back/Neck Injury (59); Bruising (109); Confusion (150); Diabetes Problems (187); Dizziness (199); Domestic Abuse (202); Extremity Injury (222); Head Injury (311); Hip Pain, Injury (334); Neck Pain (415); Neurologic Symptoms (418); Substance Abuse, Use, or Exposure (582); Weakness (649).

> *Nurse Alert:* One in every three seniors older than 75 years living at home suffers from a serious fall once a year. After a serious fracture from a fall, 25% die in 6 months to 1 year due to immobility or bedridden conditions. See Home Care Instructions (233) for fall prevention guidelines.

Reminder: Document caller response to advice, home care instructions, and when to call back.

ASSESSMENT	ACTION

A. Are any of the following present after a fall?

- Confusion or altered mental status
- Lack of coordination
- Persistent vomiting
- Slurred speech
- Weakness, tingling, or numbness in extremities
- Weakness on one side of the body
- Severe headache
- Person is unable to stand or walk
- Blurred or double vision
- Neck pain
- Seizure
- Suspicious story concerning the fall (and potential abuse suspected)
- Abdominal or chest pain
- Shortness of breath

 "Call ambulance"
or
"Seek emergency care now"

 Go to B

B. Are any of the following present?

- Blood or fluid draining from ear or nose (no known nose injury)
- Bruising behind the ear
- Limb pain, swelling, or deformity
- Back pain
- Soft spongy swelling over the skull for >12 hours in children older than 1 year
- Swelling over skull in child younger than 1 year

 YES "Seek medical care within 2 to 4 hours"

NO Go to C

C. Are any of the following present?

- Recent history of frequent falls
- Recent abrupt cessation of drugs (OTC, Rx, or street), alcohol, or caffeine

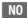 **YES** "Seek medical care within 24 hours"

NO Go to D

D. Are any of the following present?

- Swelling or bruising
- Stiffness or soreness 24 to 48 hours after a fall

YES "Call back or call PCP for appointment if no improvement" and
Follow **Home Care Instructions**

NO Follow **Home Care Instructions**

F

Home Care Instructions
Falls

- Apply ice to swollen area for 20 minutes, 4 times a day for the first 24 to 48 hours. Do not place ice directly on the skin, use a washcloth or other cloth barrier between the ice and the skin.
- Expect black and blue marks for 1 week or longer.
- Assess home for safety hazards and correct problems.
- Contact local community or senior center for information on exercise, fall prevention programs, and tips for improving home safety.
- Visit fall prevention website: www.cdc.gov/injury or www.stopfalls.org

Fall Prevention Guidelines
- Get regular exercise to improve strength and balance.
- Have eye examination annually and replace eyeglasses when change in prescription is made.
- Ask physician or pharmacist to review medications as some may alter vision, cause dizziness or confusion.
- Wear sensible shoes.
- Secure or remove loose rugs.
- Remove clutter or tripping hazards.
- Add nonslip bath-safety stickers to shower and tub floors.
- Add railings to all stairs and ensure adequate lighting.
- Add grab bars in bathrooms.
- Place a bench or place to sit in dressing area—many falls occur when trying to get dressed.

Additional Instructions

Report the Following Problems to Your PCP/Clinic/ED
- Symptoms persist or worsen
- Frequent episodes of falling
- Increasing difficulty with mobility
- Severe pain develops

Seek Emergency Care Immediately If Any of the Following Occur

- Altered mental status or confusion
- Lack of coordination
- Persistent vomiting
- Slurred speech
- Weakness, tingling, or numbness in extremities
- Weakness on one side of the body
- Severe headache
- Blurred or double vision
- Neck pain
- Seizure
- Young child does not recognize parents or caregiver

If the caller agrees with the advice given, document the call and encourage the caller to call back or see PCP if the problem worsens. If the caller does not agree with the advice given, reevaluate and advise the caller to follow up with PCP, Clinic, or ED.

F

Fatigue

 Key Questions Name, Age, Onset, Medications, History

 Other Protocols to Consider Depression (184); Fever, Adult (250), Child (253);
Postoperative Problems (457); Pregnancy Problems (481); Rectal Bleeding (510);
Vaginal Bleeding (633); Weakness (649).

Reminder: Document caller response to advice, home care instructions, and when to call back.

ASSESSMENT	ACTION
A. Is chest pain present?	
	YES Go to Chest Pain protocol (118)
	NO Go to B
B. Is there difficulty breathing?	
	YES Go to Breathing Problems protocol (101)
	NO Go to C
C. Are any of the following present?	
• Persistent black or bloody stools • Vomiting blood or dark coffee grounds–like emesis • Sudden onset of weakness on one side of the body • New onset of irregular or slow heartbeat (<50)	**YES** "Seek emergency care now" **NO** Go to D
D. Are any of the following present?	
• Sudden onset of extreme fatigue • Unexplained muscle weakness • Abnormal vaginal, rectal, or nasal bleeding	**YES** "Seek medical care within 2 to 4 hours" **NO** Go to E

E. Are any of the following present?

- Progressive fatigue that limits usual activities
- Persistent fever unresponsive to fever-reducing measures
- Sudden unexplained loss of weight

 "Seek medical care within 24 hours"

 Go to F

F. Are any of the following present?

- Depression or psychological problems
- Intermittent or persistent fatigue
- Difficulty sleeping
- Poor diet or eating habits
- Chronic allergies
- Recovering from an illness
- History of anemia, cardiac problems, kidney disease, diabetes, thyroid problems, or stroke
- Onset with recent increase in stress or activity

YES "Call back or call PCP for appointment if no improvement" and Follow **Home Care Instructions**

NO Follow **Home Care Instructions**

F

Home Care Instructions
Fatigue

- Eat a sensible, well-balanced diet. Avoid sweets to "boost energy."
- Take vitamin supplements as needed.
- Maintain a regular exercise routine. Take short walks if vigorous activity is too strenuous.
- Get an adequate amount of sleep. Try to establish a consistent sleeping pattern.
- Increase rest, relaxation, and recreation to decrease stress.
- Limit medications that contribute to fatigue, such as sleeping medications or cold and allergy medications. If prescription medication is causing fatigue, contact your PCP.
- Limit use of caffeine, smoking, and alcohol consumption.

Additional Instructions

Report the Following Problems to Your PCP/Clinic/ED

- Condition persists >2 weeks or worsens
- Fever

Seek Emergency Care Immediately If Any of the Following Occur

- Chest pain or difficulty breathing
- Black or bloody stools
- Vomiting blood or dark coffee grounds–like emesis
- Sudden onset of one-sided weakness
- New onset of irregular or slow heartbeat (<50)

If the caller agrees with the advice given, document the call and encourage the caller to call back or see PCP if the problem worsens. If the caller does not agree with the advice given, reevaluate and advise the caller to follow up with PCP, Clinic, or ED.

Feeding Tube Problems

 Key Questions Name, Age, Onset, Cause, Type of Tube, Length of Time, Tube in Place, Medications, History

 Other Protocols to Consider Abdominal Swelling (16); Wound Healing and Infection (664).

Reminder: Document caller response to advice, home care instructions, and when to call back.

ASSESSMENT	ACTION
A. Are any of the following present?	
• Severe bleeding • Severe pain • Sudden onset of difficulty breathing or shortness of breath	**YES** "Call ambulance" or "Seek emergency care now"
	NO Go to B
B. Is the following present?	
• Feeding tube removed or dislodged and pain, bleeding, or swelling	**YES** "Seek medical care within 2 to 4 hours"
	NO Go to C
C. Are any of the following present?	
• Tube frequently clogs after medication or feeding solution is added • Unable to unclog tube after trying home care measures • Feeding tube fell out • Caregiver concerned tube is displaced • Insertion site appears infected (redness, swelling, pain, red streaks, or drainage)	**YES** "Seek medical care or home health nurse visit within 24 hours"
	NO Go to D

F

247

D. Is the following present?

- Inability to pass solution into feeding tube

  YES "Call back or call PCP for appointment if no improvement" and
  Follow **Home Care Instructions**

  NO Follow **Home Care Instructions**

Home Care Instructions
Feeding Tube Problems

- To unclog feeding tube (for a caregiver who has received previous instructions; if no previous instruction, refer caller to home health nurse, PCP, Clinic, or ED):
  - Raise head of bed 45 degrees.
  - Insert the tip of a large syringe into the tube and pull back to remove as much matter from the tube as possible.
  - Fill the syringe with 30 mL (1 ounce) of water.
  - Connect syringe to tube and irrigate.
  - Remove as much matter as possible.
  - Push 5 mL of cranberry juice, cola, or tea into the tube and clamp.
  - Repeat the process until the tube is cleared.
- Flush tube with 50 mL of water after feeding, medications, or supplements are inserted into the tube.
- To check placement of feeding tube (for a caregiver who has received instruction from a nurse or PCP regarding verifying tube placement):
  - Turn off pump.
  - Using large syringe, insert tip into feeding tube and gently pull back.
- If there is concern the tube is displaced, do not use the tube until tube placement is verified.

Additional Instructions

F

Report the Following Problems to Your PCP/Clinic/ED

- Unable to unclog tube
- Signs of infection (fever, drainage, warmth, redness, red streaks, or foul-smelling drainage)
- Tube becomes dislodged or falls out

Seek Emergency Care Immediately If Any of the Following Occur

- Severe bleeding
- Severe pain
- Sudden onset of difficulty breathing or shortness of breath

If the caller agrees with the advice given, document the call and encourage the caller to call back or see PCP if the problem worsens. If the caller does not agree with the advice given, reevaluate and advise the caller to follow up with PCP, Clinic, or ED.

Fever, Adult

 Key Questions Name, Age, Onset, Temperature and Method, Allergies, Medications, History, Associated Symptoms

 Other Protocols to Consider Altered Mental Status (28); Abdominal Pain, Adult (9); Common Cold Symptoms (146); Earache, Drainage (206); Diarrhea, Adult (192); Headache (308); Heat-Exposure Problems (323); Postoperative Problems (457); Sore Throat (564); Vomiting, Adult (642); Wound Care: Sutures or Staples (660).

> *Nurse Alert:* There are many conditions that cause fever; however, it can indicate a serious problem in the elderly, immunosuppressed, and frail persons. See Appendix O (703) for Temperature Conversion chart. Provide reassurance that the cause of the fever may not be known for 24 hours until other symptoms begin to develop.

Reminder: Document caller response to advice, home care instructions, and when to call back.

ASSESSMENT	ACTION

A. Are any of the following present?

• Confusion, delirium, difficult to arouse, or difficulty breathing	"Call ambulance" or "Seek emergency care now"
• Signs of dehydration in the elderly or persons who are immunosuppressed (AIDS, chemotherapy, taking steroids): • decreased urine • sunken eyes • pinched skin does not spring back	Go to B
• excessive thirst, dry mouth	
• Rapid breathing, difficulty swallowing, or wheezing	
• Headache, neck stiffness, and/or light sensitivity	
• Purple- or blood-colored spots on skin	

B. Are any of the following present?

- Temperature >101°F (38.3°C) in the elderly or immunosuppressed
- Temperature >104°F (40°C) and unresponsive to fever-reducing measures
- Frequent or painful urination and back or flank pain
- Diabetes, steroid use, cancer, AIDS, old age, heart problems, kidney or liver disease, chronic medical condition, transplant, or pregnancy
- IV drug abuse, PICC line or peripheral IV line present

 "Seek medical care within 2 hours"

NO Go to C

C. Are any of the following present?

- Fever persists >72 hours with no known cause
- Cough with colored sputum
- Frequent or painful urination
- Vaginal bleeding, pain, or discharge
- Vomiting, diarrhea, or abdominal pain
- Earache, sore throat, and swollen glands
- Rash
- Recent surgical procedure or recent delivery
- Signs of dehydration unresponsive to home care measures

 "Seek medical care within 24 hours"

NO Go to D

D. Are any of the following present?

- Congestion, sneezing, or achiness
- Other family members are ill
- Fever responsive to self-care measures

YES "Call back or call PCP for appointment if no improvement" and Follow **Home Care Instructions**

NO Follow **Home Care Instructions**

F

Home Care Instructions
Fever, Adult

- Increase fluid intake (unless person is on a fluid-restricted diet or has CHF).
- Take usual medication (aspirin, acetaminophen, or ibuprofen) for fever and achiness. Do not give aspirin to a child. Avoid aspirin-like products if age <20 years. Avoid acetaminophen if liver disease is present. Avoid ibuprofen if kidney disease or stomach problems exist or in the case of pregnancy. Follow the directions on the label.
- Take a lukewarm sponge bath or bath soaks; do not use alcohol rubs or alcohol in water soaks.
- Wear light clothing and use light bed covering.
- Check the temperature every 2 to 4 hours. If no improvement, notify PCP or call back.
- Limit activity; rest.

Additional Instructions

Report the Following Problems to Your PCP/Clinic/ED

- No improvement in 3 days or condition worsens
- Persistent fever unresponsive to fever-reducing measures
- Vomiting, diarrhea, fatigue, lethargy, or stiff neck
- Fever or swelling

Seek Emergency Care Immediately If Any of the Following Occur

- Seizure
- Unresponsiveness
- Difficulty breathing
- Immunosuppressed and signs of dehydration
- Headache, neck stiffness, and/or photophobia
- Purple- or blood-colored spots on skin

If the caller agrees with the advice given, document the call and encourage the caller to call back or see PCP if the problem worsens. If the caller does not agree with the advice given, reevaluate and advise the caller to follow up with PCP, Clinic, or ED.

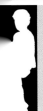

Fever, Child

 Key Questions Name, Age, Onset, Duration, Temperature, Allergies, Medications, History, Associated Symptoms

 Other Protocols to Consider Abdominal Pain, Child (13); Common Cold Symptoms (146); Earache, Drainage (206); Diarrhea, Child (195); Headache (308); Heat-Exposure Problems (323); Postoperative Problems (457); Rash, Child (500); Sore Throat (564); Sweating, Excessive (594); Vomiting, Child (645); Wound Care: Sutures or Staples (660).

> *Nurse Alert:* There are many conditions that cause fever; however, it can indicate a serious problem in newborns <1 month old, immunosuppressed, and frail children. Provide reassurance that the cause of the fever may not be known for 24 hours until other symptoms begin to develop. See Appendix O (703) for Temperature Conversion chart.

Reminder: Document caller response to advice, home care instructions, and when to call back.

ASSESSMENT	ACTION
A. Are any of the following present?	
• Difficulty breathing (for reasons other than congestion) • Skin or lips turning blue • New-onset drooling • Unable to swallow • Purple- or blood-colored spots or dots on skin • New seizure and no history of febrile seizure • Rash, red tongue and enlarged lymph nodes • Child appears very ill, lethargic, or very irritable	**YES** "Seek emergency care now" **NO** Go to B

F

B. Are any of the following present?

- Neck pain when bending head forward
- Severe headache or abdominal pain
- Difficult or rapid breathing, trouble swallowing, or wheezing
- Infant younger than 3 months (no recent immunization) and temperature >100.4°F (38.0°C)
- Fever occurs >48 hours after recent immunization
- Infant is 2 to 6 months old and has temperature >105°F (40.6°C) or diarrhea and vomiting
- Temperature >104°F (40°C) and is unresponsive to fever-reducing measures (fever decreases 2°C to 3°C 2 hours after medication)
- Seizure (history of febrile seizure)
- Signs of dehydration:
  - decreased urine
  - sunken eyes
  - pinched skin does not spring back
  - excessive thirst, dry mouth
  - crying without tears
- Difficulty drinking "adequate" amount of fluids
- Solid red rash that is tender to touch
- History of steroid use, cancer, AIDS, or cystic fibrosis

YES "Seek medical care within 2 hours"

NO Go to C

C. Are any of the following present?

- Fever >24 hours and age >2 years with no other symptoms
- Fever >72 hours that is unresponsive to fever-reducing measures or no known cause
- Yellow phlegm >72 hours
- History of diabetes, asthma, seizures
- Frequent or painful urination
- Vaginal bleeding, pain, or discharge
- Vomiting, diarrhea, or abdominal pain
- Earache, sore throat, and/or swollen glands
- Rash
- Fever lasts 2 to 3 days, 7 to 14 days after measles, mumps, and rubella (MMR) vaccine

YES "Seek medical care within 24 hours"

NO Go to D

D. Are any of the following present?

- Congestion, sneezing, or achiness
- Other family members are ill
- Fever >72 hours that is responsive to self-care measures
- Parent is comfortable with advice given

YES Follow **Home Care Instructions**

NO "Call back or call PCP for appointment if no improvement" and Follow **Home Care Instructions**

Home Care Instructions
Fever, Child

- Provide reassurance that children often eat less with a fever but need to consume adequate fluids.
- Encourage increased consumption of cold beverages, such as juices and gelatin, as well as warm tea and broth, which are soothing to the throat.
- Give acetaminophen (if infant is >2 months) or ibuprofen (if age >6 months) for fever >102°F and achiness. Do not give aspirin to a child. Avoid aspirin-like products if age <20 years. Avoid acetaminophen if liver disease is present. Avoid ibuprofen if kidney disease or stomach problems exist or in the case of pregnancy. Follow the directions on the label.
- Dress the child in light clothing. Do not bundle baby in blankets. Keep room temperature at 70°C if possible.
- Check the child's temperature every 2 to 4 hours. If no improvement, notify PCP or call back.
- Follow guidelines for antipyretic dosages: acetaminophen, 15 mg/kg every 4 hours; and ibuprofen, 10 mg/kg every 6 hours. Do not give ibuprofen if child has abdominal pain, is vomiting, or is dehydrated.
- Remember that fever is a normal body reaction to fighting infections; fevers rarely go above 104°F to 105°F (40°C to 40.6°C), even without treatment.
- Recommend return to day care or school and participation in normal activities when fever subsides.

Additional Instructions

F

Report the Following Problems to Your PCP/Clinic/ED

- Temperature >104°F (40°C)
- Rash, painful neck, or severe headache
- Frequent or painful urination
- Condition worsens or no improvement after 3 days
- Signs of dehydration
- Seizure
- Fever persists 48 hours and no other symptoms

Seek Emergency Care Immediately If Any of the Following Occur

- Unresponsiveness
- Difficulty breathing
- Stiff neck
- Purple/red spots on skin
- Skin or lips turn blue
- New onset of drooling
- Unable to swallow
- New seizure and no history of febrile seizure
- Rash, red tongue and enlarged lymph nodes

If the caller agrees with the advice given, document the call and encourage the caller to call back or see PCP if the problem worsens. If the caller does not agree with the advice given, reevaluate and advise the caller to follow up with PCP, Clinic, or ED.

Finger and Toe Problems

 Key Questions Name, Age, Onset, Contributing Cause, Allergies, Medications, History

 Other Protocols to Consider Arthritis Problems (48); Extremity Injury (222); Joint Pain/ Swelling (390); Wound Healing and Infection (664).

Reminder: Document caller response to advice, home care instructions, and when to call back.

ASSESSMENT	ACTION

A. Are any of the following present?

- Amputation or near amputation
- Deformity with break in the skin or bone protrudes through the skin
- Fingers or toes cold or blue compared with other fingers and toes

YES "Seek emergency care now"

NO Go to B

B. After an injury, are any of the following present?

- Obvious deformity or dislocation
- Severe pain
- Inability to remove rings, and digit is beginning to turn pale, white, or blue
- Fever or chills
- Nail loose or dislodged
- High-pressure nail gun injury
- Puncture wound into a joint
- Inability to stop bleeding with pressure

YES "Seek medical care within 2 hours"

NO Go to C

C. Are any of the following present?

- Swollen and tender finger pad
- Signs of infection: increased pain, swelling, redness, warmth, red streaks, or drainage
- Difficulty moving joint nearest the injury
- Fingers and toes numb compared with other fingers and toes
- Blood under nail with increased pain or pressure

YES "Seek medical care within 24 hours"

NO Go to D

F

D. Are any of the following present?

- Pain or swelling without injury
- Inability to remove rings following Home Care Instructions
- Moderate swelling
- Slow-healing wound and diabetic
- Nails discolored and thickened

YES "Call back or call PCP for appointment if no improvement" and
Follow **Home Care Instructions**

NO Follow **Home Care Instructions**

Home Care Instructions
Finger and Toe Problems

- Ice intermittently and elevate the digit for 24 to 48 hours after an injury. Do not place ice directly on the skin, use a washcloth or other cloth barrier between the ice and the skin.
- Remove rings immediately after the injury, before swelling occurs. Use soap, lotion, petroleum jelly (Vaseline), or another lubricant.
- Immobilize the injured digit by taping it to the next digit.
- Take your usual pain medication (aspirin, acetaminophen, ibuprofen). Do not give aspirin to a child. Avoid aspirin-like products if age <20 years. Avoid acetaminophen if liver disease is present. Avoid ibuprofen if kidney disease or stomach problems exist or in the case of pregnancy. Follow the directions on the label.
- For swelling or pain with no known injury, or if signs of infection are present, elevate the digit and apply warm soaks to the area for 20 minutes, 4 times a day.
- Watch for signs of infection as the nail heals. Soak digit in warm water several times a day to combat soreness and to promote healing.

Additional Instructions

Report the Following Problems to Your PCP/Clinic/ED

- Signs of infection: increased pain, swelling, redness, warmth, red streaks, fever, or drainage
- Severe pain and swelling that is unresponsive to ice and elevation measures
- Inability to remove rings, and digit is beginning to turn pale, white, or blue
- Severe pain and inability to perform procedure to release blood from under nail
- No improvement in pain, swelling, or ability to use the digit in 48 hours after home care measures
- Problem persists with treatment of >1 week

Seek Emergency Care Immediately If the Following Occurs

- Fingers or toes become cold or blue compared with other fingers or toes

F

If the caller agrees with the advice given, document the call and encourage the caller to call back or see PCP if the problem worsens. If the caller does not agree with the advice given, reevaluate and advise the caller to follow up with PCP, Clinic, or ED.

Food Allergy, Known or Suspected

 Key Questions Name, Age, Onset, Cause if Known, Allergies, Medications, History

 Other Protocols to Consider Allergic Reaction (25); Diarrhea, Adult (192), Child (195); Food Poisoning, Suspected (262); Hives (337); Itching (382); Rash, Adult (500), Child (505); Vomiting, Adult (642), Child (645).

Nurse Alert: Use this protocol only if previously diagnosed with a food allergy or prior reaction to a food substance.

Reminder: Document caller response to advice, home care instructions, and when to call back.

ASSESSMENT	ACTION
A. Are any of the following present shortly after eating?	
• Difficulty breathing • Confusion • Difficulty swallowing • Fainting • Severe dizziness	**YES** "Call ambulance" or "Seek emergency care now" **NO** Go to B
B. Is the following present within 30 minutes after eating?	
• Swelling of lips, tongue, or mouth	**YES** "Seek medical care now" **NO** Go to C
C. Are any of the following present after eating?	
• Generalized hives or itching • Sore throat • Postnasal drip and throat clearing • Congestion, sneezing, or runny nose • Fatigue • Headache • Persistent diarrhea or vomiting	**YES** "Call back or call PCP for appointment if no improvement" and Follow **Home Care Instructions** **NO** Follow **Home Care Instructions**

Home Care Instructions
Food Allergy

- Try to identify the food causing the problem and avoid it. Eggs and milk are the most common food allergies in infants. Peanuts, eggs, chocolate, cow's milk products, soybeans, tree nuts, wheat, fish, and shellfish are the most common causes of food allergies.
- Eliminate the suspected food from the diet for 2 weeks and note whether symptoms disappear. If so, avoid that food in the future. If not, observe for relationship between other foods and symptoms (hives, swelling in mouth, diarrhea).
- Try baking soda baths, Caladryl lotion, or calamine for itching or take an antihistamine (Benadryl) tablet (follow instructions on the label).

Additional Instructions

Report the Following Problems to Your PCP/Clinic/ED

- No improvement in symptoms or condition worsens
- Desire to add suspected food back to diet

Seek Emergency Care Immediately If Any of the Following Occur

- Fainting
- Difficulty breathing
- Confusion
- Difficulty swallowing
- Severe dizziness

If the caller agrees with the advice given, document the call and encourage the caller to call back or see PCP if the problem worsens. If the caller does not agree with the advice given, reevaluate and advise the caller to follow up with PCP, Clinic, or ED.

Food Poisoning, Suspected

 Key Questions Name, Age, Onset, Associated Symptoms, History, Medications, Suspected Source

 Other Protocols to Consider Abdominal Pain, Adult (9), Child (13); Abdominal Swelling (16); Avian Influenza "Bird Flu" Exposure (55); Dehydration (180); Diarrhea, Adult (192), Child (195); Rectal Bleeding (510); Vomiting, Adult (642), Child (645).

Nurse Alert: If caller suspects food poisoning after eating at a restaurant, encourage caller to notify the restaurant. Other patrons may have had the same problem. Early notification helps the restaurant to track the source and correct the problem.

Reminder: Document caller response to advice, home care instructions, and when to call back.

ASSESSMENT	ACTION

A. Sick 6 to 48 hours after eating canned, smoked, or vacuum-packed foods and are any of the following present?

- Altered mental status
- Difficulty breathing or swallowing, or blurred vision
- Vomiting blood
- Bloody stool

 "Seek emergency care now"

 Go to B

B. Are any of the following present?

- Pain is severe, worsens, or lasts >4 hours
- Nausea and vomiting >12 hours and unresponsive to home treatment or OTC medications
- Diarrhea >48 hours and unresponsive to home treatment or OTC medications
- Bloody diarrhea
- Signs of dehydration:
  - decreased urine
  - sunken eyes
  - loose dry skin
  - excessive thirst, dry mouth
- child crying without tears
- Dizziness upon standing
- Rash
- Fever

 "Seek medical care within 2 to 4 hours"

 Go to C

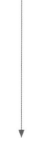

C. Are any of the following present?

- Nausea, vomiting, diarrhea, abdominal pain occurred after eating unrefrigerated meat, poultry, fish, mayonnaise, or egg products
- Others eating the same meal also are ill

YES "Call back or call PCP for appointment if no improvement"

NO Follow **Home Care Instructions**

F

Home Care Instructions
Food Poisoning, Suspected

- Drink small sips of clear fluids (apple juice, tea, broth, sports drinks, clear soda pop, ginger ale) frequently (every 5 to 10 minutes) until nausea and vomiting subside. Increase amount as tolerated during the first 24 hours after vomiting subsides.
- Avoid milk products when experiencing diarrhea.
- Avoid spicy foods, alcohol, dairy products, and coffee for 48 hours after vomiting and diarrhea have subsided.
- Avoid aspirin.
- Prevention:
  - Avoid meats, dressings, sauces, and mayonnaise-based preparations that have been at room temperature for >2 hours. Maintain a food temperature of <40°F (4.4°C) or >140°F (60°C).
  - Do not eat the contents of cans or jars with bulging lids.
  - Defrost meats in the refrigerator or microwave, rather than at room temperature.
  - Wash hands, cutting boards, and countertops frequently, especially after handling raw chicken or eggs.
  - If the food smells unusual or foul, do not eat it.

Additional Instructions

Report the Following Problems to Your PCP/Clinic/ED

- Condition persists >48 hours or worsens
- Blood in the stool or vomit (not streaks or flecks)
- Temperature >101°F (38.3°C)

Seek Emergency Care Immediately If Any of the Following Occur

- Blurred vision
- Difficulty breathing
- Difficulty swallowing
- Decreased level of consciousness
- Signs of dehydration

If the caller agrees with the advice given, document the call and encourage the caller to call back or see PCP if the problem worsens. If the caller does not agree with the advice given, reevaluate and advise the caller to follow up with PCP, Clinic, or ED.

Foot Problems

 Key Questions Name, Age, Onset, Cause, Allergies, History of Diabetes or Vascular Disease, Medications, History

 Other Protocols to Consider Ankle Problems (33); Extremity Injury (222); Finger and Toe Problems (257); Joint Pain/Swelling (390).

Reminder: Document caller response to advice, home care instructions, and when to call back.

ASSESSMENT	ACTION

A. In addition to pain after an injury, fall, or sudden movement, are any of the following present?

- Deformity
- Foot cold or blue compared with the other foot

YES "Seek emergency care now"

NO Go to B

B. Are any of the following present?

- Inability to walk or move foot
- Fever and painful, red, swollen toe joints
- Diabetic and open or infected wound unresponsive to home care measures

YES "Seek medical care within 2 to 4 hours"

NO Go to C

C. Are any of the following present?

- Nonhealing wound >1 week
- Persistent swelling >1 week
- Toe joint swollen, painful, red, and warm and there is no known injury
- Red, swollen, painful area on sole of foot

YES "Seek medical care within 24 hours"

NO Go to D

F

D. Are any of the following present?

- Pain after walking or running
- Painful, warm, swollen area around toenail
- Injured toe swollen and bruised
- Both feet ache after prolonged walking or standing
- Persistent itching
- Soft, red, peeling skin between toes or on soles of feet
- Excessive sweating or foul odor
- Painful flat hard lump of tough skin on sole of foot
- Lumps of hard skin over toes and sides of feet
- Soles of feet ache upon rising in the morning
- Heel pain
- Cracked dry skin

YES "Call back or call PCP for appointment if no improvement" and
Follow **Home Care Instructions**

NO Follow **Home Care Instructions**

Home Care Instructions
Foot Problems

- For signs of infection (pain, swelling, redness, red streaks, drainage, or warmth), apply moist hot packs or soaks to area for 20 minutes, 4 to 6 times a day.
- After an injury, elevate foot and apply ice packs to area for 20 minutes, 4 to 6 times a day. Wrap with elastic bandage to keep swelling down for the first 24 to 48 hours. Do not place ice directly on the skin, use a washcloth or other cloth barrier between the ice and the skin.
- Tape an injured toe to the next toe to provide support and promote healing for 7 to 10 days.
- Apply sponge rings around painful hard lumps to reduce the pressure of a shoe against the area.
- Wear comfortable-fitting shoes.
- Apply OTC remedies (DuoFilm, DuoPlant, Wart-Off) to warts on bottom of feet at night. Follow instructions on the label. Be careful to avoid applying treatment to surrounding sensitive skin.
- For peeling irritated skin, wash and dry frequently. Wear cotton or other natural-fiber socks and shoes with porous soles or open-toed shoes. Apply OTC antifungal cream, spray, or powder to the affected area.
- Trim toenails straight across, but do not cut them too short.
- Apply moisturizing hand or body cream (Alpha-Keri, Curel, Vaseline Intensive Care) to dry, cracked skin twice a day. Follow instructions on the label. Avoid going barefoot.
- Rest and elevate feet for discomfort and swelling. Soak aching feet in tub or basin of warm water and Epsom salt.
- Reduce weight-bearing activities until free of pain.
- Apply ice for heel pain for 20 minutes, 4 times a day and after weight-bearing activity. Do not place ice directly on the skin, use a washcloth or other cloth barrier between the ice and the skin.
- For persistent pain on sole and/or heel, perform foot exercises upon arising and throughout the day. In a sitting position, use the affected foot to create each letter in the alphabet.
- Take usual pain medication (aspirin, acetaminophen, or ibuprofen). Do not give aspirin to a child. Avoid aspirin-like products if age <20 years. Avoid acetaminophen if liver disease is present. Avoid ibuprofen if kidney disease or stomach problems exist or in the case of pregnancy. Follow the directions on the label.

F

Additional Instructions

Report the Following Problems to Your PCP/Clinic/ED

- Persistent pain, swelling, or sores
- No improvement with home care measures or condition worsens
- Inability to walk or move foot

Seek Emergency Care Immediately If the Following Occurs

- Foot turns cold or blue compared with the other foot

If the caller agrees with the advice given, document the call and encourage the caller to call back or see PCP if the problem worsens. If the caller does not agree with the advice given, reevaluate and advise the caller to follow up with PCP, Clinic, or ED.

Foreign Body, Eye

 Key Questions Name, Age, Onset, Cause, Medications, History

 Other Protocols to Consider Eye Injury (225); Eye Problems (228); Vision Problems (639).

Reminder: Document caller response to advice, home care instructions, and when to call back.

ASSESSMENT	ACTION

A. Are any of the following present?

- Object is embedded in the eyeball
- Severe pain after irrigating chemical substance from eye
- Sudden change in vision
- Bulging eyeball
- Blood in the colored part of the eye
- Clear jelly-like discharge from injured eye
- Severe pain after foreign body removed
- Unequal pupil size

YES "Seek emergency care now"

NO Go to B

B. Are any of the following present?

- Foreign object is over the colored part of the eye
- Swelling, pain, or tearing >30 minutes
- Injury caused by hot water, chemical, or foreign body and pain persists after home care treatment
- Unable to remove free-floating foreign body

YES "Seek medical care within 2 to 4 hours"
and
Follow **Home Care Instructions**

NO Go to C

C. Are any of the following present?

- Discomfort or irritation persists 24 hours after the injury or removal of a foreign body
- Signs of infection develop after an injury: pain, swelling, redness, drainage, or fever
- Unable to remove contact lens

YES "Seek medical care within 24 hours"

NO "Call back or call PCP for appointment if no improvement"
and
Follow **Home Care Instructions**

F

Home Care Instructions
Foreign Body, Eye

- Chemicals in the Eye: Immediately flush eye with cold running water for 20 to 30 minutes. Tilt head under running water with the injured eye down. While holding eyelids apart, allow water to run across the inner eye to the outer part of the eye.
- Do not try to remove
  - foreign body embedded in the eye
  - metal chip
  - foreign body over the colored part of the eye
- Foreign body removal (lint, specks of dirt, eyelashes):
  - Pull down the lower lid and remove the particle with the corner of a moistened handkerchief, tissue, or cotton-tipped swab.
  - Pull down the upper lid over the lower lid and hold in place for a moment. Release and look to see if object is visible; if so, remove it.
- Do not rub eye.
- Apply ice pack or cool compresses to reduce discomfort.
- Take your usual pain medication (aspirin, acetaminophen, or ibuprofen). Do not give aspirin to a child. Avoid aspirin-like products if age <20 years. Avoid acetaminophen if liver disease is present. Avoid ibuprofen if kidney disease or stomach problems exist or in the case of pregnancy. Follow the directions on the label.

Additional Instructions

Report the Following Problems to Your PCP/Clinic/ED
- Increased pain, swelling, drainage, or fever
- Changes in vision
- No improvement in pain after 48 hours
- Unable to remove free-floating foreign body

If the caller agrees with the advice given, document the call and encourage the caller to call back or see PCP if the problem worsens. If the caller does not agree with the advice given, reevaluate and advise the caller to follow up with PCP, Clinic, or ED.

Foreign Body, Inhaled

 Key Questions Name, Age, Onset, Object Inhaled, History, Medications

 Other Protocols to Consider Breathing Problems (106); Choking (135); Cough (170); Foreign Body, Swallowing of (280); Piercing Problems (445).

Reminder: Document caller response to advice, home care instructions, and when to call back.

ASSESSMENT	ACTION

A. Are any of the following present?

- Choking and unable to speak, cough, or breathe
- Unconscious person who is not breathing

YES "Call ambulance and begin rescue breathing"

NO Go to B

B. Are any of the following present?

- Difficulty breathing
- Lips or face turning blue
- Inability to cry or speak
- Suicide attempt

YES "Call ambulance"

NO Go to C

C. Are any of the following present?

- Aspirated foreign body into the lungs
- Coughing up blood or severe pain after dislodging foreign body from the throat
- Unable to remove foreign object from throat but no other symptoms
- Feeling of suffocation
- Drooling
- Speaking in short words
- Unable to swallow saliva or fluids

YES "Seek emergency care now"

NO Go to D

F

D. Are any of the following present?

- Fever
- Speaking in partial sentences
- Intermittent cough or wheezing after inhaling a foreign object, aerosol, or smoke

YES "Seek medical attention within 2 to 4 hours"

NO Go to E

E. Are any of the following present?

- Able to speak and cough
- No difficulty breathing
- Frequent episodes of choking on saliva, foods, or fluids
- Speaking in full sentences

YES "Call back or call PCP for appointment if no improvement" and Follow **Home Care Instructions**

NO Follow **Home Care Instructions**

Home Care Instructions
Foreign Body, Inhaled

- For frequent choking, eat slowly, taking smaller bites.
- If there is a sensation that a fish bone is stuck in the throat, try washing down the bone with bread and milk.

Additional Instructions

Report the Following Problems to Your PCP/Clinic/ED

- Fish or chicken bone in throat and persistent scratchy throat >2 hours
- Coughing up blood
- Signs of infection: persistent sore throat, fever, or drainage
- Difficulty swallowing
- No improvement or condition worsens

Seek Emergency Care Immediately If Any of the Following Occur

- Difficulty breathing, shortness of breath, or wheezing
- Unable to swallow saliva or fluids
- Feeling of suffocation

If the caller agrees with the advice given, document the call and encourage the caller to call back or see PCP if the problem worsens. If the caller does not agree with the advice given, reevaluate and advise the caller to follow up with PCP, Clinic, or ED.

Foreign Body, Nose

 Key Questions Name, Age, Onset, Cause, Object, History, Medications, Pain Scale

 Other Protocols to Consider Piercing Problems (445); Congestion (153); Nosebleed (425); Nose Injury (428).

Reminder: Document caller response to advice, home care instructions, and when to call back.

ASSESSMENT	ACTION

A. Are any of the following present?

- Sharp object embedded in nose
- Profuse bleeding
- Irritating or adhesive substance in nose
- Severe nasal pain
- Age younger than 18 months
- Foreign body may be a small disk battery

YES "Seek medical care within 2 hours"

NO Go to B

B. Body art or piercing present, and are any of the following present?

- Skin red and warm, and fever or headache
- Vomiting and abdominal pain

YES "Seek medical care within 4 to 8 hours"

NO Go to C

C. Are any of the following present?

- Unable to remove foreign object after several tries
- Swelling and tenderness
- Foul-smelling green or yellow nasal drainage from one nostril

YES "Seek medical care within 24 hours"

NO Go to D

D. Is the following present?

- Foreign substance or object in nose removed and no other symptoms

YES "Call back or call PCP for appointment if no improvement" and Follow **Home Care Instructions**

NO Follow **Home Care Instructions**

Home Care Instructions
Foreign Body, Nose

- Apply saline drops or a nasal decongestant in the affected nostril.
- Pinch the unaffected nostril and exhale through the affected nostril.
- If the object is visible, do not attempt removal if unable to hold the head absolutely still. If there is resistance or a chance of pushing the object in farther, stop and seek medical care.

Additional Instructions

Report the Following Problems to Your PCP/Clinic/ED

- Unable to remove foreign object after several tries
- Swelling and tenderness persist or worsen
- Foul-smelling green or yellow nasal drainage from one nostril
- Fever, headache, and/or stiff neck

If the caller agrees with the advice given, document the call and encourage the caller to call back or see PCP if the problem worsens. If the caller does not agree with the advice given, reevaluate and advise the caller to follow up with PCP, Clinic, or ED.

F

Foreign Body, Rectum

 Key Questions Name, Age, Onset, Object, Allergies, Medications, History, Pain Scale

 Other Protocols to Consider Child Abuse (132); Constipation (160); Rectal Bleeding (510); Rectal Problems (513); Sexual Assault (539).

Reminder: Document caller response to advice, home care instructions, and when to call back.

ASSESSMENT	ACTION
A. Are any of the following present?	
• Sharp object in rectum • Profuse bleeding • Severe pain • Victim of sexual assault • Traumatic injury • High fever, chills, nausea, or vomiting	**YES** "Seek medical care now" **NO** Go to B
B. Are any of the following present?	
• Unable to remove foreign object after several tries • Swelling and tenderness • Foul-smelling drainage • Rectal bleeding • Abdominal or shoulder pain	**YES** "Seek medical care within 2 to 4 hours" **NO** Go to C
C. Are any of the following present?	
• Sensation of rectal fullness • Rectal pain • Retained condom • Unable to pass stool	**YES** "Seek medical care within 24 hours" **NO** "Call back or call PCP for appointment if no improvement" and Follow **Home Care Instructions**

Home Care Instructions
Foreign Body, Rectum

- Do not try to remove sharp object or object that has broken inside rectum.
- Take your usual pain medication (aspirin, acetaminophen, or ibuprofen). Do not give aspirin to a child. Avoid aspirin-like products if age <20 years. Avoid acetaminophen if liver disease is present. Avoid ibuprofen if kidney disease or stomach problems exist or in the case of pregnancy. Follow the directions on the label.
- Watch for signs of infection: increased pain, discharge, fever, or swelling.

Additional Instructions

Report the Following Problems to Your PCP/Clinic/ED

- Unable to remove foreign object after several tries
- Swelling and tenderness persist or worsen
- Foul-smelling drainage or fever
- Rectal bleeding
- Unable to pass stool
- High fever, chills, nausea, or vomiting

Seek Emergency Care Immediately If Any of the Following Occur

- Profuse bleeding
- Severe pain

F

If the caller agrees with the advice given, document the call and encourage the caller to call back or see PCP if the problem worsens. If the caller does not agree with the advice given, reevaluate and advise the caller to follow up with PCP, Clinic, or ED.

Foreign Body, Skin

 Key Questions Name, Age, Onset, Object, Allergies, Medications, History

 Other Protocols to Consider Bites, Tick (87); Body Piercing Problems (445); Extremity Injury (222); Laceration (395); Puncture Wound (496); Tattoo Problems (604).

Reminder: Document caller response to advice, home care instructions, and when to call back.

ASSESSMENT		ACTION

A. Are any of the following present?

- Unable to remove embedded fishhook
- Foreign body embedded in joint space
- Deep foreign body
- Unable to remove foreign substance
- Foreign substance is adhered to the skin
- Unable to remove pierced earring back that is embedded in earlobe or other embedded body piercing or foreign object
- Signs of infection: increased redness, pain, swelling, warmth, drainage, or red streaks
- Super glue in eye
- Severe pain

YES "Seek emergency care within 2 to 4 hours"
and
Follow **Home Care Instructions**

NO Go to B

B. Are any of the following present?

- Unable to remove large splinter
- Embedded glass, plastic, or metal object
- Tetanus immunization >5 years ago
- Tick head embedded in skin and unable to remove

YES "Seek medical care within 24 hours"

NO Go to C

C. Are any of the following present?

- Unable to remove small splinter
- Persistent sensation of a foreign body under the skin

YES "Call back or call PCP for appointment if no improvement"
and
Follow **Home Care Instructions**

NO Follow **Home Care Instructions**

Home Care Instructions
Foreign Body, Skin

- Fishhook removal techniques:
  - Push barb through the skin, cut off the barb with wire cutters, and then back it out the way it entered.
  - Push barb in and down slightly to disengage the barb from the skin and pull it out of the skin.
  - Loop fishline through the bend in the fishhook. Push barb in and hold down slightly to disengage barb from skin. Jerk the fishline quickly to remove the hook.
- Remove splinter or object with tweezers or a needle sterilized with a match flame or rubbing alcohol.
- Do not soak splinter area in water or solution, which will cause the wood to swell, thus hindering removal.
- Apply hot packs or soaks 4 to 6 times a day if there are signs of infection and to aid in the removal of a foreign body.
- Apply antibiotic (Neosporin) ointment and a bandage over difficult-to-remove splinters. They often will dislodge in a couple of days.
- After removal, wash the area well with soap and water.
- Techniques for removing tar or superglue:
  - Apply petroleum jelly, Neosporin, mayonnaise, mineral oil, or nail polish remover to the involved area (except near the eyes).
  - Do not force open skin or eyelids.
  - Superglue eventually will flake.
  - If eye is glued shut, apply Neosporin and hot compresses.
  - Tar may leave a stain on the skin.
  - Reduce heat from tar by cooling the area with water or wet towels.

F

Additional Instructions

_____

_____

_____

Report the Following Problems to Your PCP/Clinic/ED

- Unable to remove foreign body after 48 hours
- Signs of infection: increased redness, pain, swelling, warmth, drainage, or red streaks
- Severe pain

If the caller agrees with the advice given, document the call and encourage the caller to call back or see PCP if the problem worsens. If the caller does not agree with the advice given, reevaluate and advise the caller to follow up with PCP, Clinic, or ED.

Foreign Body, Swallowing of

 Key Questions Name, Age, Onset, Object, Medications, History, Pain Scale

 Other Protocols to Consider Abdominal Pain, Adult (9), Child (13); Constipation (160); Diarrhea, Adult (192), Child (195); Piercing Problems (445); Rectal Bleeding (510); Rectal Problems (513); Vomiting, Adult (642), Child (645).

Reminder: Document caller response to advice, home care instructions, and when to call back.

ASSESSMENT	ACTION
A. Are any of the following present?	
• Excessive saliva, drooling, or gagging • Difficulty swallowing • Coughing, choking, or breathing difficulties • Suicide attempt	**YES** "Call ambulance" or "Seek emergency care now" **NO** Go to B
B. Are any of the following present?	
• Pain or discomfort in throat or chest • Abdominal pain • Vomiting • Object was a battery or sharp object	**YES** "Seek medical care within 2 to 4 hours" **NO** Go to C
C. Are any of the following present?	
• Metal object • Object size larger than a nickel	**YES** "Seek medical care within 24 hours" **NO** Go to D
D. Are any of the following present?	
• Wood or plastic object • Dull glass object (piece of a jar or cup) • Object size smaller than a penny • Known substance swallowed but no symptoms	**YES** "Call back or call PCP for appointment if no improvement" and Follow **Home Care Instructions** **NO** Follow **Home Care Instructions**

Home Care Instructions
Foreign Body, Swallowing of

- If no symptoms, try a sip of fluid. If no difficulty, try swallowing bread or soft food.
- A dull glass object, such as a piece of a jar, cup, or ring, should pass with stools without difficulty in 3 to 4 days.
- Do not give laxatives. Increase fiber (fruit, vegetables, whole grains) in the diet to help stimulate natural elimination.
- Check stools for swallowed object.

Additional Instructions

Report the Following Problems to Your PCP/Clinic/ED

- Intermittent choking or gagging
- Abdominal pain
- No evidence of object in stools within 7 days
- Vomiting
- Chest pain
- Fever

Seek Emergency Care Immediately If the Following Occurs

- Drooling, gagging, choking, or difficulty breathing or swallowing

F

If the caller agrees with the advice given, document the call and encourage the caller to call back or see PCP if the problem worsens. If the caller does not agree with the advice given, reevaluate and advise the caller to follow up with PCP, Clinic, or ED.

Foreign Body, Vagina

 Key Questions Name, Age, Onset, Object, Allergies, Medications, History, Pain Scale

 Other Protocols to Consider Domestic Abuse (202); Elder Abuse (216); Piercing Problems (445); Sexual Assault (539); Vaginal Bleeding (633); Vaginal Discharge/Pain/Itching (636).

Reminder: Document caller response to advice, home care instructions, and when to call back.

ASSESSMENT	ACTION
A. Are any of the following present?	
• Sharp object embedded in vagina • Profuse bleeding • Severe pain • Sexual assault • Rapid onset: rash, fever, peeling hands or feet, general ill feeling, vomiting, or diarrhea	**YES** "Seek emergency care now" **NO** Go to B
B. Are any of the following present?	
• Unable to remove foreign object after several tries • Swelling and tenderness • Foul-smelling discharge • Tampon left in vagina >24 hours and cannot be removed • Unable to remove contraceptive or pleasure device	**YES** "Seek medical care within 24 hours" **NO** "Call back or call PCP for appointment if no improvement" and Follow **Home Care Instructions**

Home Care Instructions
Foreign Body, Vagina

- Do not try to remove sharp object or object that has broken inside vagina.
- Take your usual pain medication (aspirin, acetaminophen, ibuprofen). Do not give aspirin to a child. Avoid aspirin-like products if age <20 years. Avoid acetaminophen if liver disease is present. Avoid ibuprofen if kidney disease or stomach problems exist or in the case of pregnancy. Follow the directions on the label.
- Watch for signs of infection: increased pain, discharge, fever, or swelling.

Additional Instructions

Report the Following Problems to Your PCP/Clinic/ED

- Unable to remove foreign object after several tries
- Swelling and tenderness persist or worsen
- Foul-smelling drainage or fever
- Rash, fever, peeling hands or feet, general ill feeling, vomiting, or diarrhea

Seek Emergency Care Immediately If the Following Occur

- Profuse bleeding
- Severe pain

If the caller agrees with the advice given, document the call and encourage the caller to call back or see PCP if the problem worsens. If the caller does not agree with the advice given, reevaluate and advise the caller to follow up with PCP, Clinic, or ED.

Frostbite

 Key Questions Name, Age, Onset, Exposure to Freezing Conditions, Allergies, Medication, History

 Other Protocols to Consider Cold Exposure Problems (143).

> *Nurse Alert:* Use this protocol only if exposed to freezing temperatures and skin symptoms (e.g., hard, cold, waxy, white or blue blotchy appearance, numbness, tingling, pain, or blisters) are present. Tissue damage may not be evident until after reperfusion and the extent of damage may evolve over weeks to months. Feet, hands, earlobes, nose, cheeks, and chin are the most frequently affected areas of the body.

Reminder: Document caller response to advice, home care instructions, and when to call back.

ASSESSMENT	ACTION
A. Is the following present?	
• Hard, cold, white, or blue blotchy skin (third-degree frostbite)	**YES** "Seek emergency care now" **NO** Go to B
B. Are any of the following present?	
• Symptoms of hypothermia: confusion, drowsiness, rigid muscles, or irrational behavior	**YES** "Go to Cold Exposure Problems protocol (135)" **NO** Go to C
C. Are any of the following present?	
• Frozen area with blistering or peeling skin (second-degree frostbite) • Blisters develop with rewarming • Signs of infection: increased redness, swelling, pain, drainage, red streaks, warmth, or fever	**YES** "Seek medical care within 2 to 4 hours" **NO** Go to D

D. Is the following present?

- Frozen area numb without blistering (first-degree frostbite)

  YES "Call back or call PCP for appointment if no improvement" and Follow **Home Care Instructions**

  NO Follow **Home Care Instructions**

F

Home Care Instructions
Frostbite

- Remain inside a warm shelter, away from the wind and cold.
- Protect frozen areas from continued exposure.
- Do not thaw or warm the area if there is a possibility it will refreeze; seek medical care immediately.
- Warm the body slowly, starting with the person's trunk first then the hands and feet.
- Warm chest, neck, and groin by wrapping in blankets or skin-to-skin contact under loose blankets.
- Remove from the cold exposure and avoid reexposure, if possible.
- If severe exposure is less than 24 hours, rewarm affected part in warm water for 10 to 30 minutes or apply warm wet packs. Avoid dry heat. Stop rewarming when part is warm, red, and pliable. Do not submerge the person in warm water or a warm bath. Warming the person too quickly can cause heart problems.
- Do not use direct heat to rewarm. Avoid using a radiator, campfire, hair dryer, or heating pad to rewarm as they may cause burns.
- Apply firm pressure to the area, but do not rub or massage frozen skin.
- Avoid walking on frostbitten feet, if possible.
- Keep the frostbitten area warm and elevated. Wrap the affected parts in blankets or soft material to prevent bruising.
- Blisters may develop as skin warms. Do not break open the blisters.
- Skin may become red and painful, itch, or tingle. Take usual pain medication (aspirin, acetaminophen, or ibuprofen) as tolerated for discomfort. Do not give aspirin to a child. Avoid aspirin-like products if age <20 years. Avoid acetaminophen if liver disease is present. Avoid ibuprofen if kidney disease or stomach problems exist or in the case of pregnancy. Follow the directions on the label.
- Remove wet clothing and constrictive jewelry.

Additional Instructions

Report the Following Problems to Your PCP/Clinic/ED
- Persistent hard, white, blue, or numb skin
- Swelling, blistering, or signs of infection
- If blistering occurs, may need an updated tetanus immunization

If the caller agrees with the advice given, document the call and encourage the caller to call back or see PCP if the problem worsens. If the caller does not agree with the advice given, reevaluate and advise the caller to follow up with PCP, Clinic, or ED.

Gas/Belching

 Key Questions Name, Age, Onset, Cause, Allergies, Medications, History

 Other Protocols to Consider Abdominal Pain, Adult (9), Child (13); Abdominal Swelling (16); Chest Pain (123); Constipation (160); Heartburn (316); Indigestion (368).

Reminder: Document caller response to advice, home care instructions, and when to call back.

ASSESSMENT	ACTION
A. Is the following present?	
● Chest, jaw, or neck pain or discomfort	**YES** Go to Chest Pain protocol (123)
	NO Go to B
B. Are any of the following present?	
● Severe abdominal pain	**YES** "Seek medical care within 2 hours"
● Shortness of breath	**NO** Go to C
● Excessive sweating	
● Palpitations	
● Severe nausea and/or vomiting	
C. Are any of the following present?	
● Persistent abdominal discomfort after belching	**YES** "Seek medical care within 24 hours"
● Pain radiates to back	**NO** Go to D
D. Are any of the following present?	
● Intermittent abdominal discomfort or swelling	**YES** "Call back or call PCP for appointment if no improvement" and Follow **Home Care Instructions**
● Burping, belching, or hiccups after meals	
● Belching or heartburn between meals	**NO** Follow **Home Care Instructions**

G

Home Care Instructions
Gas/Belching

- Avoid gas-forming foods (parsnips, beans, corn, cabbage, onions, fried food).
- Avoid overindulgence in sweet desserts, fatty foods, and other foods that are known to cause gas.
- Avoid eating too fast or too much.
- Avoid excessive gum chewing.
- Stop smoking if possible or reduce smoking at mealtime.
- Drink an adequate amount of fluids each day.
- Try to reduce stress or excitement, especially at mealtime.
- Sip flat, clear carbonated beverage or peppermint tea to help break up gas.
- Take your usual antacids (Di-Gel, Mylanta-II, Mylicon) to help relieve gas. Follow instructions on the label. Ask pharmacist for other product suggestions.

Additional Instructions

Report the Following Problems to Your PCP/Clinic/ED

- Symptoms persist or worsen after home care measures
- Severe pain
- Shortness of breath
- Excessive sweating
- Palpitations
- Nausea and vomiting

Seek Emergency Care Immediately If Any of the Following Occur

- Chest, neck, or jaw pain or discomfort develops
- Light-headedness

If the caller agrees with the advice given, document the call and encourage the caller to call back or see PCP if the problem worsens. If the caller does not agree with the advice given, reevaluate and advise the caller to follow up with PCP, Clinic, or ED.

Gas/Flatulence

>> **Key Questions** Name, Age, Onset, Cause, Allergies, Medications, History

>> **Other Protocols to Consider** Abdominal Pain, Adult (9), Child (13); Abdominal Swelling (16); Chest Pain (123); Constipation (160); Indigestion (368).

Reminder: Document caller response to advice, home care instructions, and when to call back.

ASSESSMENT	ACTION
A. Is severe abdominal pain present?	
	YES Go to Abdominal Pain protocols, Adult (9), Child (13)
	NO Go to B
B. Is the following present?	
• Black tarry stool	**YES** "Seek emergency care now"
	NO Go to C
C. Is the following present?	
• Severe nausea and vomiting	**YES** "Seek medical care within 2 to 4 hours"
	NO Go to D
D. Are any of the following present?	
• Persistent abdominal discomfort after passing gas	**YES** "Seek medical care within 24 hours"
• Blood in stool	**NO** Go to E
• Pain radiates to back	
E. Are any of the following present?	
• Intermittent abdominal discomfort or swelling	**YES** "Call back or call PCP for appointment if no improvement" and Follow **Home Care Instructions**
• Excessive flatulence	
• Pale, bulky, foul-smelling stools	
• Recent ingestion of high-fiber or gas-producing foods, such as beans or beer	**NO** Follow **Home Care Instructions**

G

Home Care Instructions
Gas/Flatulence

- Avoid gas-forming foods (parsnips, beans, corn, cabbage, onions, fried food).
- Avoid overindulgence in sweet desserts, fatty foods, and other foods that are known to cause gas.
- Avoid eating too fast or too much.
- Avoid laxatives.
- Drink an adequate amount of fluids each day.
- Maintain regular bowel habits.
- Exercise regularly.
- Try to reduce stress or excitement, especially at mealtime.
- Sip flat, clear carbonated beverage or peppermint tea to help break up gas.
- If lactose intolerant and unable to avoid dairy foods, ask pharmacist for OTC product suggestions.
- As an alternative, try sugar-coated fennel seeds after a meal or sip tea brewed with fennel seeds to break up and disperse gas in the intestinal tract.

Additional Instructions

Report the Following Problems to Your PCP/Clinic/ED

- Symptoms persist or worsen after home care measures
- Nausea/vomiting

Seek Emergency Care Immediately If Any of the Following Occur

- Large amount of blood in stool
- Black tarry stools
- Light-headedness

If the caller agrees with the advice given, document the call and encourage the caller to call back or see PCP if the problem worsens. If the caller does not agree with the advice given, reevaluate and advise the caller to follow up with PCP, Clinic, or ED.

Genital Lesions

 Key Questions Name, Age, Onset, Allergies, Medications, History, Pain Scale

 Other Protocols to Consider Domestic Abuse (202); Elder Abuse (216); Genital Problems, Male (294); Lice (401); Piercing Problems (445); Scrotal Problems (529); Sexually Transmitted Disease (STD) (542); Skin Lesions: Lumps, Bumps, and Sores (556); Tattoo Problems (604); Vaginal Discharge/Pain/Itching (636).

Reminder: Document caller response to advice, home care instructions, and when to call back.

ASSESSMENT	ACTION
A. Are any of the following present?	
• Severe pain • Signs of infection: increased pain, redness, swelling, drainage, warmth, fever	**YES** "Seek medical care within 4 to 12 hours" **NO** Go to B
B. Are any of the following present?	
• Open sores • New onset of scattered clustered blisters • Fever and general ill feeling • Swollen glands in groin area • Vaginal or penile discharge or bleeding • Severe itching or burning • Sores elsewhere on the body • Pelvic pain • Foreign body • Painful lump at vaginal opening • No improvement after >3 days of home treatment for yeast infection	**YES** "Seek medical care within 24 hours" **NO** Go to C
C. Are any of the following present?	
• Diagnosed herpes, genital warts, or exposure to an STD and requests treatment • Painful urination or bowel movements • Painless rash or hard bumps in genital or rectal area >24 hours	**YES** "Seek medical care within 48 hours" **NO** Go to D

G

D. Are any of the following present?

- Itchy red rash
- History of recent strenuous activity and sweating
- Pink, scaly, itchy rash on inner thighs, groin, or scrotum
- Raised red, tender, or white or hard bumps
- Painless rash or growth <24 hours

YES "Call back or call PCP for appointment if no improvement" and
Follow **Home Care Instructions**

NO Follow **Home Care Instructions**

Home Care Instructions
Genital Lesions

- Soak in a warm bath.
- Avoid bubble bath, harsh or perfumed soaps, scented toilet paper, or hygiene products.
- Avoid sexual activity until symptoms subside.
- Keep area clean and dry.
- Wear cotton underwear and loose garments. Avoid restrictive clothing.
- Try OTC cream (Lotrimin) for itchy rash. Follow instructions on the label.
- If lice are suspected by the presence of small insects or eggs on pubic hairs, see Lice protocol.
- If caller suspects an STD, refer to local public health department or clinic.

Referral Telephone Numbers

Additional Instructions

Report the Following Problems to Your PCP/Clinic/ED

- Signs of infection: pain, redness, swelling, drainage, warmth, red streaks, or swollen glands in the groin
- No improvement after 2 days or condition worsens
- Increased pain or swelling
- Discharge or fever develops
- Suspected exposure to an STD
- Severe pain

G

If the caller agrees with the advice given, document the call and encourage the caller to call back or see PCP if the problem worsens. If the caller does not agree with the advice given, reevaluate and advise the caller to follow up with PCP, Clinic, or ED.

Genital Problems, Male

 Key Questions Name, Age, Onset, Cause, Medications, History

 Other Protocols to Consider Genital Lesions (291); Piercing Problems (445); Scrotal Problems (529); Sexually Transmitted Disease (STD) (542); Skin Lesions: Lumps, Bumps, and Sores (556); Tattoo Problems (604); Urination, Difficult (624).

Reminder: Document caller response to advice, home care instructions, and when to call back.

ASSESSMENT	ACTION
A. Are any of the following present?	
• Persistent painful erection after application of ice pack for 30 minutes • Severe pain or swelling • Trauma to penis and deformity or bleeding • Foreign body in penis	**YES** "Seek emergency care now" **NO** Go to B
B. Are any of the following present?	
• Unable to pull foreskin back over head of penis • Unable to urinate • Pain with urination • Flank pain • Pain in groin after urinating and temperature >100°F (37.8°C) • Pain or swelling in scrotum or testicle(s)	**YES** "Seek medical care within 2 to 4 hours" **NO** Go to C
C. Are any of the following present?	
• Persistent swelling, hard lump, or sore in penis • Known or suspected exposure to an STD • Painful rash or sores • Penile discharge >24 hours • Redness or swelling at tip of penis • Blood in urine • Blood in semen • Rash with blisters on penis • Swollen foreskin	**YES** "Seek medical care within 24 hours" **NO** Go to D

D. Are any of the following present?

- Pain during or after intercourse
- Difficulty having or maintaining an erection and history of diabetes or taking antidepressants, antianxiety medications, blood pressure medications, or diuretics
- Premature ejaculation
- Loss of sexual interest
- Penis caught in zipper
- Swelling and cut in infant penis
- Painless rash or growth >24 hours

YES "Call back or call PCP for appointment if no improvement" and Follow **Home Care Instructions**

NO Follow **Home Care Instructions**

G

Home Care Instructions
Genital Problems, Male

- If pain during intercourse, consider using OTC lubricating jelly (K-Y jelly). Do not use petroleum jelly.
- If tip of penis is painful after intercourse, explore probable causes, such as allergy to contraceptive cream or condom, and change to alternative methods.
- If tip of penis is red from rubbing against a diaper, push penis down when diapering infant.
- If client has sexual dysfunction problems and is taking prescription medications, has diabetes, or has emotional problems, client should discuss with PCP.
- To release penis caught in zipper:
  - cut off the bottom of the zipper and pull the edges back
  - apply petroleum jelly to penis and zipper track and pull zipper in the direction that originally caused the problem
  - if unable to release penis, seek medical care immediately
- Look for hair wrapped around infant's penis and cut to release pressure. Swelling should go down. If unable to remove hair or swelling persists, seek medical care immediately.
- If an STD is suspected, partner should also be treated. Use a condom until both partners have finished taking prescription medication.

Additional Instructions

Report the Following Problems to Your PCP/Clinic/ED
- No improvement or problem worsens after home care measures
- Persistent sexual dysfunction problems

Seek Emergency Care Immediately If Any of the Following Occur
- Persistent painful erection
- Severe pain or swelling
- Inability to urinate

If the caller agrees with the advice given, document the call and encourage the caller to call back or see PCP if the problem worsens. If the caller does not agree with the advice given, reevaluate and advise the caller to follow up with PCP, Clinic, or ED.

Glands, Swollen or Tender

 Key Questions Name, Age, Onset, Allergies, Medications, History, Location

 Other Protocols to Consider Mumps (410); Rubella (German Measles) (520); Rubeola (Measles) (523); Skin Lesions: Lumps, Bumps, and Sores (556).

Reminder: Document caller response to advice, home care instructions, and when to call back.

ASSESSMENT	ACTION

A. Are any of the following present?

- Swollen node >2 inches across
- Red streaks near the swollen node
- Warmth or redness over the node
- Severe pain
- Node interferes with breathing, swallowing, or moving the neck
- Drainage from the node

YES "Seek medical care within 2 to 4 hours"

NO Go to B

B. Are any of the following present?

- Swollen node 1 to 2 inches across
- Persistent fever unresponsive to fever-reducing measures
- Swollen nodes in groin or posterior cervical or axillary area
- Signs of infection in area near or distal to swollen nodes
- Persistent rash, itching, or swelling in other parts of the body
- Persistent fatigue
- Night sweats

YES "Seek medical care within 24 hours"

NO Go to C

C. Are any of the following present?

- History of intermittent nodal swelling
- Nodal swelling in the neck with fever, sore throat, or congestion
- History of allergies
- Swelling and tenderness in underarm area before menstruation

YES "Call back or call PCP for appointment if no improvement" and Follow **Home Care Instructions**

NO Follow **Home Care Instructions**

G

Home Care Instructions
Glands, Swollen or Tender

- Do not squeeze swollen nodes.
- Take your usual pain medication (aspirin, acetaminophen, ibuprofen) as tolerated for discomfort or fever. Do not give aspirin to a child. Avoid aspirin-like products if age <20 years. Avoid acetaminophen if liver disease is present. Avoid ibuprofen if kidney disease or stomach problems exist or in the case of pregnancy. Follow the directions on the label.
- Watch for signs of infection.

Additional Instructions

Report the Following Problems to Your PCP/Clinic/ED

- Node interferes with breathing, swallowing, or moving the neck
- Persistent underarm swelling or tenderness after menstruation
- Persistent nodal swelling
- Signs of infection: increased redness, pain, swelling, warmth, red streaks, drainage

If the caller agrees with the advice given, document the call and encourage the caller to call back or see PCP if the problem worsens. If the caller does not agree with the advice given, reevaluate and advise the caller to follow up with PCP, Clinic, or ED.

Hair Loss

 Key Questions Name, Age, Onset, Location, Allergies, Medications, History

 Other Protocols to Consider Fatigue (244); Lice (401); Rash, Adult (500), Child (505); Skin Lesions: Lumps, Bumps, and Sores (556).

Reminder: Document caller response to advice, home care instructions, and when to call back.

ASSESSMENT	ACTION

A. Are any of the following present?

- New onset of hair loss and fever >101°F (38.3°C) that is unresponsive to fever-reducing measures
- Signs of infection in hair loss areas

YES "Seek medical care within 24 hours"

NO Go to B

B. Are any of the following present?

- Persistent severe fatigue
- Sudden hair loss after taking a new medication
- History of hypothyroidism
- Circular raised, rough pink patch on scalp with a clear center, ½ to 1 inch and itchy

YES "Seek medical care within 48 hours"

NO Go to C

C. Are any of the following present?

- Increased stress level
- Persistent hair loss >2 weeks
- Scaly, itchy, red bald spots
- Recent pregnancy
- Family history of hair loss
- Poor dietary habits
- History of chemotherapy, major surgery, or infection
- History of recent severe diet and weight loss
- Increased use of vitamin A, aspirin, or heparin
- Prolonged use of hair treatments or appliances
- Persistent dandruff or head lice
- History of tight braiding, use of curling iron or hot rollers, or use of chemicals (dye, bleach, or permanent wave application)
- Gradual hair loss over months/years
- Taking birth control pills

YES "Call back or call PCP for appointment if no improvement" and Follow **Home Care Instructions**

NO Follow **Home Care Instructions**

H

299

Home Care Instructions
Hair Loss

- Be reassured that hair usually grows back after sudden hair loss.
- Avoid use of rubber bands, barrettes, braids, or other styles that apply tension on the hair.
- Avoid tugging on hair. Use a cream rinse or detangler to reduce snarls when combing wet hair.
- If hair is severely damaged from chemicals or hairdressing techniques, consider a change in style.
- Eat a well-balanced diet and take diet supplements as directed. OTC Biotin is a supplement that helps to improve nail and hair growth.
- Watch for patterns of continued hair loss.
- Talk with your hairdresser for recommendations of hair growth stimulation products.
- If sudden hair loss after medications or stressful event (usually 1 to 2 months after the event), minimize hair handling. Provide reassurance hair often grows back 3 to 6 months after the event.

Additional Instructions

Report the Following Problems to Your PCP/Clinic/ED

- Persistent hair loss
- New onset of hair loss and fever >101°F (38.3°C)
- Persistent severe fatigue
- Signs of infection in hair loss areas

If the caller agrees with the advice given, document the call and encourage the caller to call back or see PCP if the problem worsens. If the caller does not agree with the advice given, reevaluate and advise the caller to follow up with PCP, Clinic, or ED.

Hand/Wrist Problems

 Key Questions Name, Age, Onset, Cause, Medications, Tetanus Immunization Status, Pain Scale, History

 Other Protocols to Consider Arm or Hand Problems (45); Arthritis Problems (48); Cast/Splint Problems (121); Extremity Injury (222); Numbness and Tingling (431); Weakness (649).

> *Nurse Alert:* Immediate first aid for hand or finger amputation: Wrap amputated part in gauze moistened with saline (if available) or water and place in plastic bag. Place bag in ice bath. Do not allow to freeze.

Reminder: Document caller response to advice, home care instructions, and when to call back.

ASSESSMENT	ACTION

A. Are any of the following present?

- Amputation
- Unable to control bleeding with pressure or spurting blood
- Bone protrudes through the skin
- Altered mental status
- No pulse distal to injury
- Difficulty breathing
- Chest pressure and pain radiates to neck, jaw, or shoulder

YES "Call ambulance"

NO Go to B

B. Are any of the following present?

- Fingers of affected limb cold, blue, and numb
- Crushing trauma
- Penetrating injury: bullet, knife, nail, etc.
- High-pressure injection injury
- Obvious deformity and distal pulse present
- Sudden onset of arm or hand pain following physical exertion

YES "Seek emergency care now"

NO Go to C

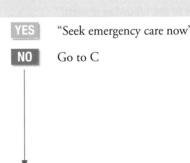

C. Are any of the following present?

- Sudden severe swelling
- Cast or splint, and decreased color, sensation, or movement
- Deep laceration, bleeding controlled
- Sudden severe pain
- Casted extremity and pain with movement of finger

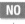 **YES** "Seek medical care immediately"

NO Go to D

D. Are any of the following present?

- Moderate pain
- Swelling
- Unable to remove dirt or other foreign body from the wound
- Pain with movement
- Fever, swelling, drainage, red streaks from a wound
- Inability to make a fist
- Inability to move joint above or below injured area
- Inability to use fingers or hand
- Suspicious explanation for injury
- Gaping laceration

 YES "Seek medical care within 2 to 4 hours"

NO Go to E

E. Are any of the following present?

- Pain increasing with repetitive movement
- Gradual swelling
- Gradual bruising
- Pain with joint movement
- Laceration or puncture wound and tetanus immunization >10 years ago or >5 years if contaminated wound
- No improvement in pain or swelling >3 days and unresponsive to home care measures
- Persistent pain or swelling >2 weeks

YES "Seek medical care within 24 hours"

NO Go to F

F. Are any of the following present?

- Chronic pain
- No known injury and pain or decreased movement >3 days
- Painful or swollen joint and limited movement
- Swelling or bruising occurred within 30 minutes of injury
- Numbness or tingling in hand at night

YES "Call back or call PCP for appointment if no improvement" and
Follow **Home Care Instructions**

NO Follow **Home Care Instructions**

Home Care Instructions
Hand/Wrist Problems

- Remove all rings from affected limb.
- Elevate hand higher than the heart to help reduce swelling.
- Apply ice pack to injured area to reduce swelling and pain for the first 24 hours. After that, alternate ice and heat. Do not apply ice directly to the skin; use a washcloth or other cloth barrier between ice and the skin.
- Apply compression bandage to wrist and hand and immobilize first 24 to 48 hours for swelling. If numbness or tingling occurs after application, loosen bandage.
- Rest the affected area.
- Wash wounds with antimicrobial soap and running water and cover with a sterile dressing.
- Take usual pain medication for discomfort. Do not give aspirin to a child. Avoid aspirin-like products if age <20 years. Avoid acetaminophen if liver disease is present. Avoid ibuprofen if kidney disease or stomach problems exist or in the case of pregnancy. Follow the directions on the label.

Additional Instructions

Report the Following Problems to Your PCP/Clinic/ED

- Increasing pain
- Decreasing range of motion
- Onset of numbness or tingling
- No improvement in pain or swelling >3 days and unresponsive to home care measures
- Persistent pain or swelling >2 weeks
- Cast or splint, and decreased color, sensation, or movement
- Fever, swelling, drainage, red streaks from a wound
- Condition worsens

H

Seek Emergency Care If Any of the Following Occur

- Altered mental status
- No pulse distal to injury
- Difficulty breathing
- Chest pressure and pain radiates to neck, jaw, or shoulder
- Fingers of affected limb cold, blue, and numb
- Sudden-onset arm or hand pain following physical exertion

If the caller agrees with the advice given, document the call and encourage the caller to call back or see PCP if the problem worsens. If the caller does not agree with the advice given, reevaluate and advise the caller to follow up with PCP, Clinic, or ED.

Hay Fever Problems

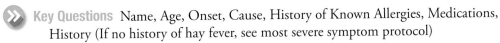

>> **Key Questions** Name, Age, Onset, Cause, History of Known Allergies, Medications, History (If no history of hay fever, see most severe symptom protocol)

>> **Other Protocols to Consider** Breathing Problems (106); Common Cold Symptoms (146); Congestion (153); Cough (170); Earache, Drainage (206); Sinus Problems (554); Sore Throat (564); Wheezing (657).

Nurse Alert: Use this protocol only if previously diagnosed with hay fever.

Reminder: Document caller response to advice, home care instructions, and when to call back.

ASSESSMENT	ACTION
A. Is there difficulty breathing for reasons other than nasal congestion?	
	YES Go to Breathing Problems protocol (106)
	NO Go to B
B. Is chest pain present?	
	YES Go to Chest Pain protocol (123)
	NO Go to C
C. Are any of the following present?	
• Wheezing in a client younger than 4 years • Persistent wheezing that is unresponsive to home care measures	**YES** Go to Wheezing protocol (657)
	NO Go to D

H

D. In addition to clear nasal discharge, sniffing, or sneezing, are any of the following present?

- Fever
- Headache and muscle aches
- Green, brown, or yellow nasal discharge or sputum for >24 hours
- Ear pain or drainage
- Persistent uncontrollable coughing

YES "Seek medical care within 24 hours"

NO Go to E

E. Are any of the following present?

- Symptoms persist, even when client avoids triggers
- Symptoms interfere with daily activities
- Intermittent coughing
- Nasal itching
- Red, itchy, or watery eyes
- Sore throat
- Clear nasal drainage

YES "Call back or call PCP for appointment if no improvement" and
Follow **Home Care Instructions**

NO Follow **Home Care Instructions**

Home Care Instructions
Hay Fever Problems

- Take OTC or prescription antihistamines of choice. Do not give aspirin to a child. Avoid aspirin-like products if age <20 years. Avoid acetaminophen if liver disease is present. Avoid ibuprofen if kidney disease or stomach problems exist or in the case of pregnancy. Follow the directions on the label.
- Avoid use of nasal sprays unless prescribed by PCP. If sprays are used, do not use >5 days.
- Shower and wash hair at night and after having exposure to pollen, dust, or known irritants.
- When pollen count is high, particularly in the morning, stay indoors with the doors and windows closed.
- For itchy eyes, apply cold compresses to the eyelids.
- Avoid pollen and other irritants that worsen the problem.

Additional Instructions

Report the Following Problems to Your PCP/Clinic/ED

- Persistent nasal discharge, sneezing, or sniffing that is unresponsive to medication
- Fever
- Sinus pressure or pain
- Green, brown, or yellow nasal discharge or sputum
- Earache
- Uncontrolled coughing
- Symptoms interfere with daily activity
- Persistent wheezing or coughing that is unresponsive to home care measures

Seek Emergency Care Immediately If Any of the Following Occur

- Chest pain
- Difficulty breathing for reasons other than nasal congestion

H

If the caller agrees with the advice given, document the call and encourage the caller to call back or see PCP if the problem worsens. If the caller does not agree with the advice given, reevaluate and advise the caller to follow up with PCP, Clinic, or ED.

Headache

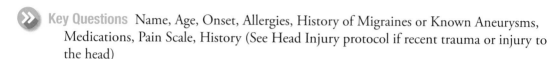

⟫ **Key Questions** Name, Age, Onset, Allergies, History of Migraines or Known Aneurysms, Medications, Pain Scale, History (See Head Injury protocol if recent trauma or injury to the head)

⟫ **Other Protocols to Consider** Alcohol Problems (21); Congestion (153); Head Injury (311); Hypertension (347); Neck Pain (415); Neurologic Symptoms (418); Sinus Problems (554); Stroke, Suspected (576); Toothache (613); Vision Problems (639).

Nurse Alert: There are many conditions that cause headaches; some can be potentially life-threatening. Error on the side of caution when triaging callers with a headache. Headache: Causes and Characteristics: Appendix T (715) is provided to help the nurse gain a better understanding of the many conditions causing headaches. It is NOT to be used to try and diagnose a caller's condition.

- Be on the alert for signs of meningitis: headache, stiff neck, fever, petechial rash, vomiting, irritability, altered mental status.
- Be on the alert for signs of a stroke: headache, weakness on one side of the body, facial drooping, difficulty talking or walking, vision changes.

Reminder: Document caller response to advice, home care instructions, and when to call back.

ASSESSMENT	ACTION

A. Are any of the following present?

- Sudden severe pain or "worst headache ever"
- Sudden onset of weakness, unsteady gait, numbness, and/or tingling on one side of the body
- Confusion, difficulty in arousing, acting differently
- Sudden onset of difficulty speaking or slurred speech
- Stiff neck and fever (pain bending head forward)
- Blurred or double vision
- Purple- or blood-colored flat spots or dots on skin
- Child with diabetes and blood glucose is high

YES "Call ambulance"
or
"Seek emergency care now"

NO Go to B

B. Are any of the following present?

- Persistent vomiting
- History of high blood pressure and light-headedness
- Fever >103°F (39.4°C) and unresponsive to fever-reducing measures
- Eye pain with redness and decreased vision
- Recent tick bite, headache, rash, and flulike symptoms
- New onset of severe persistent pain
- Change in ability to walk

YES "Seek medical care within 2 hours"

NO Go to C

C. Are any of the following present?

- Persistent migraine unresponsive to usual migraine treatment
- Migraine intensity or character different from past migraines
- Persistent headache >12 hours and no other symptoms
- Pain interferes with activity
- Pain in temporal areas and age >50 years

YES "Seek medical care within 24 hours"

NO Go to D

D. Are any of the following present?

- Congestion
- Fever and sore throat
- Muscles and joints ache
- Recent stressful event
- History of allergies
- Dull and constant pain with tender and tight neck muscles
- Recently stopped drinking coffee, eating chocolate, or smoking
- Severe dieting and weight loss
- Dental problems

YES "Call back or call PCP for appointment if no improvement" and Follow **Home Care Instructions**

NO Follow **Home Care Instructions**

Home Care Instructions
Headache

- Apply cool compresses or ice pack to forehead every 2 hours.
- Rest in a quiet darkened room.
- Take usual pain medication (aspirin, acetaminophen, ibuprofen). Do not give aspirin to a child. Avoid aspirin-like products if age <20 years. Avoid acetaminophen if liver disease is present. Avoid ibuprofen if kidney disease or stomach problems exist or in the case of pregnancy. Follow the directions on the label.
- Reduce fever with usual fever-reducing measures.
- For known migraine:
  - take medication as directed by PCP
  - rest with head elevated
  - apply heat to back of neck
  - apply cool compresses to forehead
  - consider avoiding chocolate, milk products, cheddar and blue cheeses, cured pork, caffeine, monosodium glutamate (MSG), and red wine
- If nasal congestion is present, breathe steam for 10 to 20 minutes, 4 times a day or use a vaporizer.
- Keep a migraine journal and take it to the next appointment. Try to identify triggers.

Additional Instructions

Report the Following Problems to Your PCP/Clinic/ED

- Headache persists >24 hours
- No improvement or pain worsens
- Fever is present
- Thick green or yellow nasal discharge
- High blood glucose if you have diabetes
- Persistent vomiting

Seek Emergency Care Immediately If Any of the Following Occur

- Sudden onset of weakness, numbness, or tingling on one side of the body
- Fever, stiff neck
- Confusion, severe drowsiness, or difficulty speaking
- Purple- or blood-colored flat spots or dots appear on skin
- Change in ability to walk

If the caller agrees with the advice given, document the call and encourage the caller to call back or see PCP if the problem worsens. If the caller does not agree with the advice given, reevaluate and advise the caller to follow up with PCP, Clinic, or ED.

Head Injury

 Key Questions Name, Age, Onset, Cause, Allergies, Mechanism of Injury, Medications, Associated Symptoms, History

 Other Protocols to Consider Altered Mental Status (28); Back/Neck Injury (59); Confusion (150); Falls (240); Headache (308); Vomiting, Adult (642), Child (645).

Nurse Alert:

- A neck injury should always be considered whenever there is a head injury. Assess for weakness, incoordination, numbness, neck pain.
- Altered mental status may be one of the first signs of a head injury after trauma, particularly in a child or the elderly.

Reminder: Document caller response to advice, home care instructions, and when to call back.

ASSESSMENT	ACTION

A. After a blow or injury to the head, are any of the following present?

• Difficulty moving arms or legs, weakness, incoordination, or slurred speech • Severe neck pain	**YES** "Call ambulance and do not attempt to move the person"
	NO Go to B

B. Are any of the following present?

• Abnormal breathing or difficulty in breathing • Altered mental status, difficulty in arousing, confusion, agitation • Uncontrolled bleeding • Seizure activity • Preverbal children do not recognize parents or caregiver • Persistent visual disturbance • Persistent vomiting • Persistent headache • Numbness or tingling in arm or leg	**YES** "Call ambulance" or "Seek emergency care now"
	NO Go to C

H

C. Are any of the following present?

- Persistent blood or fluid draining from the nose or ears
- Gaping, split, jagged, or deep wound
- Laceration
- Bruising behind the ears or under the eyes
- Persistent bleeding >10 minutes
- History of loss of consciousness
- Change in behavior since the injury
- Fall >2 feet in a child younger than 1 year
- Presently or recently taking blood-thinning medication

YES "Seek medical care within 2 hours"

NO Go to D

D. Is the following present?

- Child younger than 1 year with a soft spongy swollen area over the skull for >12 hours

YES "Seek medical care within 24 hours"

NO Go to E

E. Are any of the following present?

- Swollen area (goose egg) on the forehead or scalp
- Intermittent headache not responsive to pain medication

YES "Call back or call PCP for appointment if no improvement" and
Follow **Home Care Instructions**

NO Follow **Home Care Instructions**

Home Care Instructions
Head Injury

- Apply ice packs or cold compresses to area for 20 minutes every 2 hours to reduce swelling and discomfort. Place a cloth barrier between the ice and the skin.
- Allow a child to sleep after an injury. Awaken every 2 hours for 24 hours to determine level of alertness and responsiveness.
- Avoid heavy activity during first 24 hours after the injury. Rest in a quiet area with head slightly elevated.
- Take acetaminophen for discomfort. Do not give aspirin to a child. Avoid aspirin-like products if age <20 years. Avoid acetaminophen if liver disease is present. Avoid ibuprofen if kidney disease or stomach problems exist or in the case of pregnancy. Follow the directions on the label.
- Avoid aspirin and ibuprofen.
- Avoid alcohol, sleeping pills, or sedatives during the first 24 hours after the injury.
- Avoid heavy meals.

Additional Instructions

Report the Following Problems to Your PCP/Clinic/ED

- No improvement or condition worsens
- Persistent headache
- Persistent swelling >24 hours after ice pack application
- Blood or clear drainage from nose or ears

Seek Emergency Care Immediately If Any of the Following Occur

- Confusion, disorientation, agitation, or change in vision
- Altered mental status or difficulty arousing
- Numbness, tingling, or weakness in an arm or leg
- Persistent vomiting, severe headache, speech problems, seizures, or lethargy
- Child does not recognize parents or caregiver
- Persistent numbness and tingling

H

If the caller agrees with the advice given, document the call and encourage the caller to call back or see PCP if the problem worsens. If the caller does not agree with the advice given, reevaluate and advise the caller to follow up with PCP, Clinic, or ED.

Hearing Loss

Key Questions Name, Age, Onset, Cause if Known, Allergies, Medications, History

Other Protocols to Consider Earache, Drainage (206); Ear Injury, Foreign Body (209); Ear Ringing (211); Head Injury (311).

Reminder: Document caller response to advice, home care instructions, and when to call back.

ASSESSMENT	ACTION
A. Is the following present?	
• Overdose of aspirin or products containing aspirin — **YES**	"Seek emergency care now"
NO	Go to B
B. Are any of the following present?	
• Recent injury to ear or head and hearing loss, earache, swelling, or bruising behind ear or blood in ear canal — **YES**	"Seek medical care within 2 to 4 hours"
• Sudden pain, hearing loss, bleeding or discharge, and ringing in the ears	
• Dizziness, vertigo, or recent ear surgery — **NO**	Go to C
C. Are any of the following present?	
• Child shows signs of hearing loss after having measles, mumps, or meningitis: — **YES**	"Seek medical care within 24 hours"
• does not respond to a sudden sound or distracting sound — **NO**	Go to D
• Persistent hearing loss >3 days	
• Persistent earache or yellow-green drainage from ear	
• New prescription or OTC medication	
D. Are any of the following present?	
• Ringing in the ears — **YES**	"Call back or call PCP for appointment if no improvement" and Follow **Home Care Instructions**
• Prolonged exposure to loud noises	
• Sudden pain with cracking or popping noise	
• Gradual hearing loss during a period of several weeks or months	
• Feeling of fullness in one or both ears — **NO**	Follow **Home Care Instructions**

Home Care Instructions
Hearing Loss

- Do not instill liquid drops in the ear if pain is related to an injury or a ruptured eardrum is suspected (sudden pain, hearing loss, bleeding or discharge, ringing in the ears, dizziness).
- Wear earplugs when exposure to loud noises is anticipated.
- To remove excessive earwax:
  - instill Debrox as directed for as long as 3 days
  - instill two drops of mineral oil in the affected ear twice a day for 2 days
  - lie down and apply a warm damp cloth under the affected ear
  - stand under a warm shower with the ear pointed toward the shower head
- Relieve ear congestion by frequent swallowing, chewing, and swallowing with the nose pinched closed.
- Take usual pain medication (acetaminophen or ibuprofen). Do not give aspirin to a child. Avoid aspirin-like products if age <20 years. Avoid acetaminophen if liver disease is present. Avoid ibuprofen if kidney disease or stomach problems exist or in the case of pregnancy. Follow the directions on the label.
- Discontinue OTC medication if hearing loss is thought to be caused by medication.
- Do not use cotton swabs.

Additional Instructions

Report the Following Problems to Your PCP/Clinic/ED

- No improvement in 3 days or condition worsens
- Fever or swelling
- Recent injury to ear or head and hearing loss, earache, swelling, or bruising behind ear or blood in ear canal
- Sudden pain, hearing loss, bleeding or discharge, and ringing in the ears
- Dizziness, vertigo, or recent ear surgery

If the caller agrees with the advice given, document the call and encourage the caller to call back or see PCP if the problem worsens. If the caller does not agree with the advice given, reevaluate and advise the caller to follow up with PCP, Clinic, or ED.

H

Heartburn

 Key Questions Name, Age, Onset, Cause, Allergies, Medications, History, Associated Symptoms, Pain Scale

 Other Protocols to Consider Abdominal Pain, Adult (9), Child (13); Chest Pain (123); Gas/Belching (287); Indigestion (368); Vomiting, Adult (642), Child (645); Swallowing Difficulty (591).

> *Nurse Alert:* Heartburn can mimic chest pain. There are many conditions that cause chest pain; some can be potentially life-threatening. Error on the side of caution when triaging callers with chest pain. Chest Pain: Causes and Characteristics: Appendix S (712) is provided to help the nurse gain a better understanding of the many conditions causing chest pain. It is NOT to be used to try and diagnose a caller's condition.

Reminder: Document caller response to advice, home care instructions, and when to call back.

ASSESSMENT	ACTION

A. In addition to a burning or heavy sensation, are any of the following present?

- Shortness of breath
- Cool, moist skin
- Pain in the neck, jaw, shoulders, back, or arms
- Blue or gray face, lips, earlobes, or fingernails
- Fainting
- Vomiting blood or dark coffee grounds–like emesis

YES "Call ambulance"

NO Go to B

B. Are any of the following present?

- History of diabetes or cardiac disease
- Dizziness or light-headedness

YES "Seek medical care within 2 to 4 hours"

NO Go to C

C. Are any of the following present?

- Discomfort persists after taking antacids
- Condition worsening, requiring more frequent use of antacids
- Difficult or painful swallowing
- Sensation that pill is stuck in esophagus

 YES "Seek medical care within 24 hours"

 NO Go to D

D. Are any of the following present?

- Pain increased with use of medications
- Increased pain bending over, exercising, or lying down soon after eating
- Nausea or vomiting
- Pregnancy
- Frequent belching
- Burping stomach contents into mouth
- Obesity
- Heavy tobacco or alcohol use
- Increased stress

YES "Call back or call PCP for appointment if no improvement" and Follow **Home Care Instructions**

NO Follow **Home Care Instructions**

Home Care Instructions
Heartburn

- Try OTC antacids (Maalox, Mylanta, Riopan, Tums) and follow directions on bottle. Try OTC Pepcid AC, Tagamet HB, Zantac, or Prilosec. Consult with PCP if taking other prescription medications. Liquids provide faster relief than tablets. Do not give Pepto-Bismol to a child. Ask pharmacist for additional product suggestions.
- Avoid eating or drinking 2 to 3 hours before going to bed.
- Do not lie down, bend over, or exercise soon after eating.
- Elevate head of bed 4 to 6 inches using blocks or bricks, or lie on left side to help speed stomach emptying and reduce reflux.
- Eat small meals, but eat them more than three times a day.
- Avoid spicy foods, alcohol, coffee, smoking, chocolate, citrus fruits, tomatoes, vinegar, fatty foods, or any other food or drink that triggers heartburn.
- If aspirin or ibuprofen worsens the problem, try acetaminophen. Do not give aspirin to a child. Avoid aspirin-like products if age <20 years. Avoid acetaminophen if liver disease is present. Avoid ibuprofen if kidney disease or stomach problems exist or in the case of pregnancy. Follow the directions on the label.
- Avoid tight-fitting clothing, such as girdles, belts, control-top pantyhose, and pants or skirts with a tight-fitting waistband.
- Fifty minutes after dinner, sip 1 tsp apple cider vinegar, diluted in water or juice; this will help hasten digestion of food, lessening reflux when sleeping.

Additional Instructions

Report the Following Problems to Your PCP/Clinic/ED
- Discomfort occurs after taking prescribed medication
- No improvement in 3 days or condition worsens
- No relief from antacids or other OTC drugs (such as Pepcid AC or Zantac)
- Frequent use of antacids
- Difficult or painful swallowing

Call Ambulance If Any of the Following Occur

- Shortness of breath
- Dizziness
- Cool, moist skin
- Pain or discomfort in neck, jaw, shoulders, back, or arms
- Blue or gray face or lips
- Fainting
- Vomiting blood or dark coffee grounds–like emesis

If the caller agrees with the advice given, document the call and encourage the caller to call back or see PCP if the problem worsens. If the caller does not agree with the advice given, reevaluate and advise the caller to follow up with PCP, Clinic, or ED.

H

Heart Rate Problems

 Key Questions Name, Age, Onset, Cause, Rate, Medications, History, Implanted Device in Chest

 Other Protocols to Consider Alcohol Problems (21); Anxiety (36); Breathing Problems (106); Chest Pain (123); Dizziness (199); Fatigue (244); Headache (308); Hypertension (347); Hyperventilation (350); Hypotension (352); Weakness (649).

Reminder: Document caller response to advice, home care instructions, and when to call back.

ASSESSMENT	ACTION

A. Is heart rate >150 bpm and are any of the following present?

- Chest, neck, jaw, or arm pain or discomfort
- Difficulty breathing
- Skin cool and moist or hot and dry
- Face or lips blue, gray, or very pale
- Fainting

YES "Call ambulance"

NO Go to B

B. Are any of the following present?

- Persistent rapid heart rate of >150 bpm for >30 minutes
- Light-headedness, faintness, or dizziness
- Persistent rapid heart rate and history of thyroid disease or heart disease
- Repeated shocks with internal defibrillator in place
- Slow heart rate and extreme fatigue or frequent episodes of slow heart rate
- Persistent slow heart rate and pauses of >3 seconds (count 1,001, 1,002, 1,003)

YES "Seek medical care now"

NO Go to C

C. Are any of the following present?

- Frequent episodes of a rapid heart rate
- Persistent slow heart rate and history of heart disease, general ill feeling, or frequent falls
- Recent history of persistent vomiting or diarrhea

YES "Seek medical care within 24 hours"

NO Go to D

D. Are any of the following present?

- History of prior treatment for rapid heart rate
- Recent ingestion of diuretics, diet pills, decongestants, cold remedies, β-blockers, thyroid medication, a new medication, or recreational drugs
- History of bronchodilator use and new prescription or increase in dose
- Excessive use of caffeine, tobacco, alcohol, or herbal stimulants
- Difficulty sleeping or persistent fatigue
- Increase in stress
- Exercise <30 minutes before onset of symptoms
- Frequent skipped beats
- Unexplained weight gain, fatigue, and feeling cold
- Fever

YES   "Call back or call PCP for appointment if no improvement" and
Follow **Home Care Instructions**

NO   Follow **Home Care Instructions**

H

Home Care Instructions
Heart Rate Problems

- To slow down heart rate:
  - take a deep breath; hold and pinch nostrils closed. Gently try to exhale through the nose
  - take a deep breath and bear down as if having a bowel movement
  - try to blow up a balloon
  - take a cold shower and let cold water splash on the face and head
  - try to remain calm
  - rest and relax
  - try to identify the trigger and discuss it with PCP if problem persists
  - avoid medications that seem to worsen the problem
  - avoid caffeine and alcohol

Additional Instructions

Report the Following Problems to Your PCP/Clinic/ED

- Problem persists or worsens
- Light-headedness or faintness

Seek Emergency Care Immediately If Any of the Following Occur

- Chest, neck, jaw, or arm pain
- Difficulty breathing
- Cool and moist skin
- Face or lips blue, gray, or very pale
- Fainting
- Loss of consciousness or altered mental status

If the caller agrees with the advice given, document the call and encourage the caller to call back or see PCP if the problem worsens. If the caller does not agree with the advice given, reevaluate and advise the caller to follow up with PCP, Clinic, or ED.

Heat Exposure Problems

 Key Questions Name, Age, Onset, Cause, Temperature, Medications, History

 Other Protocols to Consider Altered Mental Status (28); Dehydration (180); Dizziness (199); Fainting (237); Fever, Adult (250), Child (253); Muscle Cramps (413); Sunburn (588); Sweating, Excessive (594); Weakness (649).

Nurse Alert:

- Hyperthermia may result from prolonged exposure to high temperatures or humidity, excessive exercise, infection, drug use such as amphetamines, and in the elderly who may have an impaired ability to dissipate heat.
- Elderly exposed to very warm environments are more prone to dehydration and UTIs, with altered mental status as the first sign of a problem needing prompt attention.

Reminder: Document caller response to advice, home care instructions, and when to call back.

ASSESSMENT	ACTION

A. After prolonged exposure to heat or strenuous exercise, are any of the following present?

- Temperature >102°F (38.9°C), skin is hot and dry, and any of the following:
  - flushed skin
  - no sweating
- Sudden dizziness, headache, weakness, faintness, or loss of consciousness
- Confusion, delirium, or disorientation
- Visual disturbances
- Seizures
- Rapid heart rate
- Rapid breathing
- Age <10 years or >70 years
- Low or normal temperature, skin cool and moist, and mental confusion or unconsciousness

 "Call ambulance"
or
"Seek emergency care now"
and
Follow **Emergency Home Care Instructions** while waiting for help to arrive

 Go to B

H

B. After prolonged exposure to heat or strenuous exercise, are any of the following present?

- Profuse sweating
- Dizziness, weakness, or faintness
- Severe muscle cramps or incoordination
- Slow heart rate
- Dark yellow or orange urine
- Vomiting and inability to tolerate fluids

 YES — "Follow **Home Care Instructions**, but if no immediate improvement, seek emergency care now"

NO — Go to C

C. After prolonged exposure to heat or strenuous exercise, are any of the following present?

- Temperature >100.5°F (38.1°C) and age >60 years, diabetic, bedridden, or person has weakened immune system

 YES — "Seek medical care within 2 to 4 hours"

NO — Go to D

D. After prolonged exposure to heat or strenuous exercise, are any of the following present?

- Fatigue
- Mild muscle cramps
- Flushed skin
- Slight nausea or dizziness
- Feeling hot

 YES — "Call back or call PCP if no improvement"
and
Follow **Home Care Instructions**

NO — **Home Care Instructions**

Home Care Instructions
Heat Exposure Problems

Emergency Home Care Instructions
- Help the victim to lie down in a cool, shady area and loosen clothing or remove clothes.
- Keep the victim cool while awaiting medical assistance. Apply cool towels and use a fan to help cool the victim. Do not put ice directly on the skin. Do not allow the victim to shiver, as it increases body heat. Sponge the victim with tepid water. Do not use an alcohol rub.
- Elevate legs higher than the heart.
- If alert, give the victim cold liquids (water, sports beverages, soft drinks, fruit juices) to drink. Do not drink beverages with alcohol or caffeine. Drinking too fast can cause nausea. Drink one cup every 15 minutes as tolerated and no nausea.

Moderate or Mild Heat Exposure Instructions
- Use a spray bottle or mister with lukewarm water and spray exposed skin to help cool through evaporation.
- If age <13 years, give Pedialyte or Ricelyte to rehydrate.
- Mix ¼ tsp salt in 1 quart of water. Give ½ cup every 15 minutes for 1½ hours. Do not allow person to consume salt tablets. If thirst persists, give plain water.
- If no nausea, try salty snack foods such as pretzels, potato chips.
- Do not give aspirin or acetaminophen for elevated temperature.
- Apply cool towels and use a fan to help cool down. Do not put ice directly on the skin. Do not allow the person to shiver, as it increases body heat.
- Take a cool shower or bath to reduce body temperature quickly.
- Encourage seniors living in very warm environments to go to air-conditioned or cooler places during very hot spells such as senior centers, malls, as heat exhaustion and heat stroke can develop rapidly.

Additional Instructions

Report the Following Problem to Your PCP/Clinic/ED
- No improvement after following Home Care Instructions

H

Seek Emergency Care Immediately If Any of the Following Occur

- Decreasing alertness
- Seizures
- Muscle cramps or incoordination
- Persistent unusually slow heart rate
- Persistent vomiting and inability to tolerate fluids

If the caller agrees with the advice given, document the call and encourage the caller to call back or see PCP if the problem worsens. If the caller does not agree with the advice given, reevaluate and advise the caller to follow up with PCP, Clinic, or ED.

Hemorrhoids

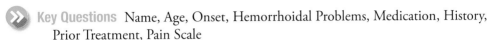

>> **Key Questions** Name, Age, Onset, Hemorrhoidal Problems, Medication, History, Prior Treatment, Pain Scale

>> **Other Protocols to Consider** Constipation (160); Diarrhea, Adult (192), Child (195); Rectal Bleeding (510); Rectal Problems (513).

Reminder: Document caller response to advice, home care instructions, and when to call back.

ASSESSMENT	ACTION

A. Are any of the following present?

- Severe persistent rectal bleeding
- Foreign body
- High fever

YES "Seek medical care within 2 to 4 hours"

NO Go to B

B. Are any of the following present?

- Severe rectal pain, interfering with activities
- Signs of infection: redness, pain, drainage, or fever
- Diabetes

YES "Seek medical care within 24 hours"

NO Go to C

C. Are any of the following present?

- Bleeding in absence of stool
- Streaks of blood on stool surface
- History of pregnancy, prolonged sitting, constipation
- Increased straining during bowel movements
- Pain, itching, or mucus discharge after bowel movement
- Small lumps around or inside the rectal area for 1 to 3 days

YES "Call back or call PCP for appointment if no improvement" and Follow **Home Care Instructions**

NO Follow **Home Care Instructions**

H

Home Care Instructions
Hemorrhoids

- Sit in a warm tub or sitz bath 10 minutes several times daily to relieve discomfort and swelling, especially after painful bowel movements.
- Clean rectal area with soft tissue or moist wipes after each bowel movement.
- To relieve itching, apply cold compresses to the area for 10 minutes, 4 times a day.
- Apply zinc oxide or petroleum jelly to the clean dry area to help reduce irritation and to ease passage of stool. Follow instructions on the label.
- If no relief with these measures, try OTC medications (hemorrhoid suppositories, hydrocortisone [0.5% strength], Tucks). Follow instructions on the label. Products with witch hazel may help to reduce discomfort. Products with hydrocortisone help to reduce itching.
- Avoid prolonged sitting, standing, lifting, or straining.
- Wear cotton clothing and loose underwear.
- Avoid straining during bowel movements. Take your time, but avoid sitting > 2 minutes. Get up, do something else, and return when it feels easier.
- To help prevent constipation, drink plenty of water and eat a diet high in fiber (fruits, vegetables, and whole grain cereals).

Additional Instructions

Report the Following Problems to Your PCP/Clinic/ED
- Hard lump develops around the rectal opening
- Excessive rectal bleeding or black stools occur (more than once)
- Severe pain is unresponsive to home care measures
- Pain or bleeding >1 week
- Signs of infection: increased redness, pain, swelling, drainage, or fever

If the caller agrees with the advice given, document the call and encourage the caller to call back or see PCP if the problem worsens. If the caller does not agree with the advice given, reevaluate and advise the caller to follow up with PCP, Clinic, or ED.

Hepatitis

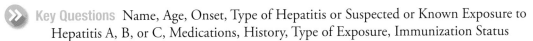 **Key Questions** Name, Age, Onset, Type of Hepatitis or Suspected or Known Exposure to Hepatitis A, B, or C, Medications, History, Type of Exposure, Immunization Status

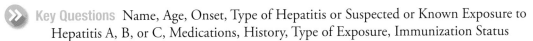 **Other Protocols to Consider** Abdominal Pain, Adult (9), Child (13); Alcohol Problems (21); Immunization Reactions (358); Jaundice (385); Vomiting, Adult (642), Child (645); Substance Abuse, Use, or Exposure (582).

> *Nurse Alert:* Use this protocol only if previously diagnosed with hepatitis, suspected or known exposure to hepatitis A, B, or C. Communicable Disease Table: Appendix M (696) is provided to help the nurse gain a better understanding of many communicable diseases, the mode of disease transmission, incubation period, and contagious period. It is NOT to be used to try and diagnose a caller's condition.

Reminder: Document caller response to advice, home care instructions, and when to call back.

ASSESSMENT	ACTION

A. Is the following present?

- Severe abdominal pain

YES Go to Abdominal Pain protocol (9)

NO Go to B

B. Are any of the following present?

- Evidence of GI bleeding
- Confusion or decreased mental alertness

YES "Seek emergency care now"

NO Go to C

C. Are any of the following present?

- Severe vomiting
- Bruises or bleeds easily
- Light-headedness upon standing
- Immunosuppressed
- Weight gain and difficulty breathing

YES "Seek medical care within 2 to 4 hours"

NO Go to D

H

D. Are any of the following present?

- Jaundiced eyes or skin
- Abdominal pain, especially in the right upper region
- Clay-colored stools
- Dark urine
- Age younger than 10 years or older than 70 years
- Diabetes
- Pregnancy
- Known exposure to hepatitis

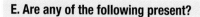 **YES** "Seek medical care within 24 hours"

NO Go to E

E. Are any of the following present?

- Decreased appetite
- Nausea or occasional or intermittent vomiting
- Symptoms of upper respiratory infections
- Flulike symptoms, generalized achiness
- Fever

YES "Call back or call PCP for appointment if no improvement" and
Follow **Home Care Instructions**

NO Follow **Home Care Instructions**

Home Care Instructions
Hepatitis

- Get plenty of rest and eat a good diet (try several small meals a day).
- Increase fluids: juices, broths, sports beverages, water, tea, and at least 8 glasses (8-ounce glasses) of water a day.
- Wash hands well after bowel movements and before eating or preparing food.
- Clean utensils in dishwasher or in 200°F (93.3°C) oven for 15 to 20 minutes, and wash clothes and bedding on hottest setting.
- Do not cook for others or share a toothbrush or utensils.
- Do not drink alcoholic beverages or take acetaminophen.
- For information about exposure and the possible need for treatment, contact your local public health department or PCP. Immunizations are available for hepatitis A and B.
- Do not engage in sexual activity without using a condom if either partner is infected with hepatitis B.
- Anyone with symptoms suspicious of hepatitis needs a medical evaluation by a PCP or local health department or clinic.
- Hepatitis A is transmitted through the fecal–oral route, usually food contamination. Individuals are contagious 2 to 3 weeks after infection.
- Hepatitis B is transmitted by blood, saliva, semen, or vaginal fluid. It is highly contagious.
- Hepatitis C is transmitted by blood and plasma, often through needle exposure. It is contagious 1 week before onset of symptoms.

Additional Instructions

Report the Following Problems to Your PCP/Clinic/ED

- White part of the eye or skin appears yellow and new onset
- Abdominal pain, clay-colored stools, or dark urine
- Signs of dehydration occur because of vomiting

H

Seek Emergency Care Immediately If Any of the Following Occur

- Evidence of GI bleeding
- Confusion or decreased mental alertness

If the caller agrees with the advice given, document the call and encourage the caller to call back or see PCP if the problem worsens. If the caller does not agree with the advice given, reevaluate and advise the caller to follow up with PCP, Clinic, or ED.

Hiccups

 Key Questions Name, Age, Onset, Allergies, Medications, History

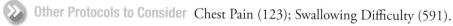 **Other Protocols to Consider** Chest Pain (123); Swallowing Difficulty (591).

Reminder: Document caller response to advice, home care instructions, and when to call back.

ASSESSMENT	ACTION

A. Are any of the following present?

- Confusion, lethargy
- Difficulty breathing
- Fainting
- Chest, neck, jaw, or arm pain or pressure

YES   "Call ambulance"
or
"Seek emergency care now"

NO   Go to B

B. Are any of the following present?

- Persistent pain
- Constant hiccups >8 hours

YES   "Seek medical care within 2 to 4 hours"

NO   Go to C

C. Are any of the following present?

- Persistent vomiting
- Pain in shoulder, abdomen, or back

YES   "Seek medical care within 24 hours"

NO   Go to D

D. Are any of the following present?

- Sudden onset after taking a new medication
- Interferes with sleep
- Anxiety or irritability
- Intermittent episodes
- Increased alcohol use
- Mild discomfort
- Recent ingestion of hot or irritating food or drink
- History of cancer

YES   "Call back or call PCP for appointment if no improvement"
and
Follow **Home Care Instructions**

NO   Follow **Home Care Instructions**

Home Care Instructions
Hiccups

- Take a deep breath and hold for 15 to 30 seconds.
- Breathe into a paper bag for 5 minutes.
- Sip ice water.
- Swallow dry bread, crackers, a teaspoon of dry sugar, or crushed ice. NOTE: Young children can choke on dry sugar. Place sugar in cloth, tie closed, and soak in water. Have the child suck on the sugar sack. May also hold a teaspoon of sugar on tongue until it melts.
- Pull on tongue.
- Apply gentle pressure to closed eyelids.
- Grasp upper lip between teeth and right side of nose and apply gentle pressure.
- Stroke back of tongue.
- Take your usual antacid (Maalox, Mylanta) as directed on container.
- Divert attention through distraction.

Additional Instructions

Report the Following Problem to Your PCP/Clinic/ED

- Persistent or worsening condition

Seek Emergency Care Immediately If Any of the Following Occur

- Chest, neck, jaw, or arm pain or pressure
- Difficulty breathing
- Confusion or lethargy
- Fainting

If the caller agrees with the advice given, document the call and encourage the caller to call back or see PCP if the problem worsens. If the caller does not agree with the advice given, reevaluate and advise the caller to follow up with PCP, Clinic, or ED.

H

Hip Pain/Injury

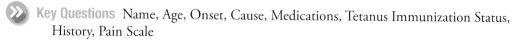

>> **Key Questions** Name, Age, Onset, Cause, Medications, Tetanus Immunization Status, History, Pain Scale

>> **Other Protocols to Consider** Arthritis Problems (48); Extremity Injury (222); Falls (240); Joint Pain/Swelling (390); Leg Pain/Swelling (398).

Reminder: Document caller response to advice, home care instructions, and when to call back.

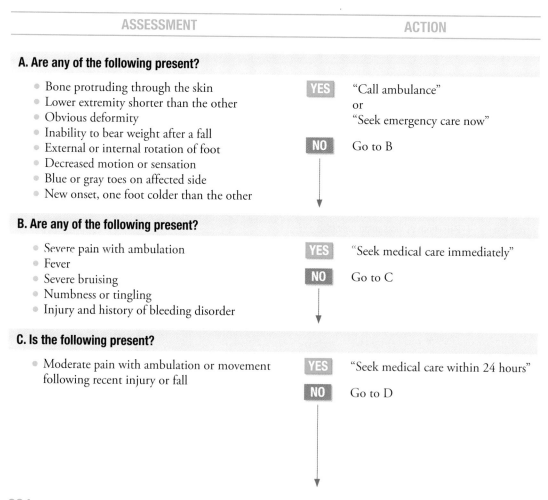

ASSESSMENT	ACTION

A. Are any of the following present?

- Bone protruding through the skin
- Lower extremity shorter than the other
- Obvious deformity
- Inability to bear weight after a fall
- External or internal rotation of foot
- Decreased motion or sensation
- Blue or gray toes on affected side
- New onset, one foot colder than the other

YES "Call ambulance"
or
"Seek emergency care now"

NO Go to B

B. Are any of the following present?

- Severe pain with ambulation
- Fever
- Severe bruising
- Numbness or tingling
- Injury and history of bleeding disorder

YES "Seek medical care immediately"

NO Go to C

C. Is the following present?

- Moderate pain with ambulation or movement following recent injury or fall

YES "Seek medical care within 24 hours"

NO Go to D

D. Are any of the following present?

- Chronic pain unrelieved with usual pain control measures
- Intermittent pain following injury, exercise, or fall

YES   "Call back or call PCP for appointment if no improvement" and
Follow **Home Care Instructions**

NO   Follow **Home Care Instructions**

H

Home Care Instructions
Hip Pain/Injury

- Rest injured part as much as possible for 48 hours.
- Elevate leg on pillow for the first 24 hours.
- Apply ice pack to injured area 20 to 30 minutes every 3 to 4 hours for the first 24 to 48 hours, then alternate with heat. Do not apply ice directly on the skin; use a washcloth or other cloth barrier between the ice and the skin.
- Take your usual pain medication. Do not give aspirin to a child. Avoid aspirin-like products if age <20 years. Avoid acetaminophen if liver disease is present. Avoid ibuprofen if kidney disease or stomach problems exist or in the case of pregnancy. Follow the directions on the label.
- Avoid activity that causes pain.
- Warm up and stretch before exercising.
- If pain increases with exercise, take frequent breaks.

Additional Instructions

Report the Following Problems to Your PCP/Clinic/ED

- Painful ambulation
- Fever
- Severe bruising
- Numbness or tingling
- No improvement or condition worsens
- Change in color, sensation, or ability to ambulate
- Pain unresponsive to home care measures

Seek Emergency Care Immediately If Any of the Following Occur

- Difficulty breathing
- Decreased motion or sensation
- Blue or gray toes on affected side
- New onset, one foot colder than the other

If the caller agrees with the advice given, document the call and encourage the caller to call back or see PCP if the problem worsens. If the caller does not agree with the advice given, reevaluate and advise the caller to follow up with PCP, Clinic, or ED.

Hives

 Key Questions Name, Age, Onset, Suspected Cause, Red Raised Itchy Patches on Skin, Allergies, Medications, History, Associated Symptoms

 Other Protocols to Consider Allergic Reaction (25); Bee Stings (72); Bites, Insect (79); Breathing Problems (106); Immunization Reactions (358); Itching (382); Rash, Adult (500), Child (505); Skin Lesions: Lumps, Bumps, and Sores (556); Wheezing (657).

Nurse Alert: A sudden onset of hives can precede an anaphylactic reaction, a severe life-threatening allergic reaction, and can occur within seconds to an hour after exposure to the offending substance such as food, medication, or a bee sting. An anaphylactic reaction involves the respiratory, cardiovascular, and central nervous systems. Sudden onset of symptoms may include difficulty breathing; feeling faint; swelling of the tongue, throat, or lips; hives; wheezing or coughing; or a feeling of impending doom. The sooner symptoms occur after exposure to the antigen, the more severe the anaphylaxis.

Reminder: Document caller response to advice, home care instructions, and when to call back.

ASSESSMENT	ACTION
A. Hives, and are any of the following present?	
• Difficulty breathing, chest tightness, or wheezing • Difficulty swallowing or swelling of tongue or back of throat • Confusion, agitation, or decreasing level of consciousness • Fainting • History of bee sting(s) and bee sting allergy • Previous severe allergic reaction to same allergen	**YES** "Call ambulance" **NO** Go to B
B. Are any of the following present?	
• Faintness or dizziness • Severe abdominal pain • Nausea or vomiting • Rapid onset of cough • Sudden onset of hoarseness	**YES** "Seek emergency care now" **NO** Go to C

H

C. Are any of the following present?

- Rapid progression of red, raised, itchy rash on several areas of the body
- Swelling in face or limbs
- Hives after 2 days of antihistamine therapy

 "Seek medical care within 2 to 4 hours"

NO Go to D

D. Are any of the following present?

- Diarrhea or fever
- Joint swelling or pain
- Exposure to plants in the woods (such as poison ivy, poison oak, or poison sumac) that required steroid therapy in the past

 "Seek medical care within 24 hours"

NO Go to E

E. Are any of the following present?

- New medication
- New foods in diet
- New soaps, shampoos, laundry detergent, clothing, cosmetics, toothpaste, or other toiletries
- Recent new contact with plants or animals or new insect bites
- Intermittent hives
- Hives >7 days and interfering with activity

YES "Call back or call PCP for appointment if no improvement" and

Follow **Home Care Instructions**

NO Follow **Home Care Instructions**

Home Care Instructions
Hives

- For widespread hives, take an OTC antihistamine (e.g., Benadryl, Claritin, Alavert) until hives have disappeared. Follow instructions on the label. Do not drive or engage in activities that require concentration. Ask pharmacist for other product suggestions.
- If medications are suspected as the cause of the reaction, discontinue use and contact PCP.
- Cool baths of plain water, baking soda and water, or oatmeal powder and water may help to relieve itching and discomfort.
- Apply Caladryl or calamine lotion to help control itching and dry lesions. Follow instructions on the label. Limit use of Caladryl on small children because it may cause sedation.
- Avoid the sun. Seek cool areas and take cool showers to help relieve discomfort.

Additional Instructions

Report the Following Problems to Your PCP/Clinic/ED

- Persistent hives >7 days
- Persistent itching >24 hours after taking antihistamines

Seek Emergency Care Immediately If Any of the Following Occur

- Difficulty breathing, chest tightness, or wheezing
- Difficulty swallowing, or swelling of tongue or back of throat
- Confusion, agitation, or decreasing level of consciousness
- Fainting
- Difficulty breathing
- Swelling of lips or mouth

If the caller agrees with the advice given, document the call and encourage the caller to call back or see PCP if the problem worsens. If the caller does not agree with the advice given, reevaluate and advise the caller to follow up with PCP, Clinic, or ED.

HIV Exposure

 Key Questions Name, Age, Onset, Cause, Medications, History, HIV Status

 Other Protocols to Consider Blood/Body Fluid Exposure (93); Sexually Transmitted
Disease (STD) (542).

> *Nurse Alert:* Use this protocol only if known exposure to blood or body fluids of someone suspected
> with or diagnosed with HIV infection or concerned about exposure and HIV status unknown.

Reminder: Document caller response to advice, home care instructions, and when to call back.

ASSESSMENT	ACTION

A. Are exposure and any of the following present?

- Open wounds (sores, cuts, scrapes), eyes, or mouth exposed to infected person's blood or body fluids
- Puncture with a contaminated needle
- Unprotected sexual contact

 YES "Seek medical care now to discuss options"

 NO Go to B

B. Blood or body fluid exposure to a person whose HIV status is unknown, and did any of the following occur?

- Persistent fever and night sweats
- Persistent diarrhea
- Persistent swollen nodes in neck, underarm, or groin
- Unusual sores and increased number of sores
- Dry cough

YES "Seek medical care in 24 hours"

NO Go to C

C. Blood or body fluid exposure to a person whose HIV status is unknown, and did any of the following occur?

- Unprotected sexual contact
- Open wounds (sores, cuts, or scrapes), eyes, or mouth exposed to another person's blood or body fluids
- Weight loss
- Numbness or pain in hands or feet

YES "Call back or call PCP within 24 hours to discuss options" and
Follow **Home Care Instructions**

NO Follow **Home Care Instructions**

Home Care Instructions
HIV Exposure

- If wound is present, wash with soap and water and watch for signs of infection: increased redness, pain, drainage, fever, warmth, red streaks from the wound.
- Rinse exposed eyes or mouth with running water for 5 minutes.
- Consult with PCP or health department (# _____) for HIV testing on self and contact person.
- Understand that casual contact cannot transmit disease.
- If caller suspects HIV/AIDS infection, encourage to follow up with PCP or Clinic or call National AIDS Hotline at 1-800-232-4636.

Additional Instructions

Report the Following Problems to Your PCP/Clinic/ED

- Known blood or body fluid exposure to person with HIV infection; hepatitis A, B, or C; or an STD
- Persistent fever and night sweats
- Persistent diarrhea
- Persistent swollen nodes in neck, underarm, or groin
- Unusual sores and increased number of sores
- Dry cough
- Severe fatigue
- Weight loss

If the caller agrees with the advice given, document the call and encourage the caller to call back or see PCP if the problem worsens. If the caller does not agree with the advice given, reevaluate and advise the caller to follow up with PCP, Clinic, or ED.

H

Hoarseness

 Key Questions Name, Age, Onset, Contributing Factors, Medications, History

 Other Protocols to Consider Allergic Reaction (25); Breathing Problems (106); Cough (170); Croup (173); Hay Fever Problems (305); Hives (337); Foreign Body, Inhaled (271); Sore Throat (564).

Reminder: Document caller response to advice, home care instructions, and when to call back.

ASSESSMENT	ACTION

A. Sudden onset of hoarseness, and are any of the following present?

- Sore throat, drooling, and difficulty breathing
- Sensation of swelling tongue or throat
- Recent trauma to neck
- Speaking in short three-word sentences

YES "Seek emergency care now"

NO Go to B

B. Are any of the following present?

- Sudden onset of swelling in face
- Speaking in partial sentences

YES "Seek medical care within 2 to 4 hours"

NO Go to C

C. Are any of the following present?

- High fever and feels or looks ill
- Persistent hoarseness >1 week
- History of tobacco use, recent weight loss, and decreased appetite
- Dry skin or hair, increased sensitivity to cold, increased fatigue, or unexplained weight gain

YES "Seek medical care within 24 hours"

NO Go to D

D. Are any of the following present?

- Recent sore throat, cough, cold, or fever
- Frequent use of voice in work (such as teacher or singer)
- Heavy use of tobacco or alcohol
- Recently used voice more than usual (yelling, cheering, singing)
- Speaking in complete sentences

YES "Call back or call PCP for appointment if no improvement" and Follow **Home Care Instructions**

NO Follow **Home Care Instructions**

Home Care Instructions
Hoarseness

- Avoid tobacco or alcohol.
- Rest voice as much as possible.
- Drink plenty of fluids.
- Take your usual pain medication (aspirin, acetaminophen, ibuprofen) as tolerated for discomfort or fever. Do not give aspirin to a child. Avoid aspirin-like products if age <20 years. Avoid acetaminophen if liver disease is present. Avoid ibuprofen if kidney disease or stomach problems exist or in the case of pregnancy. Follow the directions on the label.
- Use honey or throat lozenges for throat discomfort or cough.

Additional Instructions

_____

_____

_____

Report the Following Problems to Your PCP/Clinic/ED

- Condition persists >1 week or worsens
- High fever and appears ill

Seek Emergency Care Immediately If Any of the Following Occur

- Sore throat, drooling, and difficulty breathing
- Sensation of swelling tongue or throat
- Speaking in short three-word sentences

If the caller agrees with the advice given, document the call and encourage the caller to call back or see PCP if the problem worsens. If the caller does not agree with the advice given, reevaluate and advise the caller to follow up with PCP, Clinic, or ED.

H

Hospice Problems

 Key Questions Name, Age, Onset, Terminal Condition, Verify Hospice Client, Medications, History

 Other Protocols to Consider Altered Mental Status (28); Breathing Problems (106); Dehydration (180); Depression (184); Feeding Tube Problems (247); Fever, Adult (250), Child (253).

Nurse Alert: Use this protocol only if under hospice care.

Reminder: Document caller response to advice, home care instructions, and when to call back.

ASSESSMENT	ACTION
A. Are any of the following present?	
• Severe uncontrolled pain unresponsive to pain-relieving measures • Unexpected death at home and no do-not-resuscitate (DNR) order	**YES** "Call ambulance" or "Seek emergency care now" **NO** Go to B
B. Are any of the following present?	
• Difficulty breathing, decreased level of consciousness, decreased or absent urine output, and family wishes to revoke plans for home death • No DNR order and family wants to care for the dying at home or is unsure what to do • Inability to take medications • New onset of restlessness, agitation, or confusion • Fever and symptoms of infection • Fever and antibiotic use recently stopped • Persistent discomfort after taking medication	**YES** "Contact PCP or hospice nurse immediately" **NO** Go to C

C. Are any of the following present?

- Caregiver anxious and having difficulty coping or unable to maintain pain control
- Planned death and DNR order in place
- Lethargy and possible overmedication

YES "Contact hospice nurse immediately"

NO Go to D

D. Are any of the following present?

- Depression
- Dehydration
- Lack of interest in eating
- Cracked lips and dry mouth
- High fever, unconsciousness, and respiratory changes

YES "Call back or call PCP/hospice nurse if no improvement" and Follow **Home Care Instructions**

NO Follow **Home Care Instructions**

H

Home Care Instructions
Hospice Problems

- Give pain and antianxiety medications as prescribed to ensure optimal comfort. Check pump to ensure proper functioning.
- Contact pastoral services or spiritual community leader.
- Remember that it is a normal part of the dying process to lose interest in food.
- Remember that dehydration helps the person to feel more comfortable when near death.
- Provide mouth and skin care as directed by nurse.
- Raise head of bed 45 degrees to help breathing.
- Open windows or use fans to increase circulation of air in the room.
- If oxygen is in use, check tubing and tank to ensure proper functioning.
- If fever and changes in breathing and consciousness are present, contact and inform those who have expressed a desire to be at the bedside at the time of death.
- Apply cool packs to armpit, groin, and back of the neck.
- Reposition to assist with breathing and comfort.
- If lethargic and overmedication is suspected, lower the dose unless pain, restlessness, or agitation recurs.
- If changing condition is worrisome to caregiver or caregiver has questions, call back.

Additional Instructions

Report the Following Problems to Your PCP/Hospice Nurse/ED

- Unable to take medications
- New onset of restlessness, agitation, or confusion
- Fever and symptoms of infection
- Fever and antibiotic use recently stopped
- Persistent discomfort after taking medication

Seek Emergency Care Immediately If Any of the Following Occur

- Severe uncontrolled pain unresponsive to pain-relieving measures
- Unexpected death at home and no DNR order

If the caller agrees with the advice given, document the call and encourage the caller to call back or see PCP if the problem worsens. If the caller does not agree with the advice given, reevaluate and advise the caller to follow up with PCP, Clinic, or ED.

Hypertension

Key Questions Name, Age, Onset, Known Hypertension, Last Elevated Blood Pressure Reading, Medications, History (If pregnant, see Pregnancy, Hypertension protocol)

Other Protocols to Consider Dizziness (199); Headache (308); Hypotension (352); Nosebleed (425); Pregnancy, Hypertension (471); Pregnancy Problems (481).

Nurse Alert: Use this protocol only if caller has questions about high blood pressure, has been diagnosed with hypertension, is taking medication for hypertension, or regularly takes blood pressure readings and is concerned about elevated reading.

Reminder: Document caller response to advice, home care instructions, and when to call back.

ASSESSMENT	ACTION
A. Is the following present?	
● Chest pain in addition to high blood pressure	**YES** Go to Chest Pain protocol (123)
	NO Go to B
B. Elevated blood pressure (diastolic >100 mm Hg), and are any of the following present?	
● History of thoracic or abdominal dissection	**YES** "Seek emergency care now"
● Severe headache, blurred vision, nausea, or vomiting	**NO** Go to C
● Drowsiness or confusion	
● Persistent numbness and tingling in hands and feet	
● Coughing up blood or blood-tinged sputum	
● Difficulty breathing	
● Persistent nosebleed unresponsive to home care measures	
● Diastolic blood pressure of >110 mm Hg	
● Severe weakness	
● Under medical care for blood pressure control, and persistent blood pressure >160/100 mm Hg	
● Dizziness or light-headedness	

H

C. Are any of the following present?

- Periods of dizziness after starting new blood pressure medication
- Intermittent nosebleed
- Blood pressure elevation and recent change in blood pressure medications
- Blood pressure elevation and taking OTC cold medications

YES "Seek medical care within 24 hours"

NO Go to D

D. Are any of the following present?

- Persistent blood pressure readings >140/90 mm Hg
- Recent increase in stress
- Increased use of alcohol
- Blood pressure elevation and missed a dose of medication

YES "Call back or call PCP for appointment if no improvement" and Follow **Home Care Instructions**

NO Follow **Home Care Instructions**

Home Care Instructions
Hypertension

- Measure blood pressure weekly if >140/90 mm Hg.
- Avoid smoking and alcohol consumption.
- Eat a well-balanced, low-fat, low-salt diet. If overweight, start a weight reduction program. Discontinue use of caffeine, nicotine, and licorice.
- Exercise regularly. Start with walking.
- Learn how to manage stress effectively. Read, exercise, take classes on stress reduction, meditate, do yoga.
- If taking blood pressure medication, avoid cold remedies with antihistamines and decongestants. Consult with PCP before taking such medications.
- Take blood pressure medication regularly. Do not skip doses. Do not stop or change medication without consulting PCP.
- When experiencing symptoms of high blood pressure, do not drive.

Additional Instructions

Report the Following Problems to Your PCP/Clinic/ED

- Periods of dizziness, constipation, impotence, or tongue swelling after starting new blood pressure medication
- Under medical care for blood pressure control and persistent elevated blood pressure >160/100 mm Hg
- Blood pressure >140/90 mm Hg consistently for >3 months

Seek Emergency Care Immediately If Blood Pressure Is Very High and Any of the Following Occur

- Severe headache or blurred vision
- Drowsiness or confusion
- Persistent numbness and tingling in hands and feet
- Coughing up blood or blood-tinged sputum
- Difficulty breathing
- Chest pain or heart palpitations
- Persistent nosebleed

H

If the caller agrees with the advice given, document the call and encourage the caller to call back or see PCP if the problem worsens. If the caller does not agree with the advice given, reevaluate and advise the caller to follow up with PCP, Clinic, or ED.

Hyperventilation

 Key Questions Name, Age, Onset, Cause, Medications, History, Associated Symptoms

 Other Protocols to Consider Anxiety (36); Breathing Problems (106); Chest Pain (123); Numbness and Tingling (431).

Reminder: Document caller response to advice, home care instructions, and when to call back.

ASSESSMENT	ACTION

A. Is chest pain present?

YES	See Chest Pain protocol (123)
NO	Go to B

B. In addition to breathing rapidly, are any of the following present?

- Blue lips or fingernails
- Unable to talk
- Must sit up to breathe

YES	See Breathing Problems protocol (106)
NO	Go to C

C. In addition to rapid breathing, are any of the following present?

- Severe pain
- High fever unresponsive to fever-reducing measures
- Abnormal drowsiness

YES	"Seek medical care within 2 to 4 hours"
NO	Go to D

D. In addition to rapid deep breathing, are any of the following present?

- Numbness and tingling around the face, mouth, fingers, or toes
- Weakness
- Feeling faint
- Twitching in the hands and feet
- Anxiety or emotional upset
- History or prior episodes of similar symptoms

YES	"Call back or call PCP for appointment if no improvement" and Follow **Home Care Instructions**
NO	Follow **Home Care Instructions**

Home Care Instructions
Hyperventilation

- Sit down and focus on slowing breathing, one breath every 5 seconds.
- Cover mouth and nose with a paper bag and breathe in and out 10 times.
- If no improvement, continue breathing in the bag for 5 to 15 minutes.
- Breathe without the bag for a few minutes.
- Repeat breathing with and without the bag until condition improves.

Additional Instructions

Report the Following Problems to Your PCP/Clinic/ED

- No improvement or condition worsens
- Sudden fever occurs during an attack
- Frequent attacks

Seek Emergency Care Immediately If Any of the Following Occur

- Fainting
- Seizure
- Blue lips or fingernails
- Chest pain

If the caller agrees with the advice given, document the call and encourage the caller to call back or see PCP if the problem worsens. If the caller does not agree with the advice given, reevaluate and advise the caller to follow up with PCP, Clinic, or ED.

H

Hypotension

 Key Questions Name, Age, Onset, Last Systolic Blood Pressure Reading, Medications, History

 Other Protocols to Consider Abdominal Pain, Adult (9), Child (13); Chest Pain (123); Cold Exposure Problems (143); Confusion (150); Dizziness (199); Fainting (237); Heart Rate Problems (320); Weakness (649).

> *Nurse Alert:* Use this protocol only if caller has questions about low blood pressure, regularly takes blood pressure readings and is concerned about low blood pressure reading, or known low blood pressure reading and symptoms of concern.

Reminder: Document caller response to advice, home care instructions, and when to call back.

ASSESSMENT	ACTION

A. In addition to low blood pressure, is chest pain present?

YES	Go to Chest Pain protocol
NO	Go to B

B. Systolic pressure <90 mm Hg, sudden onset, and are any of the following present?

- Cool, pale, moist skin
- Drowsiness or confusion
- Hot dry skin and rapid pulse
- Shoulder or abdominal pain
- Recent injury, fall, or blunt force
- Rapid pulse >120 bpm
- Fainting
- Fever, rapid pulse, hypotension

YES	"Call ambulance" or "Seek emergency care now"
NO	Go to C

C. Are any of the following present?

- Feeling faint when sitting or rising from seated position
- Persistent bleeding

 "Seek medical care within 2 to 4 hours"

NO Go to D

D. Are any of the following present?

- Periods of dizziness after starting new blood pressure medication
- While taking blood pressure medication or diuretics, hypotension and symptoms persist
- Pregnancy

 "Seek medical care within 24 hours"

NO Go to E

E. Are any of the following present?

- Persistent systolic blood pressure readings <90 mm Hg and no other symptoms
- Caller concerned about low blood pressure and no other symptoms

YES "Call back or call PCP for appointment if no improvement" and Follow **Home Care Instructions**

NO Follow **Home Care Instructions**

H

Home Care Instructions
Hypotension

- Change positions slowly when rising to a sitting or standing position.
- Take prescribed medications as directed.
- Avoid sudden significant weight loss while dieting or use of diuretics in weight control.
- If taking blood pressure medication, avoid cold remedies with antihistamines and decongestants. Consult with PCP before taking such medications.
- Take blood pressure medication regularly and do not skip doses.

Additional Instructions

Report the Following Problems to Your PCP/Clinic/ED

- Periods of dizziness after starting new blood pressure medication
- Under medical care for blood pressure control and systolic persistent blood pressure <90 mm Hg
- Repeated fainting episodes

Seek Emergency Care Immediately If Any of the Following Occur

- Cool, pale, moist skin
- Drowsiness or confusion
- Hot dry skin and rapid pulse
- Chest or abdominal pain
- Rapid pulse >120 bpm
- Fever, hypotension, or rapid pulse
- Fainting

If the caller agrees with the advice given, document the call and encourage the caller to call back or see PCP if the problem worsens. If the caller does not agree with the advice given, reevaluate and advise the caller to follow up with PCP, Clinic, or ED.

Immunization, Tetanus

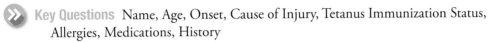

>> **Key Questions** Name, Age, Onset, Cause of Injury, Tetanus Immunization Status, Allergies, Medications, History

>> **Other Protocols to Consider** Allergic Reaction (25); Fever, Adult (250), Child (253); Immunization Reactions (358); Laceration (395); Puncture Wound (496).

> *Nurse Alert:* Use this protocol if concerns about a recent tetanus immunization reaction or questions about immunization status and recent injury. If the puncture or wound is dirty, another immunization is recommended within 5 years. Wounds are defined as clean or dirty. A wound is considered dirty if it is contaminated with dirt, feces, saliva, or soil; puncture wounds; avulsions; caused by flying or crushing objects, animal bites, burns, or frostbite.

Reminder: Document caller response to advice, home care instructions, and when to call back.

ASSESSMENT	ACTION
A. After tetanus immunization, are any of the following present?	
• Difficulty breathing, speaking, or swallowing • Sudden swelling in back of throat or tongue • Chest pain • Fainting • Confusion, agitation, or decreased level of consciousness (LOC) • Palpitations	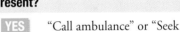 "Call ambulance" or "Seek emergency care now" Go to B
B. After tetanus immunization, are any of the following present?	
• Rash or flushing • Generalized hives	"Seek medical care within 2 to 4 hours" Go to C

C. Sustained injury within 48 hours, and are any of the following present?

- No prior tetanus immunization
- >10 years since last immunization
- Puncture or dirty wound and >5 years since last tetanus immunization
- Fewer than four tetanus immunizations since birth
- Fever, pain, redness, swelling at injection site >48 hours after injection

 YES   "Seek medical care within 24 hours"

NO   Go to D

D. Is the following present?

- Fever, pain, redness, swelling at DT injection site <48 hours after injection

YES   "Call back or call PCP for appointment if no improvement" and Follow **Home Care Instructions**

NO   Follow **Home Care Instructions**

Home Care Instructions
Immunization, Tetanus

- Apply ice pack to injection site for 20 minutes every 2 hours throughout a 24-hour period to help reduce swelling and discomfort. Place a cloth barrier between ice and skin.
- Take your usual pain medication (aspirin, acetaminophen, ibuprofen) if needed for fever or discomfort. Do not give aspirin to a child. Avoid aspirin-like products if age <20 years. Avoid acetaminophen if liver disease is present. Avoid ibuprofen if kidney disease or stomach problems exist or in the case of pregnancy. Follow the directions on the label.
- Record date of booster. A booster provides protection for 10 years. If the puncture or wound is dirty, another immunization is recommended within 5 years.
- Tetanus immunization should be given within 72 hours of injury.
- Monitor injection site for signs of infection.
- Provide reassurance; pain and swelling are normal reactions for first 48 hours.

Additional Instructions

Report the Following Problems to Your PCP/Clinic/ED

- Child cries >3 hours after injection
- Redness, swelling, pain, or fever occurs >48 hours after injection

Seek Emergency Care Immediately If Any of the Following Occur

- Difficulty breathing, speaking, or swallowing
- Sudden swelling in back of throat or tongue
- Chest pain or fainting
- Palpitations
- Confusion, agitation, or decreased LOC

If the caller agrees with the advice given, document the call and encourage the caller to call back or see PCP if the problem worsens. If the caller does not agree with the advice given, reevaluate and advise the caller to follow up with PCP, Clinic, or ED.

Immunization Reactions

 Key Questions Name, Age, Onset, Cause, Allergies, Medications, History, Date and Type of Immunization

 Other Protocols to Consider Allergic Reaction (25); Fever, Adult (250), Child (253); Immunization, Tetanus (355).

> *Nurse Alert:* Use this protocol if concerns about a recent immunization and possible reaction or questions about immunization reactions. Serious reactions are rare but do occur.
>
> - Minor reaction: pain or swelling at the site of injection (usually within 2 days); fever, headache, or muscle aches (usually occur within 7 days).
> - Severe reaction: anaphylaxis; difficulty breathing; feeling faint; swelling of the tongue, throat, or lips; hives; wheezing or coughing; or a feeling of impending doom (can occur within seconds to an hour after exposure). The sooner the symptoms occur after exposure to the antigen, the more severe the anaphylaxis.
> - VAERS—Vaccine Adverse Event Reporting System is a national program for monitoring vaccine safety. Call for reporting forms: 1-800-822-7967, or locate on the Internet at http://www.vaers.hhs.gov
> - National Vaccine Injury Compensation Program provides compensation to individuals whose injuries may have been caused by certain vaccines. Call 1-800-338-2382.
> - National Immunization Hotline provides vaccine information. Call 1-800-232-2522.
> - Vaccine website information: www.cdc.gov/vaccines

Reminder: Document caller response to advice, home care instructions, and when to call back.

ASSESSMENT	ACTION
A. After an immunization, are any of the following present?	
- Difficulty breathing or speaking - Sudden swelling in back of throat - Chest pain or fainting - Palpitations - Confusion, agitation, or decreased level of consciousness	**YES** "Call ambulance" or "Seek emergency care now" **NO** Go to B

B. Are any of the following present?

- Rash or flushing
- Hives
- Temperature >105°F (40.6°C)

 "Seek medical care within 2 to 4 hours"

NO Go to C

C. Are any of the following present?

- Persistent fever and rash >24 hours 7 to 10 days after measles immunization
- Child cries constantly >3 hours after immunization
- Increasing redness, swelling, pain, fever >48 hours after immunization

 "Seek medical care within 24 hours"

NO Go to D

D. Are any of the following present?

- Temperature >101°F to 103°F (38.3°C to 39.4°C) and pink rash 7 to 10 days after measles vaccine
- Fever, pain, redness, or swelling at DPT injection site
- Swollen glands in neck after mumps immunization
- Rash or swollen glands 7 to 14 days after rubella immunization and painful joints 2 to 4 weeks afterward

YES "Call back or call PCP for appointment if no improvement" and Follow **Home Care Instructions**

NO Follow **Home Care Instructions**

I

Home Care Instructions
Immunization Reactions

- Take usual pain medication (aspirin, acetaminophen, ibuprofen) for fever. Do not give aspirin to a child. Avoid aspirin-like products if age <20 years. Avoid acetaminophen if liver disease is present. Avoid ibuprofen if kidney disease or stomach problems exist or in the case of pregnancy. Follow the directions on the label.
- Women should avoid pregnancy for 4 weeks after rubella immunization.
- Discuss with your PCP the safety of immunizations if the child is ill or taking immune suppressors or cortisone.
- Expect side effects to include fever, fussiness, and redness at injection site.

Additional Instructions

 Report the Following Problems to Your PCP/Clinic/ED

- Persistent fever and rash >3 days after measles immunization
- Child cries constantly >3 hours after immunization
- Temperature >105°F (40.5°C)
- Redness, swelling, pain, fever >48 hours

 Seek Emergency Care Immediately If Any of the Following Occur

- Difficulty breathing or speaking
- Sudden swelling in back of throat
- Chest pain or fainting
- Confusion, agitation, or decreased level of consciousness

If the caller agrees with the advice given, document the call and encourage the caller to call back or see PCP if the problem worsens. If the caller does not agree with the advice given, reevaluate and advise the caller to follow up with PCP, Clinic, or ED.

Impetigo

 Key Questions Name, Age, Onset, Known Diagnosis or Exposure to Impetigo, Sores with Honey-Colored Crusts, Medications, History

 Other Protocols to Consider Rash, Adult (500), Child (505); Skin Lesions (556).

> *Nurse Alert:* Use this protocol only if new skin lesions, known diagnosis of impetigo, questions about impetigo, or exposure to person with known impetigo lesions.

Reminder: Document caller response to advice, home care instructions, and when to call back.

ASSESSMENT	ACTION
A. Are any of the following present?	
• Red or cola-colored urine • Bright red and tender face • Flank pain • Very rapid spread • Abdominal swelling	**YES** "Seek emergency care now" **NO** Go to B
B. Are any of the following present?	
• Blister or sore >1 inch across • Red streak extends from sore • History of diabetes, steroid therapy, cancer, HIV, or other immunosuppression	**YES** "Seek medical care within 2 to 4 hours" **NO** Go to C
C. Are any of the following present?	
• Child younger than 1 year • Two or more household members have sores • More than two sores • Sores in nostril, ear canal, or around mouth • Swollen nodes in area near sores • Temperature >100°F (37.8°C) or sore throat • Sores increase in number after >2 days of treatment • Red, yellow, brown, green, or white drainage from sore	**YES** "Seek medical care within 24 hours" **NO** Go to D

I

361

D. Are any of the following present?

- Sore <1 inch across
- Small red bump changed to a cloudy blister or pimple and then a sore with a yellow-brown scab

YES "Call back or call PCP for appointment if no improvement" and Follow **Home Care Instructions**

NO Follow **Home Care Instructions**

Home Care Instructions
Impetigo

- To remove scabs, apply a cloth soaked in a solution of bleach and water to the scab (1 tbsp bleach in 1 quart of water). Rub scab gently; do not scrub.
- Wash sores with antibacterial soap.
- Apply antibiotic (Mycitracin, Neosporin, Polysporin) ointment 3 times a day after sores are washed. Follow instructions on the label.
- Avoid touching, scratching, or picking at sores to help prevent spreading and infection.
- Wash hands after touching sores.
- Keep fingernails short, and wash hands frequently with antibacterial soap.
- Do not share towels with other family members. Impetigo is highly contagious and can spread easily to other household members.
- Keep child out of school until he/she has taken antibiotics for >24 hours, or for mild infections, wash well with soap and water and cover the scabs with antibiotic ointment and a bandage before sending the child to school or day care.

Additional Instructions

Report the Following Problems to Your PCP/Clinic/ED

- Blister or sore >1 inch across
- Red streak extends from sore
- Temperature >100°F (37.8°C) or sore throat
- Other family members experience similar symptoms
- Sores increase in number after 2 days of home treatment
- No improvement after 1 week of treatment

Seek Emergency Care Immediately If Any of the Following Occur

- Red or colored urine
- Bright red and tender face
- Flank pain
- Abdominal swelling

If the caller agrees with the advice given, document the call and encourage the caller to call back or see PCP if the problem worsens. If the caller does not agree with the advice given, reevaluate and advise the caller to follow up with PCP, Clinic, or ED.

Incontinence, Stool

 Key Questions Name, Age, Onset, Allergies, Medications, History

 Other Protocols to Consider Abdominal Pain, Adult (9), Child (13); Constipation (160); Diarrhea, Adult (192), Child (195); Neurologic Symptoms (418);Rectal Bleeding (510); Rectal Problems (513); Stroke, Suspected (576); Stools, Abnormal (573).

Reminder: Document caller response to advice, home care instructions, and when to call back.

ASSESSMENT	ACTION
A. Are any of the following present?	
• Incontinence of urine and stool after a seizure, faint, or loss of consciousness	**YES** "Call ambulance"
• Sudden loss of bowel control and slurred speech, muscle weakness, blurred or double vision, or decreased level of consciousness	**NO** Go to B
B. Are any of the following present?	
• Recent back injury, trauma, or fall, severe pain, and several episodes of incontinence	**YES** "Seek emergency care now"
• Black or bloody stool with clots	**NO** Go to C
C. Are any of the following present?	
• Recent history of childbirth, vaginal or rectal surgery, hemorrhoids, or anal fistula or fissure	**YES** "Seek medical care within 24 hours"
• Abdominal pain	**NO** Go to D
• Several incontinent episodes	
D. Are any of the following present?	
• Lump felt inside anal opening	**YES** "Call back or call PCP for appointment if no improvement" and Follow **Home Care Instructions**
• Sudden onset of diarrhea and unable to make it to the toilet	
• Frequent involuntary seepage of stool and recent history of no bowel movements or several hard stools	**NO** Follow **Home Care Instructions**
• Recurrence of stool incontinence in child previously toilet-trained	

Home Care Instructions
Incontinence, Stool

- Avoid constipation. Increase fiber, bulk, and fluids (fresh fruit, vegetables, whole grains, cereals, and brown rice). Try Metamucil to add bulk. Drink 6 to 8 glasses of water daily. Exercise regularly.
- In a child previously toilet-trained:
  - Allow child to determine time for toileting. Do not force child to sit on toilet.
  - Provide praise when toilet is used.
  - Discuss with child a reward for staying clean all day.
  - If child is soiled, have the child clean self and change clothes (if old enough).
  - Do not scold or punish for accidents or allow other siblings to tease the child.
- If an elderly or disabled adult is having difficulty making it to the toilet in time, do not show anger. Discuss ways to identify warning signs and get to the bathroom as soon as signs occur.
- Consider renting or buying a portable toilet for use when sudden diarrhea attacks occur.
- Review diet and medications, such as use of laxatives, new medications, prune juice, or castor oil.

Additional Instructions

Report the Following Problems to Your PCP/Clinic/ED

- Bloody stool
- Abdominal pain
- Several incontinent episodes
- No improvement or condition worsens

If the caller agrees with the advice given, document the call and encourage the caller to call back or see PCP if the problem worsens. If the caller does not agree with the advice given, reevaluate and advise the caller to follow up with PCP, Clinic, or ED.

I

Incontinence, Urine

 Key Questions Name, Age, Onset, Medications, History

 Other Protocols to Consider Bed-Wetting (70); Pregnancy Problems (481); Seizure (531); Seizure, Febrile (533); Stroke, Suspected (576); Urinary Catheter/Nephrostomy Tube Problems (621); Urination, Difficult (624); Urination, Excessive (626); Urination, Painful (628).

Reminder: Document caller response to advice, home care instructions, and when to call back.

ASSESSMENT	ACTION
A. Are any of the following present?	
• History of recent back injury or weakness in legs • Sudden inability to control urination • Postseizure faintness or loss of consciousness	**YES** "Seek emergency care now" **NO** Go to B
B. Are any of the following present?	
• Signs of urinary tract infection: painful urination, frequency, or urgency • Blood in urine • Abdominal pain	**YES** "Seek medical care within 24 hours" **NO** Go to C
C. Are any of the following present?	
• Leakage of urine when coughing, sneezing, lifting, straining, laughing, or running • Pregnancy • Obesity • Sensation of heaviness in genitals • Sudden urge to urinate and inability to control urine before making it to the toilet • Difficulty starting urination • Unable to tolerate the problem any longer	**YES** "Call back or call PCP for appointment if no improvement" and Follow **Home Care Instructions** **NO** Follow **Home Care Instructions**

Home Care Instructions
Incontinence, Urine

- Practice exercises to strengthen and tighten muscles supporting the bladder and reproductive organs.
  - Tighten the muscles to stop the flow of urine midstream. Hold for a count of six, then release urine for a count of six. Stop and hold the flow of urine and count to six. Release remaining urine.
  - Practice tightening and releasing the muscles that control urine and the muscles around the anus several times a day while sitting, standing, and walking.
- Drink plenty of fluids, including cranberry juice, to help avoid urinary tract infections.
- Wear a pad or absorbent underpants.
- Observe incidence and frequency of incontinence. Avoid medications, foods, or drinks (such as caffeine or alcohol) that seem to cause or worsen incontinence.

Additional Instructions

Report the Following Problems to Your PCP/Clinic/ED

- Condition persists or worsens after practicing exercises for 3 months
- Unable to tolerate the problem any longer
- Signs of urinary tract infection: painful urination, frequency, or urgency
- Blood in urine
- Sudden inability to control urination
- Abdominal pain

If the caller agrees with the advice given, document the call and encourage the caller to call back or see PCP if the problem worsens. If the caller does not agree with the advice given, reevaluate and advise the caller to follow up with PCP, Clinic, or ED.

I

Indigestion

 Key Questions Name, Age, Onset, Symptoms Usually Occur Soon After Eating, Allergies, Medications, History

 Other Protocols to Consider Abdominal Pain, Adult (9), Child (13); Abdominal Swelling (16); Chest Pain (123); Diarrhea, Adult (192), Child (195); Gas/Belching (287); Gas/Flatulence (289); Heartburn (316); Rectal Bleeding (510); Vomiting, Adult (642), Child (645); Swallowing Difficulty (591).

Nurse Alert: Indigestion and heartburn can mimic chest pain. There are many conditions that cause chest pain; some can be potentially life-threatening. Err on the side of caution when triaging callers with symptoms like chest pain. Chest Pain: Causes and Characteristics, Appendix S (712) is provided to help the nurse gain a better understanding of the many conditions causing chest pain. It is NOT to be used to try and diagnose a caller's condition.

Reminder: Document caller response to advice, home care instructions, and when to call back.

ASSESSMENT	ACTION

A. Is there a burning or heavy sensation in the chest, and are any of the following present?

- Shortness of breath
- Cool moist skin
- Pain in the neck, jaw, shoulders, back, or arms
- Blue or gray face, lips, earlobes, or fingernails
- History of cardiac disease or diabetes
- Pain occurs with exertion
- Feeling of impending doom
- Chest pain and palpitations

YES "Call ambulance"

NO Go to B

B. Are any of the following present?

- Belching blood
- Vomiting blood or dark coffee grounds–like emesis
- Black tarry stool
- Severe abdominal pain

YES "Seek emergency care now"

NO Go to C

C. Are any of the following present?

- Discomfort persists after taking medication
- Condition worsening, requires more frequent use of medication
- Frequent vomiting, weight loss, or decreased appetite
- Difficult or painful swallowing

 "Seek medical care within 24 hours"

 Go to D

D. Are any of the following present?

- Pain increased with use of aspirin, ibuprofen, or steroids
- Increased pain when bending, exercising, or lying down soon after eating
- Frequent belching or gas
- Acid taste in mouth
- Bloated or full feeling
- Recent increase in stress
- Symptoms appear soon after eating or drinking
- Mild nausea or diarrhea after eating
- Previously diagnosed with reflux esophagitis
- Recently started new medication

 "Call back or call PCP for appointment if no improvement" and Follow **Home Care Instructions**

 Follow **Home Care Instructions**

I

Home Care Instructions
Indigestion

- Try OTC medications (Maalox, Mylanta, Riopan, Tums, Pepcid, Prilosec) and follow instructions on the label. Liquids often provide faster relief than tablets. Consult with PCP if taking other prescription medications.
- Do not give Pepto-Bismol to a child.
- Avoid eating 2 to 3 hours before bed.
- Do not lie down for 2 to 3 hours after eating or bend over or exercise soon after eating.
- Elevate head of bed 4 to 6 inches using blocks or bricks.
- Eat small, frequent meals.
- Avoid spicy foods, alcohol, coffee, smoking, chocolate, citrus fruits, tomatoes, vinegar, fatty foods, and carbonated beverages.
- If aspirin or ibuprofen worsens the problem, try acetaminophen. Do not give aspirin to a child. Avoid aspirin-like products if age <20 years. Avoid acetaminophen if liver disease is present. Avoid ibuprofen if kidney disease or stomach problems exist or in the case of pregnancy. Follow the directions on the label.
- Avoid tight-fitting clothing, such as girdles, belts, control-top panty hose, or pants or skirts with a tight waistband.
- Take time to eat and drink, thoroughly chewing food.
- Avoid chewing gum or other activities that result in swallowing air.
- Avoid foods and drinks known to cause stomach upset and heartburn. Try taking OTC medications (Pepcid AC, Pepto-Bismol, or Prilosec) before eating foods causing symptoms. Follow instructions on the label.
- Try Gas-X for belching and follow instructions on the label.
- Sip a tonic made of 4 ounces ginger ale, 1 tsp grated ginger root, 1 tsp honey to soothe an upset stomach.
- Avoid straining during bowel movements, urinating, and lifting.

Additional Instructions

Report the Following Problems to Your PCP/Clinic/ED

- Persistent discomfort unresponsive to home care measures after >3 days or condition worsens
- No relief from antacids
- Difficult or painful swallowing

Seek Emergency Care Immediately If Persistent Discomfort and Any of the Following Occur

- Shortness of breath
- Cool moist skin
- Pain in the neck, jaw, shoulders, back, or arms
- Blue or gray face, lips, earlobes, or fingernails
- Belching or vomiting blood or dark coffee grounds–like emesis
- Severe abdominal pain
- Chest pain
- Pain occurs with exertion

If the caller agrees with the advice given, document the call and encourage the caller to call back or see PCP if the problem worsens. If the caller does not agree with the advice given, reevaluate and advise the caller to follow up with PCP, Clinic, or ED.

Influenza

 Key Questions Name, Age, Onset, Symptoms, Known Exposure or Community Outbreak, Medications, History

 Other Protocols to Consider Avian Influenza ("Bird Flu") (55); Common Cold Symptoms (146); Congestion (153); Cough (170); Fever, Adult (250), Child (253); Headache (308); Swine Flu (H1N1 Virus) Exposure (600); Sore Throat (564); West Nile Virus (653).

Nurse Alert: Use this protocol if exposure to influenza is known or suspected, there is a community outbreak, or previously diagnosed with influenza.

Reminder: Document caller response to advice, home care instructions, and when to call back.

ASSESSMENT	ACTION

A. Are any of the following present?

- Altered mental status
- Difficulty breathing for reasons other than congestion
- Fever >104.9°F (40.5°C)
- Flat purple or dark red spots on face or trunk and stiff or painful neck
- Severe headache
- Skin or lips turning blue
- New onset of drooling or unable to swallow
- Age <6 weeks

YES "Seek emergency care now"

NO Go to B

B. Are any of the following present?

- Stiff or painful neck
- Fever >103.1°F (39.5°C)
- Fever, and child or older adult appears very ill, lethargic, or very irritable
- Signs of dehydration

YES "Seek medical care immediately"

NO Go to C

C. Are any of the following present?

- Known exposure and any of the following: fatigue, fever <103.1°F (39.5°C), dry cough, sore throat, GI symptoms, runny nose or congestion, muscle aches
- History of CHF, immunosuppression, 6 weeks to 23 months of age, age >65 years, pregnancy, long-term care resident, asthma, COPD, metabolic disorders

YES   "Seek medical care within 24 hours"

NO   Go to D

D. Are any of the following present?

- Mild symptoms
- No symptoms but parent or person concerned

YES   "Call back or call PCP for appointment if no improvement" and Follow **Home Care Instructions**

NO   Follow **Home Care Instructions**

Home Care Instructions
Influenza

- Wash hands frequently with soap and water or alcohol-based hand rubs.
- Reinforce that influenza is highly contagious. Maintain good respiratory etiquette; cover mouth and nose with a tissue when coughing or sneezing.
- Avoid contact with sick individuals.
- If sick, avoid contact with other people. If coughing and sneezing, wear a surgical mask during close contact with others to prevent the spread of droplets. Change the mask if it becomes soiled or moist.
- Get plenty of rest and drink plenty of fluids.
- Do not give aspirin to a child. Avoid aspirin-like products if age <20 years. Avoid acetaminophen if liver disease is present. Avoid ibuprofen if kidney disease or stomach problems exist or in the case of pregnancy. Follow the directions on the label.
- Give antivirals within 48 hours of symptom onset.

Additional Instructions

Report the Following Problems to Your PCP/Clinic/ED

- Stiff or painful neck
- Fever >103.1°F (39.5°C)
- Fever, and child or older adult appears very ill, lethargic, or very irritable
- Signs of dehydration

Seek Emergency Care If Any of the Following Occur

- Altered mental status
- Difficulty breathing
- Fever >104.9°F (40.5°C)
- Flat purple or dark red spots on face or trunk and stiff or painful neck
- Severe headache
- Skin or lips turning blue
- New onset of drooling or unable to swallow

If the caller agrees with the advice given, document the call and encourage the caller to call back or see PCP if the problem worsens. If the caller does not agree with the advice given, reevaluate and advise the caller to follow up with PCP, Clinic, or ED.

Insomnia

 Key Questions Name, Age, Onset, Cause, Allergies, Medications, History

 Other Protocols to Consider Alcohol Problems (21); Anxiety (36); Depression (184); Heartburn (316); Substance Abuse, Use, or Exposure (582); Suicide Attempt, Threat (585).

Reminder: Document caller response to advice, home care instructions, and when to call back.

ASSESSMENT	ACTION

A. Is the following present?

- Suicidal ideation

YES "Seek emergency care now"

NO Go to B

B. Are any of the following present?

- Persistent pain, itching, coughing, or fever that interferes with sleep and is unresponsive to home care measures
- Persistent depression, anxiety, or stress

YES "Seek medical care within 24 hours"

NO Go to C

C. Are any of the following present?

- Persistent difficulty sleeping >7 days
- Consistently unable to sleep >2 to 3 hours
- Requesting medication for sleep
- Urinary or bowel problems that frequently interrupt sleep
- Problem interferes with work, school, or other daily activity
- Ingestion of caffeine products
- Intermittent episodes lasting 3 to 5 days
- Recent withdrawal from drugs or alcohol
- Prescribed sleep medication ineffective
- Taking a new medication
- Ingestion of OTC products
- Feeling overwhelmed

YES "Call back or call PCP for appointment if no improvement" and Follow **Home Care Instructions**

NO Follow **Home Care Instructions**

Home Care Instructions
Insomnia

- Increase daily exercise. Avoid strenuous exercise 2 to 3 hours before bedtime. Do gentle stretching exercises for 10 minutes before retiring.
- Read non–work-related materials or listen to soothing music at bedtime.
- Avoid caffeine and other stimulants 11 hours before bedtime.
- Take a warm bath or shower 2 hours before retiring.
- Drink warm milk before bed.
- Drink 8 ounces of orange juice before bedtime if alcoholic beverages have been consumed earlier; this helps to speed the breakdown of alcohol and reduces reawakening after a few hours of sleep.
- Try relaxation techniques, such as deep breathing exercises or visualizing flower-filled meadows.
- Identify stress factors and try to reduce them. If awakening prompts worry about things to be done, devise a plan of action, list the items, and try to go back to sleep.
- Avoid eating 3 hours before bedtime. Sip 1 tbsp of apple cider vinegar diluted with water or juice 30 minutes after dinner to help speed gastric flow through the stomach and reduce gastric reflux.
- If difficulty sleeping is due to gastric reflux, sleep lying on the left side as tolerated to help speed stomach emptying and prevent reflux into the esophagus.
- If stress, anxiety, or depression interferes with sleep, seek help from a local counseling center or mental health services.
- Consider taking Benadryl or melatonin on a short-term basis. Follow the instructions on the label.
- If taking supplements, choose energizing supplements like B-complex vitamins in the morning and soothing minerals such as calcium and magnesium at night.
- Plug in a red, blue, or green nightlight to avoid turning on bright lights to use the restroom at night.
- Keep the bedroom dark, cool, and quiet. Use a fan or other appliance to block noise.
- Wear loose-fitting nightclothes.
- Call back immediately if feeling overwhelmed.

Additional Instructions

Report the Following Problems to Your PCP/Clinic/ED

- No improvement with home care measures or problem worsens
- Problem interferes with work, school, or other daily activity
- Feeling overwhelmed

Seek Emergency Care Immediately If the Following Occurs

- Suicidal ideation

If the caller agrees with the advice given, document the call and encourage the caller to call back or see PCP if the problem worsens. If the caller does not agree with the advice given, reevaluate and advise the caller to follow up with PCP, Clinic, or ED.

Intravenous Therapy Problems

>> **Key Questions** Name, Age, Onset, Cause, Location and Type of Intravenous (IV), Length of Time in Place, Medications, History

>> **Other Protocols to Consider** Wound Healing and Infection (664).

> *Nurse Alert:* Use this protocol for questions or problems with an existing IV.

Reminder: Document caller response to advice, home care instructions, and when to call back.

ASSESSMENT	ACTION
A. Are any of the following present?	
• IV site painful and antineoplastic agents are infusing • Catheter tip possibly broken or sheared • Obvious central line dislodgement • Central line and sudden onset of shortness of breath or chest pain	**YES** "Call ambulance" or "Seek emergency care now" Stop the infusion by clamping the tubing, and apply ice pack to the site **NO** Go to B
B. Are any of the following present?	
• Inability to flush central line after home care advice • Persistent fever unresponsive to home care measures • Redness, swelling, pain, red streaks, and warmth at IV insertion site • Swelling at central line insertion site	**YES** "Seek medical care within 2 to 4 hours" and See **Home Care Instructions** **NO** Go to C
C. Are any of the following present?	
• IV will not flush, and there are no tubing or clamp problems • IV site cold to touch or swollen and painful • IV running slowly or not running • No blood return when tubing is pinched • Blood backed up in tubing	**YES** "Seek medical care within 24 hours" and Follow **Home Care Instructions** **NO** Go to D

378

D. Are any of the following present?

- Painful IV site and no swelling or signs of infection or infiltration
- IV leaking

YES "Call back or call PCP for appointment if no improvement" and Follow **Home Care Instructions**

NO Follow **Home Care Instructions**

I

Home Care Instructions
Intravenous Therapy Problems

- Do not wear a watch or other restrictive jewelry above the IV site.
- Do not wear clothing that fits tightly above the IV site.
- Central line problems:
  - Check tubing for kinks and clamps.
  - Change positions of body or arm.
  - Raise bag if not on a pump.
  - Check pump to make sure it is functioning properly.
  - If instruction in flushing has been received, flush the line slowly. If the line flushes easily, flush it more forcibly with 10 mL normal saline, then restart the infusion.
  - If line is broken externally, clamp the tube and secure it with a rubber band to prevent backflow and clotting, and contact the PCP for repair.
- IV problems:
  - If IV is running sluggishly or not at all and site is cool to the touch, clamp the tubing.
  - If there is no swelling or pain at the site, check the tubing, pump, and clamp for problems. Change position of the extremity or body. Raise bag if it is not on a pump.
  - Check pump for proper functioning. Is pump connected to electrical source (plugged in)?
  - If instruction in flushing has been received, flush the line with 3 mL normal saline.
  - If no signs of infection or infiltration, run the IV more slowly and apply cold packs to the insertion site. Check the site every 10 minutes for swelling, redness, or pain.
  - If IV is leaking, dry the area and recheck for leaks. Tighten all connections, replace the cap, change and prime the tubing (if instruction has been received in changing the tubing), and restart the infusion.
  - If IV is dislodged or has pulled out, apply pressure at the bleeding site and contact PCP for a restart.
  - If leaking persists after home care measures, contact the PCP for a restart.

Report the Following Problems to Your PCP/Clinic/ED

- Problem persists after home care measures taken
- Signs of infiltration (site cool to touch, swelling, redness, painful)
- Signs of infection (site warm to touch, swelling, redness, pain, streaks)
- Persistent discomfort

Seek Emergency Care Immediately If Any of the Following Occur

- IV site painful, and antineoplastic agents are infusing
- Catheter tip possibly broken or sheared
- Obvious central line dislodgement
- Central line and sudden onset of chest pain or shortness of breath

If the caller agrees with the advice given, document the call and encourage the caller to call back or see PCP if the problem worsens. If the caller does not agree with the advice given, reevaluate and advise the caller to follow up with PCP, Clinic, or ED.

Itching

 Key Questions Name, Age, Onset, Medications, History, Associated Symptoms

 Other Protocols to Consider Allergic Reaction (25); Bedbug Exposure or Concerns (67); Chickenpox (129); Genital Problems, Male (294); Hemorrhoids (327); Lice (401); Pinworms (452); Rash, Adult (500), Child (505); Rubella (German Measles) (520); Rubeola (Measles) (523); Vaginal Discharge/Pain/Itching (636); Wound Healing and Infection (664).

Reminder: Document caller response to advice, home care instructions, and when to call back.

ASSESSMENT	ACTION

A. Is the following present?

- Severe itching in several areas of the body, generalized hives, difficulty breathing, or swelling in the face, mouth, or throat

YES "Seek emergency care now"

NO Go to B

B. Are any of the following present?

- Generalized itching, or yellow skin and eyes
- Itching rash started after taking a new medication
- Intense itching, particularly at night; red dots in folds of skin; and other household members have similar symptoms
- Persistent itching interferes with activity
- Itching scalp and bald spots
- Persistent itchy rash and recent exposure to poison oak or ivy and unresponsive to home care measures

YES "Seek medical care within 24 hours"

NO Go to C

C. Are any of the following present?

- Multiple insect bites
- Itching around anus, vagina, or genitals
- Itching scalp or pubic area, and white round spots along hair shaft will not detach
- Itching hands that are frequently exposed to moisture or chemicals
- Itching after wearing new clothing
- New-onset itchy rash and recent exposure to poison oak or ivy

YES "Call back or call PCP for appointment if no improvement" and Follow **Home Care Instructions**

NO Follow **Home Care Instructions**

I

Home Care Instructions
Itching

- Apply cool compress to affected area. Soak cloth in ice water.
- Soak in baking soda or oatmeal bath or Aveeno Bath, make an oatmeal sponge using a cotton cloth and cooked oatmeal, or apply baking soda paste mixed with white vinegar.
- Apply Caladryl lotion or Domeboro solution to insect bites and poison oak or ivy rashes. Follow instructions on the label.
- Itching around the anus may be caused by hemorrhoids or pinworms. See Hemorrhoids or Pinworms protocol, as appropriate.
- Apply OTC NIX Creme Rinse or Rid treatments for lice. Follow instructions on the label. See Lice protocol.
- If sensitivity to clothing exists, wash clothes before wearing and rinse twice. Wear cotton clothing. Avoid wool and synthetic clothing next to skin.
- Take OTC antihistamines (Benadryl, Chlor-Trimeton) for severe, persistent itching. Follow instructions on the label.
- Wrap a young child's hands or place in gloves to prevent scratching at night. Keep nails short.
- Apply OTC hydrocortisone creams to rash for short periods of time. Do not use longer than 3 days.
- Apply moisturizing cream (Curel, Vaseline Intensive Care) to dry, itching skin. Follow instructions on the label.
- For itching feet, wash frequently and dry well. Expose to air as much as possible. Wear cotton, rather than synthetic, socks.

Additional Instructions

_____

_____

_____

Report the Following Problems to Your PCP/Clinic/ED

- No improvement or condition worsens after >3 days of home care measures
- Other household members have the same symptoms

Seek Emergency Care Immediately If the Following Occur

- Severe itching over several areas of the body, generalized hives, swelling in the face or throat, and difficulty breathing

If the caller agrees with the advice given, document the call and encourage the caller to call back or see PCP if the problem worsens. If the caller does not agree with the advice given, reevaluate and advise the caller to follow up with PCP, Clinic, or ED.

Jaundice

 Key Questions Name, Age, Onset, Yellow Tint to Skin or Eyes, Medications, History, Associated Symptoms

 Other Protocols to Consider Abdominal Pain, Adult (9), Child (13); Abdominal Swelling (16); Hepatitis (329); Itching (382); Newborn Problems (421); Stools, Abnormal (573).

Reminder: Document caller response to advice, home care instructions, and when to call back.

ASSESSMENT	ACTION

A. Are any of the following present?

- Yellow-tinted skin in newborn within first 24 hours of life
- Yellow tint involves arms or legs
- Rectal temperature >100.4°F (38°C) or <96.8°F (36°C)
- Newborn with yellow tint below waistline
- Unable to awaken infant for two feedings in a row (4 to 6 hours)
- Newborn and no wet diapers for >8 hours

YES "Seek medical care within 2 to 4 hours"

NO Go to B

B. Are any of the following present?

- Dark urine
- Yellow skin
- White, yellow, or clay-colored stools
- Fatigue
- Headache
- Nausea, vomiting, or loss of appetite
- Abdominal pain
- Newborn >7 days of age with yellow skin
- Newborn 2 to 4 days old and no stool for >24 hours
- Wet diapers <6 per day or <3 per day if breastfeeding
- Newborn and yellow skin persists >14 days of age

YES "Seek medical care within 24 hours"

NO "Call back or call PCP for appointment if no improvement" and Follow **Home Care Instructions**

Home Care Instructions
Jaundice

Newborn

- If newborn is breastfed, feed every 1½ to 2½ hours (8 or more times in 24 hours).
- If newborn is bottle-fed, feed every 2 to 3 hours during the day.
- Place newborn near a window during sleep periods, with the skin exposed during the day to absorb the sun's rays.
- If supplement is offered, use formula or breast milk. Do not use water.
- Remember that jaundice occurs in many newborns and usually peaks at 3 to 5 days and disappears in 1 to 2 weeks. Newborns excrete bilirubin through stool. (The more they feed, the more stool they excrete.)
- Tips for awakening a sleepy newborn:
  - Unwrap blankets and undress the newborn.
  - Change the diaper.
  - Massage the newborn's legs, back, and arms.
  - Give the newborn a back rub by walking fingers down the spine.
  - Perform "sit-ups" by holding the newborn away from you and gently lifting the newborn toward your face.
- If newborn has not eaten in 6 hours, feed pumped breast milk or formula.

Additional Instructions

Report the Following Problems to Your PCP/Clinic/ED

- Persistent yellowing of the skin with or without symptoms
- Unable to awaken newborn for feeding

If the caller agrees with the advice given, document the call and encourage the caller to call back or see PCP if the problem worsens. If the caller does not agree with the advice given, reevaluate and advise the caller to follow up with PCP, Clinic, or ED.

Jaw Pain

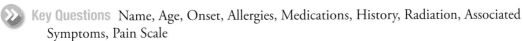

Key Questions Name, Age, Onset, Allergies, Medications, History, Radiation, Associated Symptoms, Pain Scale

Other Protocols to Consider Chest Pain (123); Heartburn (316); Indigestion (368); Mouth Problems (407); Neck Pain (415); Toothache (613); Tooth Injury (616).

> *Nurse Alert:* There are many conditions that cause jaw pain; some can be potentially life-threatening. Err on the side of caution when triaging callers with jaw pain. Women with jaw, neck, or back pain, nausea, and/or shortness of breath may be experiencing a heart attack.

Reminder: Document caller response to advice, home care instructions, and when to call back.

ASSESSMENT	ACTION
A. Are any of the following present?	
• Chest pain • Difficulty breathing	**YES** Go to Chest Pain protocol (123) or Breathing Problems protocol (106)
	NO Go to B
B. Are any of the following present?	
• Intermittent jaw pain and history of hypertension, cardiovascular disease, high cholesterol, obesity, heavy smoker, or age >30 years • New onset and pain radiates to neck, shoulders, or arms	**YES** "Seek emergency care now" **NO** Go to C
C. Are any of the following present?	
• Severe pain • Recent trauma to the area • Teeth do not align as usual	**YES** "Seek medical or dental care within 2 to 4 hours" **NO** Go to D

D. Are any of the following present?

- Jaw locks in certain positions
- Signs of infection (increased pain, swelling, drainage, red streaks, or warmth)

YES "Seek medical or dental care within 24 hours"

NO Go to E

E. Are any of the following present?

- Pain >2 weeks
- Headache, neck, and shoulder pain
- Clicking, snapping, or popping sound with jaw movement
- Difficulty opening mouth wide
- Pain in jaw joint
- Ear or eye pain
- Intermittent swelling over the area

YES "Call back or call PCP or dentist for appointment if no improvement" and Follow **Home Care Instructions**

NO Follow **Home Care Instructions**

Home Care Instructions
Jaw Pain

- Avoid chewing gum or tough foods.
- Alternate cold and hot packs to the jaw 6 times a day.
- Avoid cradling the telephone receiver between the jaw and shoulder.
- Take your usual pain medication (aspirin, acetaminophen, ibuprofen) for discomfort and swelling, as tolerated. Do not give aspirin to a child. Avoid aspirin-like products if age <20 years. Avoid acetaminophen if liver disease is present. Avoid ibuprofen if kidney disease or stomach problems exist or in the case of pregnancy. Follow the directions on the label.
- Massage muscles around the jaw.

Additional Instructions

Report the Following Problems to Your PCP/Dentist/Clinic

- Persistent pain unrelieved by home care measures
- Condition worsens
- Signs of infection: increased pain, swelling, drainage, red streaks, warmth, or fever

Seek Emergency Care Immediately If Any of the Following Occur

- Chest pain
- Difficulty breathing
- New pain radiates to neck, shoulders, or arms

If the caller agrees with the advice given, document the call and encourage the caller to call back or see PCP if the problem worsens. If the caller does not agree with the advice given, reevaluate and advise the caller to follow up with PCP, Clinic, or ED.

Joint Pain/Swelling

 Key Questions Name, Age, Onset, Cause, Allergies, Medications, History, Pain Scale

 Other Protocols to Consider Ankle Injury (31); Ankle Problems (33); Arthritis Problems (48); Bone, Joint, and Tissue Injury (95); Extremity Injury (222); Hip Pain/Injury (334); Knee Pain/Swelling/Injury (393); Leg Pain/Swelling (398); Pregnancy Problems (481); Sickle Cell Disease Problems (551).

Reminder: Document caller response to advice, home care instructions, and when to call back.

ASSESSMENT	ACTION
A. Are any of the following present?	
• Ankle swelling with chest pain, coughing up blood, or shortness of breath • Dislocation or deformity • Fingers or toes of affected part are cold or blue	**YES** "Call ambulance" or "Seek emergency care now" **NO** Go to B
B. Are any of the following present?	
• Swelling and pain in thigh or calf • New onset and unable to walk or bear weight • Joint, calf, or thigh painful, swollen, warm, or red with no known injury • Child with purple rash on the arms and/or legs • Swelling in one extremity and a recent long trip, pregnant, history of cancer, prolonged bed rest, or history of blood clots in legs	**YES** "Seek medical care within 2 to 4 hours" **NO** Go to C

C. Are any of the following present?

- Pregnant and recent onset of symptoms
- Pain persists or worsens with:
  - walking or standing
  - rest
  - raising the leg
  - flexing the foot
  - using hand, arm, or shoulder
- History of heart, liver, kidney disease, immunosuppression, diabetes, or recent illness, such as sore throat or skin infection
- New prescription medication
- Severe pain in joint or base of big toe
- Skin over joint red or shiny
- Child with pain in knee or hip and limping
- Child with two of the following: headache, sore throat, cough
- Child not using arm or hand
- Fever
- Recent weight gain of >10 lb(4.5 kg)

YES   "Seek medical care within 24 hours"

NO   Go to D

D. Are any of the following present?

- Pregnancy
- Pain in other joints
- General ill feeling
- Sudden onset with no known injury
- Mild swelling
- Chronic pain unrelieved with home care measures

YES   "Call back or call PCP for appointment if no improvement" and Follow **Home Care Instructions**

NO   Follow **Home Care Instructions**

Home Care Instructions
Joint Pain/Swelling

- Elevate the affected limb higher than the heart. Place pillows under the calves to elevate swollen ankles.
- For ankle swelling, reduce salt in diet.
- Apply heat to area (if no known injury): use caution when applying heat and diabetic. Do not fall asleep on a heating pad.
- Do not massage painful thighs or calves.
- Take your usual pain medication (aspirin, acetaminophen, ibuprofen). Do not give aspirin to a child. Avoid aspirin-like products if age <20 years. Avoid acetaminophen if liver disease is present. Avoid ibuprofen if kidney disease or stomach problems exist or in the case of pregnancy. Follow the directions on the label. Check with PCP before taking aspirin if on anticoagulant therapy.
- Rest.
- For known injury, apply ice pack to joint for 20 to 30 minutes every 2 hours for first 24 to 48 hours. Do not apply ice directly on skin; place a washcloth or other cloth barrier between ice and skin.

Additional Instructions

Report the Following Problems to Your PCP/Clinic/ED

- No improvement or condition worsens
- Increased pain
- Decreased mobility
- Fever

Seek Emergency Care Immediately If Any of the Following Occur

- Ankle swelling with chest pain, coughing up blood, or shortness of breath
- Fingers or toes of affected part are cold or blue

If the caller agrees with the advice given, document the call and encourage the caller to call back or see PCP if the problem worsens. If the caller does not agree with the advice given, reevaluate and advise the caller to follow up with PCP, Clinic, or ED.

Knee Pain/Swelling/Injury

>> **Key Questions** Name, Age, Onset, Cause, Allergies, History of Arthritis or Gout, Medications, History, Pain Scale

>> **Other Protocols to Consider** Arthritis Problems (48); Bone, Joint, and Tissue Injury (95); Extremity Injury (222); Joint Pain/Swelling (390); Leg Pain/Swelling (398).

Reminder: Document caller response to advice, home care instructions, and when to call back.

ASSESSMENT	ACTION

A. Are any of the following present?

- Sudden onset and extremity is cold, blue, or numb
- Obvious deformity or dislocation

YES "Seek emergency care now"

NO Go to B

B. Are any of the following present?

- Severe pain
- Unable to bear weight
- Extreme swelling
- Signs of infection: increased pain, swelling, redness, red streaks, warmth, or fever
- Trauma to knee

YES "Seek medical care within 2 to 4 hours"

NO Go to C

C. Are any of the following present?

- Moderate swelling
- Increased pain with knee movement or weight bearing and interferes with activity
- History of recent knee injury
- Persistent numbness
- Knee buckles or locks in place
- History of diabetes

YES "Seek medical care within 24 hours"

NO Go to D

D. Are any of the following present?

- Intermittent pain and swelling but does not interfere with activity
- Persistent pain but does not interfere with activity
- Knee prosthesis

YES "Call back or call PCP for appointment if no improvement" and Follow **Home Care Instructions**

NO Follow **Home Care Instructions**

393

Home Care Instructions
Knee Pain/Swelling/Injury

- For known injury
  - Apply ice pack to knee for 20 to 30 minutes every 2 hours for the first 24 to 48 hours, then alternate heat and ice. Do not apply ice directly to injured area. Place a cloth barrier between the skin and the ice. Use caution when applying heat and cold if diabetic.
  - Elevate the extremity above the heart.
  - Rest and decrease weight-bearing activities.
  - Immobilize the knee or apply an elastic bandage or soft splint when active.
  - Take your usual pain medication (aspirin, acetaminophen, ibuprofen). Do not give aspirin to a child. Avoid aspirin-like products if age <20 years. Avoid acetaminophen if liver disease is present. Avoid ibuprofen if kidney disease or stomach problems exist or in the case of pregnancy. Follow the directions on the label.
- If no known injury
  - Apply moist heat to the knee for 20 to 30 minutes every 2 hours. Soak a towel in warm water and apply over the knee.
  - Elevate the extremity on pillows so that feet are higher than the heart.
  - Rest and decrease activity.
  - Take aspirin, acetaminophen, ibuprofen, or pain medication of choice for discomfort. Do not give aspirin to a child. Avoid aspirin-like products if age <20 years. Avoid acetaminophen if liver disease is present. Avoid ibuprofen if kidney disease or stomach problems exist or in the case of pregnancy. Follow the directions on the label.
  - Avoid prolonged standing.

Additional Instructions

Report the Following Problems to Your PCP/Clinic/ED
- Persistent pain and swelling after following home care measures
- Continued mobility problems after following home care measures
- Signs of infection: increased pain, swelling, redness, red streaks, warmth, or fever

Seek Emergency Care Immediately If the Following Occurs
- Extremity is cold or blue

If the caller agrees with the advice given, document the call and encourage the caller to call back or see PCP if the problem worsens. If the caller does not agree with the advice given, reevaluate and advise the caller to follow up with PCP, Clinic, or ED.

Laceration

>> **Key Questions** Name, Age, Onset, Cause, Allergies, Pain Scale, Medications, Tetanus Immunization Status, Location (If caused by a bite, see Bites, Animal/Human (76), Marine Animal (83), and Snake (85).)

>> **Other Protocols to Consider** Foreign Body, Skin (278); Immunization, Tetanus (355); Piercing Problems (445); Puncture Wound (496); Wound Care: Sutures or Staples (660); Wound Healing and Infection (664).

Nurse Alert: If the puncture or wound is dirty, another immunization is recommended within 5 years. Wounds are defined as clean or dirty. A wound is considered dirty if it is contaminated with dirt, feces, saliva, or soil; puncture wounds; avulsions; caused by flying or crushing objects, animal bites, burns, or frostbite.

Reminder: Document caller response to advice, home care instructions, and when to call back.

ASSESSMENT	ACTION

A. Are any of the following present?

- Large gaping wound
- Partial or complete amputation
- Deep wound to the head, back of mouth or throat, chest, neck, genitals, or abdomen
- Difficulty breathing
- Pulsating or squirting blood
- Visible bone in laceration
- Penetrating injury (knife, bullet, metal object)

YES "Call ambulance" or "Seek emergency care now" and "Do not remove knife or other penetrating cause of injury"

NO Go to B

B. Are any of the following present?

- Gaping, split, jagged, or deep wound
- Newly sutured, stapled, or glued wound now split open
- Severe pain
- Unable to move or limited movement of injured part
- History of diabetes
- Persistent bleeding after 10 minutes of direct pressure
- Numbness
- Laceration through eyelid, lip border, or eyebrow
- High-pressure injection injury
- Unable to remove dirt or other foreign material from wound
- Taking a steroid or a blood-thinning medication
- Signs of infection: increased redness, drainage, fever, increased pain, red streaks, or swelling in a healing wound

YES "Seek medical care within 2 to 4 hours"

NO Go to C

C. Are any of the following present?

- Persistent pain unrelieved by home care measures
- No tetanus immunization, immunization status unknown, or last tetanus immunization >5 years ago
- Wound over a joint and difficulty keeping edges of wound together
- Wound not healing well after 7 to 10 days

YES "Seek medical care within 24 hours"

NO Go to D

D. Are any of the following present?

- Small laceration in the mouth
- Edges of wound stay together and bleeding is controlled
- No history of tetanus immunization
- Headache, muscle aches, general ill feeling, or fever
- Parent or caller concerned about scarring

YES "Call back or call PCP for appointment if no improvement" and Follow **Home Care Instructions**

NO Follow **Home Care Instructions**

Home Care Instructions
Laceration

- Apply direct pressure over the wound with a clean bandage or cloth to control the bleeding.
- Clean the wound with soap and water.
- Pull edges of the wound together and hold in place with a butterfly or sterile strip bandage. Do not overlap skin edges. Leave butterfly or sterile strip in place until it falls off.
- May apply antibiotic ointment 2 to 3 times a day.
- Cover the wound with a clean, dry dressing.
- Check the wound daily for signs of infection. Replace soiled dressings daily or more often, as needed.
- For lacerations in the mouth, suck on an ice cube or flavored ice to reduce swelling and control bleeding.

Additional Instructions

Report the Following Problems to Your PCP/Clinic/ED

- Increase in pain, swelling, or bleeding
- Headache, muscle aches, general ill feeling, or fever
- Signs of infection, numbness, or tingling
- Laceration is not healing well after 1 week to 10 days
- Newly sutured, stapled, or glued wound now split open
- Unable to move or limited movement of injured part

Seek Emergency Care Immediately If Any of the Following Occur

- Difficulty breathing

If the caller agrees with the advice given, document the call and encourage the caller to call back or see PCP if the problem worsens. If the caller does not agree with the advice given, reevaluate and advise the caller to follow up with PCP, Clinic, or ED.

Leg Pain/Swelling

 Key Questions Name, Age, Onset, Cause, History, Medications (If pain and swelling are caused by a recent injury, see Extremity Injury protocol.)

 Other Protocols to Consider Ankle Injury (31); Ankle Problems (33); Bone, Joint, and Tissue Injury (95); Congestive Heart Failure Problems (157); Extremity Injury (222); Knee Pain/Swelling/Injury (393); Pregnancy Problems (481); Tattoo Problems (604).

Reminder: Document caller response to advice, home care instructions, and when to call back.

ASSESSMENT	ACTION

A. In addition to leg swelling, are any of the following present?

- Chest pain
- Coughing up blood or pink frothy sputum
- Severe shortness of breath
- Sudden onset and cold or blue foot or toe(s)
- Sudden onset and no pulse in foot of affected leg and numbness or tingling

YES "Call ambulance" or "Seek emergency care now"

NO Go to B

B. Are any of the following present?

- Severe swelling and pain in thigh, calf, ankle, or toes
- Unable to walk
- Child is reluctant to use or move the leg
- Fever
- Area over the ankle, calf, or thigh is warm to touch; red streaks extending from area
- Sudden swelling in one leg or ankle
- Signs of infection and immunosuppressed

YES "Seek medical care within 2 to 4 hours"

NO Go to C

C. Are any of the following present?

- Pain persists or worsens with
  - walking or standing
  - rest
  - raising the leg
  - flexing the foot
- New prescription medication
- Swelling increases at night
- Pregnancy and recent onset of symptoms
- No improvement with home care
- Recent weight gain of >10 lb (4.5 kg)
- History of blood clots, cancer, diabetes, cardiac disease, immunosuppression, liver or kidney disease
- Signs of infection, swelling, pain, warmth, drainage, red streaks
- Fever
- Child limping and pain in knee or hip
- Increased pain with movement or weight bearing and interferes with activity

YES   "Seek medical care within 24 hours"

NO   Go to D

D. Are any of the following present?

- Pain in other joints
- General ill feeling
- Pain over the shin bone in the lower leg after exercising
- Persistent pain but does not interfere with activity
- Muscle cramps that awaken during sleep
- Persistent phantom pain postamputation

YES   "Call back or call PCP for appointment if no improvement" and Follow **Home Care Instructions**

NO   Follow **Home Care Instructions**

L

Home Care Instructions
Leg Pain/Swelling

- Elevate legs on pillows so that the feet are higher than the heart. Do not place anything under the knees. Place pillows under the calves.
- Reduce salt in the diet.
- Rest and decrease activity.
- Apply heat to the area. If shins become painful after exercising, apply ice. Do not apply ice directly to the skin. Use a washcloth or other cloth barrier between ice and the skin.
- Do not massage area.
- Avoid sitting or standing for long periods of time, but if such activity is unavoidable, move toes and calf muscles frequently.
- Try elastic support stockings during the day.
- Try usual medication for discomfort. Do not give aspirin to a child. Avoid aspirin-like products if age <20 years. Avoid acetaminophen if liver disease is present. Avoid ibuprofen if kidney disease or stomach problems exist or in the case of pregnancy. Follow the directions on the label.
- Talk with provider about phantom pain after an amputation. There are a variety of treatment options including medications, acupuncture, spinal stimulator, mirror box therapy, injections, implanted devices, biofeedback, massage therapy.
- Contact the Amputee Coalition @ www.amputee-coalition.org for information on the National Peer Network.

Additional Instructions

Report the Following Problems to Your PCP/Clinic/ED

- No improvement or condition worsens
- Increased pain
- Decreased mobility
- Fever

Seek Emergency Care Immediately If Any of the Following Occur

- Chest pain
- Severe shortness of breath
- Blood in sputum
- Cold or blue foot or toe(s)
- No pulse in foot of affected leg

If the caller agrees with the advice given, document the call and encourage the caller to call back or see PCP if the problem worsens. If the caller does not agree with the advice given, reevaluate and advise the caller to follow up with PCP, Clinic, or ED.

Lice

 Key Questions Name, Age, Onset, Cause, Allergies, Medications

Other Protocols to Consider Bedbug Exposure or Concerns (67); Itching (382); Rash, Adult (500), Child (505); Skin Lesions: Lumps, Bumps, and Sores (556).

> *Nurse Alert:* Use this protocol if undergoing treatment for lice, history of lice (small gray or brown bugs), and lice or nits (white eggs) are present and attached to the hair shaft on the scalp, groin, underarm, or eyelashes.
>
> - If symptoms of an allergic reaction develop after using a lice treatment medication (rash, swelling of the lips, tongue, or throat or difficulty breathing), go to the Allergic Reaction protocol (25).

Reminder: Document caller response to advice, home care instructions, and when to call back.

ASSESSMENT	ACTION
A. Lice present and are any of the following present?	
<ul><li>Persistent rash and itch that interfere with sleep</li><li>Rash persists after 1 week of treatment</li><li>Sores spread or show signs of infection</li><li>New eggs appear after treatment</li><li>Rash clears, then returns</li><li>Local skin reaction to OTC or prescribed treatment medication</li><li>Pregnancy</li><li>Fever, malaise, or enlarged nodes</li></ul>	**YES** "Seek medical care within 24 to 48 hours" See Allergic Reaction protocol (25) if suspected allergic reaction to medication **NO** Go to B
B. No lice seen and are any of the following present?	
<ul><li>Undergoing treatment for lice and has questions regarding medication or preventing the spread to others</li><li>Known exposure to someone with lice or suspicion of infestation</li></ul>	**YES** "Call back or call PCP for appointment if no improvement" and Follow **Home Care Instructions** **NO** Follow **Home Care Instructions**

Home Care Instructions
Lice

- Search for lice when hair is wet and comb through small sections at a time with a fine comb, louse comb, or flea comb used on cats and dogs. Repeat every 2 to 3 days for 2 weeks.
- Check the scalps and bodies of other household members for rash or itching. If present, treat with antilice shampoo.
- If lice are found, apply antilice product (prescribed or OTC—Rid, Nix, or Pronto shampoos) to dry hair for 10 minutes and follow instructions on the label. Do not use Rid on children who are allergic to ragweed. Do not use Nix on children with asthma. Be sure to read the label for warnings and contraindications. Retreat in 7 to 10 days. Ask pharmacist for additional product suggestions.
- Rinse over a sink with cool water (Nix kills eggs).
- Use a fine-toothed comb to remove eggs from the shaft of the hairs. Scotch tape applied to the shaft of the hair is also effective in removing nits.
- To remove eggs on eyelashes, apply petrolatum to lashes twice a day for 8 days.
- Soak brushes and combs in antilice shampoo for 1 hour.
- Wash clothing and linens in hot water. Wash clothing inside out to destroy lice or eggs hiding in the seams. Dry on high heat (if possible) and iron seams. Place clothing and items that cannot be washed in a plastic bag for 3 days.
- Clean furniture, carpets, and mattresses. Vacuum and immediately throw away the vacuum bag.
- Avoid sharing personal items, such as combs, brushes, hats, or towels.
- Lice are highly contagious. Avoid head-to-head contact.
- Blow-dry hair every day to help remove and prevent lice infestation.
- If lice are resistant to antilice medications, apply real mayonnaise or olive oil liberally to the hair and cover the hair with plastic wrap or a shower cap for at least 3 hours. The mayonnaise or olive oil will help to smother the lice.
- A child can return to school after one application of antilice shampoo.

Additional Instructions

Report the Following Problems to Your PCP/Clinic/ED

- The rash, lice, or nits disappear, then return
- Signs of infection: redness, pain, drainage, or fever
- Questions concerning the medication for the ill, elderly, infants, children, or pregnant women
- Mild allergic reaction to the medication
- Rash itching >1 week after treatment

Seek Emergency Care Immediately If Any of the Following Occur

- Severe allergic reaction to medication

If the caller agrees with the advice given, document the call and encourage the caller to call back or see PCP if the problem worsens. If the caller does not agree with the advice given, reevaluate and advise the caller to follow up with PCP, Clinic, or ED.

Menstrual Problems

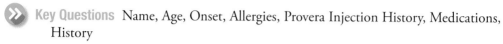

Key Questions Name, Age, Onset, Allergies, Provera Injection History, Medications, History

Other Protocols to Consider Abdominal Pain, Adult (9), Child (13); Sexually Transmitted Disease (542); Vaginal Bleeding (633); Vaginal Discharge/Pain/ Itching (636).

Reminder: Document caller response to advice, home care instructions, and when to call back.

ASSESSMENT	ACTION

A. Are any of the following present?

- Persistent severe bleeding that requires use of more than one full-size sanitary pad or tampons per hour for 8 hours
- Passage of large blood clots or tissue and different than usual menstrual cycle
- Severe pain and possible pregnancy
- Sexually active and last menstrual period is 6 to 8 weeks ago and abdominal or shoulder pain or vaginal bleeding

YES "Seek emergency care now"

NO Go to B

B. Are any of the following present?

- Unusually severe pain and no possibility of pregnancy
- Unexplained fever (temperature >100°F or 37.8°C) and abdominal pain
- Fainting or dizziness sitting up or standing
- Use of tampons and sudden high fever, sunburn-type rash, general ill feeling, dizziness, vomiting, watery diarrhea, rapid pulse, or headache

YES "Seek medical care within 2 to 4 hours"

NO Go to C

C. Are any of the following present?

- Cramping interferes with school, work, or daily activity
- Persistent vaginal discharge
- Persistent vaginal bleeding for >10 days or <21 days since last period
- Possible pregnancy and bleeding and no pain

YES "Seek medical care within 24 hours"

NO Go to D

D. Are any of the following present?

- Persistent pain after bleeding stops
- Late period and history of increased stress, strenuous activity, significant weight loss, recent illness, stopped taking birth control pills, or older than 40 years
- Light bleeding or mild abdominal discomfort mid-cycle
- Irritability, bloating, headaches, or breast tenderness before period
- Vaginal bleeding occurs after menopause
- Breakthrough bleeding and taking birth control pills
- Irregular periods
- Postcoital bleeding

YES "Call back or call PCP for appointment if no improvement" and Follow **Home Care Instructions**

NO Follow **Home Care Instructions**

Home Care Instructions
Menstrual Problems

- Take usual pain medication (aspirin, acetaminophen, ibuprofen, naproxen). Avoid aspirin and ibuprofen if pregnant. Do not give aspirin to a child. Avoid aspirin-like products if age <20 years. Avoid acetaminophen if liver disease is present. Avoid ibuprofen if kidney disease or stomach problems exist. Follow the directions on the label.
- Apply heating pad or hot water bottle to abdomen for 20 to 30 minutes for abdominal discomfort or take a warm bath. Do not fall asleep on a heating pad.
- Change tampons frequently, at least every 4 hours. Use pads at night. Avoid using tampons if skin infection is present and near the genitals.
- If period is >2 weeks late, use home pregnancy kit on first morning urine sample.
- For premenstrual symptoms, decrease salt, caffeine, and sugar in the diet and alcohol and cigarette use before menstruation.
- Increase exercise to help reduce cramping and premenstrual symptoms.

Additional Instructions

Report the Following Problems to Your PCP/Clinic/ED

- No improvement in 3 days or condition worsens
- Menstrual cramps interfere with school, work, or daily activity
- Fainting or dizziness sitting up or standing
- Unexplained fever and abdominal pain

Seek Emergency Care Immediately If Any of the Following Occur

- Persistent severe bleeding requiring use of more than one full-size sanitary pad or tampons per hour for 8 hours
- Passage of blood clots or tissue

If the caller agrees with the advice given, document the call and encourage the caller to call back or see PCP if the problem worsens. If the caller does not agree with the advice given, reevaluate and advise the caller to follow up with PCP, Clinic, or ED.

Mouth Problems

 Key Questions Name, Age, Onset, Allergies, Medications, History

 Other Protocols to Consider Bad Breath (65); Jaw Pain (387); Piercing/Pocketing
Problems (445); Skin Lesions: Lumps, Bumps, and Sores (556); Sore Throat (564);
Swallowing Difficulty (591); Toothache (613); Tooth Injury (616).

Reminder: Document caller response to advice, home care instructions, and when to call back.

ASSESSMENT	ACTION

A. Are any of the following present?

- Sudden swelling in back of throat or tongue
- Jaw feels locked in place, inability to open mouth
- Unable to swallow own saliva

YES "Seek emergency care now"

NO Go to B

B. Are any of the following present?

- Penetrating injury to mouth with sharp object
- Persistent bleeding
- Severe pain
- Gaping laceration to lip, tongue, or inside mouth
- Pain with facial swelling
- Sensation of bone or food stuck in throat

YES "Seek medical care within 2 to 4 hours"

NO Go to C

C. Are any of the following present?

- Fever and mouth sores
- Blisters
- White patches on tongue, gums, or inner cheeks
- General ill feeling
- Pain with biting, chewing, or opening mouth
- Persistent mouth pain unresponsive to home care measures
- History of phenytoin (Dilantin) use
- Long history of smoking or use of chewing tobacco
- Foul odor despite regular hygiene
- Red, swollen, tender gums with fever
- Difficulty swallowing

YES "Seek medical care within 24 hours"

NO Go to D

M

407

D. Are any of the following present?

- History of oral herpes, canker sores, recent viral illness, or new medication
- Taking large doses of vitamins
- Red, swollen, tender gums and no fever
- Sore spot on tongue
- Poor eating habits or change in diet
- Recent increase in stress
- Dental caries

YES "Call back or call PCP for appointment if no improvement" and Follow **Home Care Instructions**

NO Follow **Home Care Instructions**

Home Care Instructions
Mouth Problems

- Iced fluids may soothe mouth sores but will worsen a toothache.
- Rinse mouth with warm water and ½ tsp salt or baking soda 4 times a day, or rinse with an antiseptic mouthwash.
- Avoid spicy, citrus, or salty foods until sores are healed.
- Avoid touching sores.
- Brush, floss, and rinse teeth and mouth at least twice daily.
- Take usual pain medication (acetaminophen or ibuprofen) for fever and discomfort. Do not give aspirin to a child. Avoid aspirin-like products if age <20 years. Avoid acetaminophen if liver disease is present. Avoid ibuprofen if kidney disease or stomach problems exist or in the case of pregnancy. Follow the directions on the label.
- Use OTC product containing Orabase to provide protective coating and diminish discomfort.

Additional Instructions

M

Report the Following Problems to Your PCP/Clinic/ED

- Mouth lesion persists >2 weeks
- Persistent pain or bleeding
- Signs of infection: pain, swelling, drainage, warmth, or fever
- Difficulty swallowing
- No improvement or condition worsens

Seek Emergency Care Immediately If Any of the Following Occur

- Sudden swelling in back of throat or tongue
- Jaw feels locked in place, inability to open mouth
- Unable to swallow own saliva

If the caller agrees with the advice given, document the call and encourage the caller to call back or see PCP if the problem worsens. If the caller does not agree with the advice given, reevaluate and advise the caller to follow up with PCP, Clinic, or ED.

Mumps

 Key Questions Name, Age, Onset, Known or Suspected Mumps, History, Medications

 Other Protocols to Consider Fever, Adult (250), Child (253); Glands, Swollen or Tender (297); Neck Pain (415).

> *Nurse Alert:* Use this protocol if diagnosed with mumps or caller has known exposure to mumps, has swollen glands, and has questions about mumps.

Reminder: Document caller response to advice, home care instructions, and when to call back.

ASSESSMENT	ACTION

A. Person has diagnosed mumps and are any of the following present?

- Stiff neck or severe headache
- Repeated vomiting
- Severe abdominal pain
- Confusion
- Decreased level of consciousness
- Difficulty breathing
- Severe dizziness on standing

YES "Seek emergency care now"

NO Go to B

B. Are any of the following present?

- Swollen gland >8 days
- Fever >5 days
- Skin red over swollen gland
- Painful testicle
- Severe pain

YES "Seek medical care within 24 hours"

NO Go to C

C. Are any of the following present?

- Swollen and tender gland in front of ear and around jaw
- Chewing increases pain
- Fever
- No prior mumps vaccine
- Exposure to mumps 16 to 18 days earlier

YES   "Call back or call PCP for appointment if no improvement" and Follow **Home Care Instructions**

NO   Follow **Home Care Instructions**

M

Home Care Instructions
Mumps

- Isolate person with mumps until the swelling is gone.
- Rest until fever subsides.
- Apply an ice collar or ice pack to swollen glands for discomfort. Do not place ice directly on skin; place a cloth barrier between the ice and the skin.
- Take usual pain medication (aspirin, acetaminophen, ibuprofen). Do not give aspirin to a child. Avoid aspirin-like products if age <20 years. Avoid acetaminophen if liver disease is present. Avoid ibuprofen if kidney disease or stomach problems exist or in the case of pregnancy. Follow the directions on the label.
- Eat a liquid or soft diet until pain subsides. Avoid sour or citrus foods.
- Avoid mumps exposure to people who are immunosuppressed (including individuals receiving chemotherapy or those with AIDS).

Additional Instructions

Report the Following Problems to Your PCP/Clinic/ED
- Swollen gland >8 days
- Fever >5 days
- Skin red over swollen gland
- Painful testicle

Seek Emergency Care Immediately If Any of the Following Occur
- Stiff neck or severe headache
- Repeated vomiting
- Severe abdominal pain
- Confusion
- Decreased level of consciousness
- Difficulty breathing
- Severe dizziness on standing

If the caller agrees with the advice given, document the call and encourage the caller to call back or see PCP if the problem worsens. If the caller does not agree with the advice given, reevaluate and advise the caller to follow up with PCP, Clinic, or ED.

Muscle Cramps

 Key Questions Name, Age, Onset, Cause, Allergies, History, Pain Scale, Medications

 Other Protocols to Consider Back Pain (62); Bone, Joint, and Tissue Injury (95); Extremity Injury (222); Joint Pain/Swelling (390); Leg Pain/Swelling (398).

Reminder: Document caller response to advice, home care instructions, and when to call back.

ASSESSMENT	ACTION

A. Are any of the following present?

- Cramping following an injury and inability to move or use limb
- Tender, swollen calf with no known injury
- Extremity pale, blue, or cool compared with other limb, or extremity numb

YES "Seek medical care within 2 to 4 hours"

NO Go to B

B. Are any of the following present?

- Tender red area on calf with no known injury
- Sudden onset after taking new medication
- Cramping interferes with activity
- Frequent use of diuretics

YES "Seek medical care within 24 hours"

NO Go to C

C. Are any of the following present?

- Cramping occurs during or several hours after strenuous exercise
- Excessive sweating and inadequate fluid replacement
- Calf pain frequently occurs with exercise and disappears with rest
- Prolonged sitting, standing, or lying in an awkward position
- Leg cramps occur at night

YES "Call back or call PCP for appointment if no improvement" and Follow **Home Care Instructions**

NO Follow **Home Care Instructions**

M

413

Home Care Instructions
Muscle Cramps

- Perform stretching exercises for 15 to 20 minutes before strenuous exercise.
- After strenuous exercise or excessive sweating, rest in a cool place and replace lost fluid. Drink a mixture of ¼ tsp salt in 1 quart of water, a sports drink, juice, soda, or water.
- Discuss diuretic use with physician. When taking OTC diuretics, make sure lost fluid is adequately replaced. Follow instructions on the label.
- Stretch the muscle cramp after prolonged sitting, standing, or lying in an awkward position by extending the leg and pulling the foot back, or stand and press the foot against the floor.
- Apply moist heat for cramping or an ice pack for injury for 20 minutes, 4 to 6 times a day, for the first 24 hours. Do not apply ice directly to the skin. Use a washcloth or other barrier to protect the skin from burning. Do not fall asleep on a heating pad. If diabetic, use caution when applying heat or cold.
- Take your usual pain medication (aspirin, acetaminophen, ibuprofen). Do not give aspirin to a child. Avoid aspirin-like products if age <20 years. Avoid acetaminophen if liver disease is present. Avoid ibuprofen if kidney disease or stomach problems exist or in the case of pregnancy. Follow the directions on the label.

Additional Instructions

Report the Following Problems to Your PCP/Clinic/ED

- Persistent and frequent cramping
- Cramping after taking prescribed medication
- Increased pain, swelling, redness, or inability to use limb
- Persistent discomfort interferes with activity
- Extremity becomes pale, blue, or cool compared with other limb, or extremity numb
- No improvement or condition worsens

If the caller agrees with the advice given, document the call and encourage the caller to call back or see PCP if the problem worsens. If the caller does not agree with the advice given, reevaluate and advise the caller to follow up with PCP, Clinic, or ED.

Neck Pain

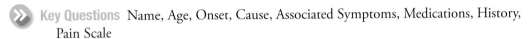

>> **Key Questions** Name, Age, Onset, Cause, Associated Symptoms, Medications, History, Pain Scale

>> **Other Protocols to Consider** Back/Neck Injury (59); Chest Pain (123); Glands, Swollen or Tender (297); Jaw Pain (387); Mumps (410); Numbness and Tingling (431).

> *Nurse Alert:* There are many conditions that can cause neck pain. When neck pain is associated with several other symptoms, triage with caution and note signs that may be an indication of a more serious condition such as meningitis (pain bending head forward, headache, fever, vomiting, confusion, photophobia) or a heart attack (chest, neck, back or jaw pain, sweating, palpitations, nausea, and/or vomiting).

Reminder: Document caller response to advice, home care instructions, and when to call back.

ASSESSMENT	ACTION
A. Is neck pain related to an injury?	
	YES Go to Back/Neck Injury protocol (59)
	NO Go to B
B. Is chest pain present?	
	YES Go to Chest Pain protocol (123)
	NO Go to C

N

C. Sudden onset of pain, and are any of the following present?

- History of cardiac disease or angina
- Jaw pain
- Sweating, palpitations, nausea, and/or vomiting
- Difficulty breathing
- Pain worsens when head is bent toward chest and any of the following:
  - confusion/drowsiness
  - severe headache
  - light sensitivity
  - fever
  - purple- or blood-colored rash
- Numbness, tingling, weakness in both arms and legs
- Changes in bowel or bladder control
- Head involuntarily turns to side

 YES "Seek emergency care now"

NO Go to D

D. Are any of the following present?

- Weakness or numbness in one arm
- Signs of infection: pain, swelling, redness, drainage, warmth, or red streaks
- Fever >103°F (39.4°C)
- Fever >101°F (38.3°C) and history of diabetes, elderly, immunosuppressed, or IV drug abuse
- Swollen, painful lymph nodes >1 inch (2.5 cm)
- Swollen, painful nodes and difficulty swallowing

YES "Seek medical care within 2 to 4 hours"

NO Go to E

E. Are any of the following present?

- Rash
- Sore throat associated with neck pain
- Pain interferes with sleep or activity
- Swelling on one or both sides of the neck

YES "Seek medical care within 24 hours"

NO Go to F

F. Are any of the following present?

- Slept in an awkward position
- New exercise or activity
- Recently carried heavy bag, purse, or other object using a shoulder strap
- Pain worsens with lateral movement
- History of prolonged sitting at a computer terminal or workstation
- Intermittent pain and history of prior neck problems

YES "Call back or call PCP for an appointment if no improvement" and Follow **Home Care Instructions**

NO Follow **Home Care Instructions**

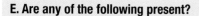

Home Care Instructions
Neck Pain

- Apply heat to neck for 20 minutes every 2 hours. Be careful with heat if diabetic. Do not sleep on a heating pad.
- Sleep with a towel folded around neck to lessen neck movement.
- Carry purse or briefcase under arm, rather than over the shoulder.
- Avoid prolonged sitting. Frequently stretch and move around.
- Exercise regularly to develop strong neck muscles.
- Soak in hot bath or whirlpool.
- Take usual pain medication (aspirin, acetaminophen, ibuprofen) as directed by your physician. Do not give aspirin to a child. Avoid aspirin-like products if age <20 years. Avoid acetaminophen if liver disease is present. Avoid ibuprofen if kidney disease or stomach problems exist or in the case of pregnancy. Follow the directions on the label.
- Maintain good posture and proper body alignment.

Additional Instructions

Report the Following Problems to Your PCP/Clinic/ED

- Rash, fever, or increased pain bending neck forward
- No improvement or condition worsens

Seek Emergency Care Immediately If Any of the Following Occur

- Chest pain
- Difficulty breathing
- Numbness, tingling, or weakness in both arms and legs
- Severe headache and confusion
- Sweating, palpitations, nausea, and/or vomiting
- Swelling to one side of the neck with pain on palpation with or without fever
- Loss of bowel or bladder control
- Pain worsens when head is bent toward chest, confusion/drowsiness, severe headache, light sensitivity, fever, purple- or blood-colored rash

If the caller agrees with the advice given, document the call and encourage the caller to call back or see PCP if the problem worsens. If the caller does not agree with the advice given, reevaluate and advise the caller to follow up with PCP, Clinic, or ED.

Neurologic Symptoms

 Key Questions Name, Age, Onset, Medications, History

 Other Protocols to Consider Altered Mental Status (28); Back/Neck Injury (59); Confusion (150); Dizziness (199); Falls (240); Headache (308); Head Injury (311); Numbness and Tingling (431); Stroke, Suspected (576); Vision Problems (639); Weakness (649).

Nurse Alert:

- Sudden changes in vision, weakness, numbness, speech, or mental status may be signs of a stroke or other serious neurologic disorder. Prompt treatment may prevent extensive damage to the brain or spinal cord and reduce permanent disability. Medications used to break up a clot in the brain need to be administered within 3 hours of symptom onset.
- Ask how current condition is different from normal.

Reminder: Document caller response to advice, home care instructions, and when to call back.

ASSESSMENT	ACTION

A. Did any of the following symptoms suddenly occur?

- Numbness or weakness in face, arm, or leg on one side of the body
- Unexplained dizziness or falls
- Difficulty breathing
- Altered mental status
- Inability to stand, walk, or bear weight
- Difficulty speaking
- Facial drooping on one side
- Difficulty swallowing
- Unable to move a limb
- Visual changes
- Sudden, severe headache
- Recent history of head trauma and elevated blood pressure

YES "Call ambulance" or "Seek emergency care now"

NO Go to B

418

B. Are any of the following present?

- Transient focal neurologic deficits that completely resolve within hours
- New and sudden onset of bladder or bowel incontinence
- New onset of back pain and numbness to groin or rectal area
- Unable to urinate and bladder full
- Headache worse than prior headaches
- Low blood glucose and weakness, confusion, dizziness, headache, tremors, or vision problems, and unresponsive to usual home remedies

YES "Seek medical care immediately"

NO Go to C

C. Is the following present?

- Tremors and history of heavy alcohol use

YES "Seek medical care within 24 hours"

NO Go to D

D. Are any of the following present?

- Poor attention span
- Transient tingling in hands or feet
- New onset of tremors and no history of diabetes, alcohol abuse, Parkinson disease, or seizures

YES "Call back or call PCP for appointment if no improvement" and Follow **Home Care Instructions**

NO Follow **Home Care Instructions**

Home Care Instructions
Neurologic Symptoms

- Provide reassurance that foot or hand tingling after prolonged sitting or pressure to the area will resolve with movement and stretching.
- Avoid crossing legs at the knees or ankles.
- Avoid smoking.
- Take medications as prescribed.
- Avoid driving or operating machinery when experiencing transient symptoms.
- Take fall precautions. Remove safety hazards. Place bell or other communication device within reach of person to summon help before trying to get up.

Additional Instructions

Report the Following Problems to Your PCP/Clinic/ED

- Weakness or numbness in the face, arms, or legs
- Difficulty understanding
- Persistent vision changes
- Persistent dizziness
- No improvement or condition worsens

Seek Emergency Care Immediately If Any of the Following Suddenly Occur

- Weakness on one side of the body
- Unexplained dizziness or falls
- Difficulty breathing
- Altered mental status
- Inability to stand, walk, or bear weight
- Difficulty speaking or swallowing
- Facial drooping on one side
- Unable to move a limb
- Severe headache
- Visual changes

If the caller agrees with the advice given, document the call and encourage the caller to call back or see PCP if the problem worsens. If the caller does not agree with the advice given, reevaluate and advise the caller to follow up with PCP, Clinic, or ED.

Newborn Problems

 Key Questions Name, Age, Onset, Cause, Birth History, Medications

 Other Protocols to Consider Breastfeeding Problems (98); Circumcision Care (141); Crying, Excessive, in Infants (176); Fever, Child (253); Jaundice (385); Sleep Apnea, Infant (562).

> *Nurse Alert:* There are many conditions that affect newborns. When there are multiple associated symptoms, use the protocol that is the primary concern and has the highest probability of a referral to a higher level of care. Ask how the baby's current condition is different from the usual pattern and how the baby is acting at time of call.

Reminder: Document caller response to advice, home care instructions, and when to call back.

ASSESSMENT	ACTION

A. Are any of the following present?

- Seizure
- Unresponsiveness
- Rectal temperature >100.4°F (38°C)
- Temperature <96.8°F (36°C) and unresponsive to warming
- Bulging soft spot with vomiting, fever, or acting sick
- Fall onto a hard surface with obvious injury
- Nonblanching rash
- Rash or bruising

YES "Call ambulance" or "Go to Emergency Department now"

NO Go to B

N

B. Are any of the following present?

- Fall onto a hard surface with no obvious injury
- Refuses to drink >6 hours
- Umbilical cord bleeding >10 minutes of direct pressure
- Red streaks or red area around umbilicus
- Clumps of blisters on one part of body
- Chicken pox
- Breathing quickly
- Distressed and grunting with breathing
- Difficult to comfort
- Nasal flaring
- Pale or blue skin, lips, or nail beds
- Yellow tint below waistline, arms, or legs
- Yellow skin and <24 hours old

 YES — "Seek medical care immediately"

NO — Go to C

C. Are any of the following present?

- Bulging soft spot and infant acting normally
- Umbilical cord intermittently bleeding >3 days
- Pimples or blisters near the cord
- Moderate amount of drainage from navel but no fever
- Yellow sticky discharge from eye
- Red eyes or swollen eyelids
- Newborn >7 days of age with yellow skin
- Yellow or green penile discharge after circumcision (no fever)
- No stool >24 hours
- White-, yellow-, or clay-colored stools

YES — "See medical care within 24 hours"

NO — Go to D

D. Are any of the following present?

- Intermittent bulging soft spot with no signs or symptoms of illness
- Scant bleeding from umbilical cord
- Pink tissue inside the navel
- Foul odor from cord for >2 days (with no fever or redness)
- Grunting with breathing and no distress

YES — "Call back or call PCP for appointment if no improvement" and Follow **Home Care Instructions**

NO — Follow **Home Care Instructions**

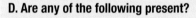

Home Care Instructions
Newborn Problems

Provide Reassurance
- Swollen breasts are normal in the first week of life.
- Red streaks in the white part of the eye are related to the birthing process and will resolve in 2 to 3 weeks.
- Watery eyes are often a result of a blocked tear duct and will resolve within a year. Watch for signs of infection, redness, swelling, and drainage.
- A clear, white, or pink-tinged vaginal discharge is normal and will resolve in 2 to 3 days.
- Swelling in the scrotum will resolve in 6 to 12 months.
- Tips for awakening a sleepy newborn:
  - Unwrap blankets and undress the newborn.
  - Change the diaper.
  - Massage the newborn's legs, back, and arms.
  - Give the newborn a back rub by walking fingers down the spine.
  - Perform "sit-ups" by holding the newborn away from you and gently lifting the newborn toward your face.
- See "Other Protocols to Consider" (421) for associated symptoms or conditions and additional home care instructions.

Additional Instructions

N

Report the Following Problems to Your PCP/Clinic/ED
- Refusal to drink >6 hours
- Umbilical cord bleeding >10 minutes of direct pressure
- Red streaks or red area around umbilicus
- Clumps of blisters on one part of body
- Breathing quickly, grunting when breathing, or nasal flaring
- Difficult to comfort
- Newborn >7 days of age with yellow skin
- Pale or blue skin, lips, or nail beds
- No stool >24 hours or white-, yellow-, or clay-colored stools
- No improvement or condition worsens
- Newborn looks or acts sick

Seek Emergency Care Immediately If Any of the Following Occur

- Seizure
- Unresponsiveness
- Temperature >100.4°F (38°C)
- Bulging soft spot with vomiting, fever, or a newborn that acts sick
- Nonblanching rash of dark red or purple spots

If the caller agrees with the advice given, document the call and encourage the caller to call back or see PCP if the problem worsens. If the caller does not agree with the advice given, reevaluate and advise the caller to follow up with PCP, Clinic, or ED.

Nosebleed

 Key Questions Name, Age, Onset, Cause, Medications, History

 Other Protocols to Consider Bleeding, Severe (90); Foreign Body, Nose (274); Headache (308); Head Injury (311); Hypertension (347); Nose Injury (428); Piercing Problems (445).

Reminder: Document caller response to advice, home care instructions, and when to call back.

ASSESSMENT	ACTION
A. Are any of the following present?	
• Unable to stop the bleeding after 30 minutes of constant pressure • Altered mental status • Rapid heart rate, pale skin, or shortness of breath	**YES** "Seek emergency care now" **NO** Go to B
B. Are any of the following present?	
• Difficulty breathing (for reasons other than a stuffy nose) • Light-headedness, dizziness • Nosebleed follows a severe headache • History of high blood pressure or bleeding disorder • Taking blood-thinning medications, aspirin, or nonsteroidal anti-inflammatory drugs and persistent nosebleeds • Foreign body in nose and profuse bleeding • Recent head injury and bloody or fluid nasal drainage	**YES** "Seek medical care within 2 hours" **NO** Go to C
C. Are any of the following present?	
• Recent injury and persistent deformity or obstruction • More than three nosebleeds in the past 48 hours • Recent nasal surgery, bleeding has stopped and restarted • Recent nasal surgery and persistent bleeding	**YES** "Seek medical care within 24 hours" **NO** Go to D

N

D. Are any of the following present?

- History of allergies or hay fever
- History of frequent controlled nosebleeds
- History of repetitive use of nasal sprays
- Frequent use of cocaine

YES   "Call back or call PCP for appointment if no improvement" and Follow **Home Care Instructions**

NO   Follow **Home Care Instructions**

Home Care Instructions
Nosebleed

- In a sitting position, with the head bent forward, firmly pinch the nose closed for 15 minutes with an ice-cold washcloth. Breathe through the mouth.
- If the bleeding stops but then recurs, pinch the nose closed for another 15 minutes.
- Do not blow nose.
- Avoid aspirin and anti-inflammatory products.
- Avoid smoking and strenuous activity for 24 hours after a nosebleed.
- Keep mucous membranes moist. Use saline nasal drops or spray several times a day.
- Avoid hot liquids (such as soup, coffee, or tea).
- Use a humidifier in your bedroom to help keep nasal passages moist.

Additional Instructions

Report the Following Problems to Your PCP/Clinic/ED
- Difficulty breathing, light-headedness, or dizziness
- Problem persists or worsens

Seek Emergency Care Immediately If Any of the Following Occur
- Change in mental status
- Rapid heart rate, pale skin, or shortness of breath
- Bleeding persists after >30 minutes of pressure

If the caller agrees with the advice given, document the call and encourage the caller to call back or see PCP if the problem worsens. If the caller does not agree with the advice given, reevaluate and advise the caller to follow up with PCP, Clinic, or ED.

Nose Injury

 Key Questions Name, Age, Onset, Cause, Associated Symptoms, Medications, History, Pain Scale

 Other Protocols to Consider Headache (308); Head Injury (311); Laceration (395); Nosebleed (425); Piercing Problems (445).

Nurse Alert:

- A neck injury should always be considered whenever there is a blow to the head. Assess for weakness, incoordination, numbness, and neck pain.
- Altered mental status may be one of the first signs of a head injury after trauma to the head, particularly in a child or the elderly.

Reminder: Document caller response to advice, home care instructions, and when to call back.

ASSESSMENT	ACTION

A. Blow to the nose, and are any of the following present?

- Persistent bleeding for >30 minutes
- Signs of head injury:
  - lethargy
  - confusion/combativeness
  - difficulty speaking
  - visual disturbance
  - severe headache
  - coordination problems
  - nausea and/or vomiting
- Sudden onset of neck pain, numbness, tingling, or weakness in arms
- Persistent clear or pink nasal drainage

YES "Call ambulance" or "Seek emergency care now"

NO Go to B

B. Are any of the following present?

- History of sinus surgery
- Gaping, split or jagged, or deep wound

YES "Seek medical care within 2 to 4 hours"

NO Go to C

C. Are any of the following present?

- Deformity after 72 hours and home care measures
- Difficulty breathing through one or both nostrils after swelling has subsided

YES "Seek medical care within 24 hours"

NO Go to D

↓

D. Are any of the following present?

- Nasal swelling
- Pain
- Controlled nosebleed
- Abrasion or bruising around nose and eyes
- Nose appears deformed the first 24 to 72 hours after injury

YES "Call back or call PCP for appointment if no improvement" and Follow **Home Care Instructions**

NO Follow **Home Care Instructions**

Home Care Instructions
Nose Injury

- Apply ice pack to nose for 20 to 30 minutes every 2 hours for the first 48 hours to help reduce swelling and pain. Do not apply ice directly to the skin. Wrap ice in a towel or washcloth.
- To stop a nosebleed, apply continuous pressure to the soft part of the nose for 15 minutes. Sit up and lean forward. Avoid swallowing blood; spit it out. Breathe through mouth.
- If bleeding stops but then recurs, pinch the nose closed for another 15 minutes.
- Expect swelling, bruising, and deformity for the first 48 to 72 hours.

Additional Instructions

Report the Following Problems to Your PCP/Clinic/ED

- Deformity lasting >72 hours after swelling subsides
- Difficulty breathing through one or both nostrils
- No improvement or condition worsens

Seek Emergency Care Immediately If Any of the Following Occur

- Persistent bleeding for >30 minutes
- Signs of head injury:
  - lethargy
  - confusion, combativeness
  - difficulty speaking
  - visual disturbance
  - severe headache
  - coordination problems
  - nausea and/or vomiting
- Sudden onset of neck pain, numbness, tingling, or weakness in arms
- Persistent clear or pink nasal drainage

If the caller agrees with the advice given, document the call and encourage the caller to call back or see PCP if the problem worsens. If the caller does not agree with the advice given, reevaluate and advise the caller to follow up with PCP, Clinic, or ED.

Numbness and Tingling

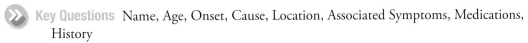

Key Questions Name, Age, Onset, Cause, Location, Associated Symptoms, Medications, History

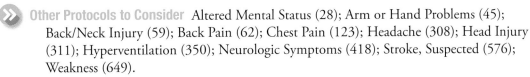

Other Protocols to Consider Altered Mental Status (28); Arm or Hand Problems (45); Back/Neck Injury (59); Back Pain (62); Chest Pain (123); Headache (308); Head Injury (311); Hyperventilation (350); Neurologic Symptoms (418); Stroke, Suspected (576); Weakness (649).

Nurse Alert:

- Sudden changes in vision, weakness, numbness, speech, or mental status may be signs of a stroke or other serious neurologic disorder. Prompt treatment may prevent extensive damage to the brain or spinal cord and reduce permanent disability. Medications used to break up a clot in the brain need to be administered within 3 hours of symptom onset.
- Ask how current condition is different from normal.

Reminder: Document caller response to advice, home care instructions, and when to call back.

N

ASSESSMENT	ACTION

A. Are any of the following present?

- Confusion
- Change in mental status

YES Go to Altered Mental Status protocol (28)

NO Go to B

B. Is the following present?

- Severe headache

YES Go to Headache protocol (308)

NO Go to C

C. Are any of the following present?

- One side of the body affected
- Sudden weakness in arms and/or legs
- Difficulty speaking, slurred speech
- Blurred vision
- Loss of bladder or bowel control
- Fingers or toes are cold or blue compared with the other fingers or toes
- Headache prior to onset of symptoms
- Chest pain

YES → "Call ambulance" or "Seek emergency care now"

NO → Go to D

D. Are any of the following present?

- History of recent heavy lifting or strenuous exercise
- Area painful, swollen, and/or warm
- Severe pain

YES → "Seek medical care within 2 to 4 hours"

NO → Go to E

E. Are any of the following present?

- Numbness, tingling, and/or a sharp pain in the hand or arm at night
- History of recent illness or surgery
- Gradual onset
- Stiff or painful neck and no known injury
- Diagnosed carpal tunnel and worsening symptoms
- Pregnant

YES → "Seek medical care within 24 hours"

NO → Go to F

F. Are any of the following present?

- Symptoms followed prolonged sitting or lying in one position
- Rapid breathing, dizziness, and hands, face, or lips affected

YES → "Call back or call PCP for appointment if no improvement" and Follow **Home Care Instructions**

NO → Follow **Home Care Instructions**

Home Care Instructions
Numbness and Tingling

- Avoid sitting in one position for long periods of time.
- Periodically tighten and release muscles in affected area to stimulate circulation.
- Protect numb area from injury.
- To slow rapid breathing and control numbness and tingling, see next page.
- Avoid repetitive motions; take breaks and do stretching exercises.
- Apply heat or cold to stiff neck.
- Sit down and focus on slowing breathing, one breath every 5 seconds.
- Cover mouth and nose with a paper bag and breathe in and out 10 times.
- If no improvement, continue breathing in the bag for 5 to 15 minutes.
- Breathe without the bag for a few minutes.
- Repeat breathing with and without the bag until condition improves.

Additional Instructions

Report the Following Problems to Your PCP/Clinic/ED

- No improvement in 20 to 30 minutes or condition worsens
- Symptoms interfere with daily activities

Seek Emergency Care Immediately If Any of the Following Occur

- Change in mental status
- Sudden weakness on one side of body
- Difficulty speaking or slurred speech
- Loss of bowel or bladder control
- Chest pain
- Vision changes
- Fingers or toes are blue

If the caller agrees with the advice given, document the call and encourage the caller to call back or see PCP if the problem worsens. If the caller does not agree with the advice given, reevaluate and advise the caller to follow up with PCP, Clinic, or ED.

Ostomy Problems

>> **Key Questions** Name, Age, Onset, Cause, Type of Ostomy or Reason for Pouch, Medications, History

>> **Other Protocols to Consider** Abdominal Pain, Adult (9), Child (13); Bleeding, Severe (90); Constipation (160); Wound Healing and Infection (664).

Nurse Alert: Use this protocol if the person has an ostomy and has concerns or questions.

Reminder: Document caller response to advice, home care instructions, and when to call back.

ASSESSMENT	ACTION
A. Are any of the following present?	
• Severe bleeding from stoma • Severe abdominal pain or swelling • Persistent vomiting • Fever and abdomen tender or rigid • Constipation, abdominal pain, swelling, and vomiting	**YES** "Call ambulance" or "Seek emergency care now" **NO** Go to B
B. Are any of the following present?	
• Urostomy and temperature >100.4°F (38°C) and urine is pink, red, or unusually cloudy • Nausea, loss of appetite, and abdominal pain • Drainage leaking into a surgical wound • Taking blood-thinning medication and new onset of bleeding at stoma site or urine is pink or red • No ostomy drainage • Blood in stool	**YES** "Seek medical care within 2 to 4 hours" **NO** Go to C
C. Are any of the following present?	
• No bowel movement for >4 days and constipation unresponsive to home care measures • Unable to manage the ostomy or pouch wound	**YES** "Seek medical care within 24 hours" **NO** Go to D

D. Are any of the following present?

- Small amount of bleeding at the stoma site
- New onset of itching and burning at ostomy or pouch site
- Decreased ostomy drainage
- Mild constipation
- New medication and change in normal bowel habits

YES "Call back or call PCP for appointment if no improvement" and Follow **Home Care Instructions**

NO Follow **Home Care Instructions**

0

Home Care Instructions
Ostomy Problems

Ostomy Care
- Check appliance and make sure parts are snapped securely together.
- If the ostomy is leaking, remove the appliance, clean the skin with water, dry well, and prepare the skin as directed by a nurse or PCP; apply the new appliance. Hold in place for 5 minutes to ensure pouch seals to the skin.
- Take prescribed medications as directed.
- Empty ileostomy pouch when 1/3-1/2 full.
- Soap can interfere with skin barrier adhesive; discuss with the ET nurse or the provider before using soap to cleanse area around the stoma.
- Change skin barrier regularly—usually every 3 to 4 days or as directed by the provider.
- Skin around the stoma should be clean and dry before applying a skin barrier and new appliance.

Bleeding Stoma
- Remember that a small amount of bleeding is normal, and tissues bleed easily, similar to the bleeding of the gums after brushing teeth.

Constipation
- Make sure the diet is adequate in volume, bulk (high fiber), and fluids (6 to 8 glasses a day, unless on a fluid-restricted diet).
- Drink a hot beverage each morning, such as coffee, tea, hot water with lemon, or prune juice.
- Follow the prescribed plan for using stool softeners, laxatives, and irrigation.
- When taking medications with codeine or other medications that increase constipation, follow the constipation prevention plan prescribed by the PCP.

Additional Instructions

Report the Following Problems to Your PCP/Clinic/ED

- Fever or bleeding persists or worsens
- Constipation persists or worsens after home care measures
- Drainage leaking into a surgical wound
- Persistent leakage after home care measures
- Itching and burning persist after use of prescribed medication
- Blood in stool
- Persistent diarrhea
- New buldge in skin around the stoma.
- Persistent skin irritation unresponsive to home care measures.

Seek Emergency Care Immediately If Any of the Following Occur

- Severe bleeding
- Severe abdominal pain or swelling
- Persistent vomiting
- Fever and abdomen is tender and rigid

If the caller agrees with the advice given, document the call and encourage the caller to call back or see PCP if the problem worsens. If the caller does not agree with the advice given, reevaluate and advise the caller to follow up with PCP, Clinic, or ED.

Overdose

Key Questions Name, Age, Onset, Name of Medication(s) or Substance(s), Amount, History, Medications

Other Protocols to Consider Depression (184); Diarrhea, Adult (192), Child (195); Mental Health Challenges in Telephone Triage (App V, 720) Poisoning, Suspected (454); Substance Abuse, Use, or Exposure (582); Suicide Attempt, Threat (585); Vomiting, Adult (642), Child (645).

Reminder: Document caller response to advice, home care instructions, and when to call back.

ASSESSMENT	ACTION

A. Suspected overdose, and are any of the following present?

- Severe difficulty breathing or respiratory rate
  <10 breaths per minute
- Chest pain
- Suicide attempt
- Seizure activity
- Combined alcohol and drug overdose
- Intoxication in a victim younger than 17 years
- Cocaine/crack use and chest pain
- Change in mental status

YES "Call ambulance"

NO Go to B

B. Possible drug ingestion, and are any of the following present?

- Wheezing or shortness of breath
- Severe abdominal pain

YES "Seek emergency care now" and
Follow **Home Care Instructions**

NO Go to C

C. Possible ingestion, no symptoms, and are any of the following present?

- Nausea, vomiting, or diarrhea
- Ingestion of aspirin, acetaminophen, or other OTC medication, hallucinogen, or unknown mushroom
- Victim is a child in the presence of open spilled containers, such as pill bottles, or has substance on face, skin, or clothes
- Smell of suspected ingested product on breath or clothes

YES "Call Poison Control Center" (Telephone number: 1-800-222-1222) and Follow **Home Care Instructions**

NO "Call back or call PCP for appointment if no improvement" and Follow **Home Care Instructions**

0

Home Care Instructions
Overdose

- Follow instructions as directed by the Poison Control Center (Telephone number: 1-800-222-1222). Provide the Center with the following information:
  - Identify the substance ingested. Read the exact name off the label on the container, including the strength, or describe the markings on the pill or capsule.
  - Describe how much was ingested or is missing from the container.
  - Indicate time the substance was ingested.
- Read the instructions on the container for accidental ingestion.
- Take the container or mushroom with you to the hospital.
- If the Poison Control Center's telephone number is not readily available, call an ambulance.
- Do not induce vomiting if the person has an altered level of consciousness or has difficulty swallowing. Do not induce vomiting until directed to do so by the Poison Control Center. Do not induce vomiting if acid, alkalis, or petroleum products were ingested, including battery, sulfuric or hydrochloric acid; bleach; Drano; drain or oven cleaners; gasoline; furniture polish; kerosene; or lighter fluid. Neutralize with milk, water, or milk of magnesia.
- All overdoses should be evaluated by a physician unless told by the Poison Control Center that the ingestion is nothing to be concerned about.
- Do not try to arouse an overdose victim by placing him/her in the shower or forcing coffee.
- Do not give anything to eat or drink unless instructed to do so by the Poison Control Center, or as instructed above when the Poison Control Center is unavailable.

Additional Instructions

Report the Following Problems to Your PCP/Clinic/ED

- Persistent problems or illness after initial treatment
- Suicide attempt or threat
- Unsure whether or not a substance was ingested and nausea or vomiting occurs

If the caller agrees with the advice given, document the call and encourage the caller to call back or see PCP if the problem worsens. If the caller does not agree with the advice given, reevaluate and advise the caller to follow up with PCP, Clinic, or ED.

Pertussis (Whooping Cough)

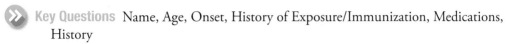 **Key Questions** Name, Age, Onset, History of Exposure/Immunization, Medications, History

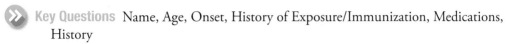 **Other Protocols to Consider** Breathing Problems (106); Common Cold Symptoms (146); Congestion (153); Cough (170); Croup (173); Fever, Adult (250), Child (253).

Nurse Alert:

- Use the protocol if previously diagnosed with pertussis, for known or suspected exposure to pertussis, recent local community outbreak of pertussis, and severe cough. Pertussis is highly contagious.
- Communicable Disease Table in Appendix M (696) is provided to help the nurse gain a better understanding of many communicable diseases, the mode of disease transmission, incubation period, and contagious period. It is NOT to be used to try and diagnose a caller's condition.

Reminder: Document caller response to advice, home care instructions, and when to call back.

ASSESSMENT	ACTION

A. Are any of the following present?

- Altered mental status
- Severe difficulty breathing
- Difficulty breathing and unable to speak
- Seizures
- Apnea
- New onset of drooling
- Unable to swallow
- Nonblanching dark red or purple rash, headache, pain bending head forward, or fever

YES "Call ambulance" or "Seek emergency care now"

NO Go to B

P

B. Are any of the following present?

- Skin, lips, or tongue turns blue during coughing spells
- Productive or severe cough
- High fever unresponsive to fever-reducing measures
- Infant unable to feed due to coughing
- Persistent nosebleed
- Fever and signs of dehydration
- Infant, 3 months old or younger (no recent immunization) and temperature >100.4°F (38°C)
- Cough and cold symptoms >1 week and chest pain, weakness, fever

YES "Seek medical care immediately"

NO Go to C

C. Are any of the following present?

- Family members and classmates exposed to person with known pertussis and request prophylaxis
- Cough lasting >2 weeks
- Subconjunctival hemorrhage
- Rectal prolapse or abdominal hernia and persistent coughing
- Fever >72 hours and unresponsive to fever-reducing measures
- Taking antibiotics for pertussis and persistent fever or worsening condition
- Green, brown, or yellow sputum >72 hours
- Coughing up blood

YES "Seek medical care within 24 hours"

NO Go to D

D. Is the following present?

- Community epidemic and recent onset of runny nose, cough, watery eyes

YES "Call back or call PCP for appointment if no improvement" and Follow **Home Care Instructions**

NO Follow **Home Care Instructions**

Home Care Instructions
Pertussis

- Practice good respiratory hygiene. Cover mouth when coughing or sneezing. Discard tissues in a paper bag. Cough into sleeve to help prevent droplets from contaminating others. Bend elbow and raise upper arm to cover mouth.
- Practice good handwashing to help prevent transmission of the disease. Wash with soap and water or alcohol-based hand rub.
- Take antibiotics as prescribed, and finish the complete course.
- Sip warm liquids to soothe coughing spasms.
- Give small frequent feedings.
- Avoid cough triggers (smoke, pollutants, etc.).
- Give acetaminophen (if infant older than 2 months) or ibuprofen (if older than 6 months) for fever and achiness. Do not give aspirin to a child. Avoid aspirin-like products if age <20 years. Avoid acetaminophen if liver disease is present. Avoid ibuprofen if kidney disease or stomach problems exist or in the case of pregnancy. Follow the directions on the label.
- Increase fluid consumption (juices, tea, broths, gelatin).
- Expected course: 1 to 2 weeks of cold symptoms followed by severe coughing spells. Can last up to 6 weeks. Chronic cough can last for 1 to 2 months.
- Once diagnosed, avoid public contact until on antibiotics for at least 3 days. Pertussis is highly contagious.

Additional Instructions

Report the Following Problems to Your PCP/Clinic/ED
- No improvement or condition worsens
- Fever >72 hours
- Green, brown, or yellow sputum develops and lasts >72 hours
- Coughing up blood
- Signs of dehydration

Seek Emergency Care Immediately If Any of the Following Occur
- Breathing worsens
- Skin, lips, or tongue blue or gray
- Chest pain
- New onset of drooling or unable to swallow
- Altered mental status
- Seizures
- Nonblanching dark red or purple rash, headache, pain bending head forward, or fever

If the caller agrees with the advice given, document the call and encourage the caller to call back or see PCP if the problem worsens. If the caller does not agree with the advice given, reevaluate and advise the caller to follow up with PCP, Clinic, or ED.

Piercing/Pocketing Problems

 Key Questions Name, Age, Onset, Cause, Allergies, Type, Location and Age of Piercing or Pocketing, Medications, Pain Scale, History

 Other Protocols to Consider Ear Injury, Foreign Body (209); Foreign Body, Skin (278); Genital Lesions (291); Genital Problems, Male (294); Lacerations (395); Mouth Problems (407); Skin Lesions: Lumps, Bumps, and Sores (556); Wound Healing and Infection (664).

Reminder: Document caller response to advice, home care instructions, and when to call back.

ASSESSMENT	ACTION
A. Are any of the following present 2 to 4 days after the piercing/pocketing?	

- Rapidly increasing pain, swelling, or redness
- Red streaks extending from wound
- White, yellow, or green foul-smelling wound drainage
- Fever
- Enlarged nodes (>1 inch in diameter) and overlying redness
- Gaping laceration to earlobe, eyelid, eyebrow, tongue, nipple, or genitals
- Unable to remove embedded piercing or other foreign object

YES "Seek medical care within 2 to 4 hours"

NO Go to B

P

445

B. Are any of the following present?

- Increased pain or swelling
- Increased redness or red streaks extending from inflamed area
- Enlarged nodes (>1 inch in diameter)
- Thick white, yellow, or green foul-smelling drainage
- Temperature >100.4°F (38°C)
- Chills, feeling of illness, or headache
- No improvement with home care measures
- Warmth over the area
- Darkened hard and painful area around the piercing
- Minor tear from piercing and last tetanus shot >10 years
- No improvement after 3 days of home care

YES "Seek medical care within 24 hours"

NO Go to C

C. Are any of the following present?

- Small blisters, redness, and/or itching around the piercing
- Bleeding, bruising, discoloration, or swelling
- White-yellow crust at jewelry opening
- White thick secretion at opening
- Tongue turns yellow-white

YES "Call back or call PCP for appointment if no improvement" and Follow **Home Care Instructions**

NO Follow **Home Care Instructions**

Home Care Instructions
Piercing/Pocketing Problems

- Apply a cotton ball or gauze pad saturated in salt water solution (¼ tsp in 1 cup water) to pierced area several times a day for at least 1 minute. Rinse with clear water and pat dry with paper products.
- Apply salt water soaks before cleaning the piercing and before activity to prevent the crust from being pulled into the piercing, and remove matter.
- Remember that healing times can vary and that stinging, burning, or aching may persist for several days. Itching usually is a sign of healing.
- Avoid aspirin during the healing period. OTC medication (ibuprofen or acetaminophen) can help to relieve the discomfort and reduce swelling. Do not give aspirin to a child. Avoid aspirin-like products if age <20 years. Avoid acetaminophen if liver disease is present. Avoid ibuprofen if kidney disease or stomach problems exist or in the case of pregnancy. Follow the directions on the label.
- Elevate head of the bed for above-the-neck piercing.
- Do not use alcohol, povidone–iodine (Betadine), peroxide, or other harsh cleaners on piercing. They will cause excessive drying.
- Do not apply ointments to the piercing. They may trap bacteria in the piercing and delay healing.

Cleaning Body Piercing

- Using recommended cleaning solution, clean the piercing 1 to 2 times a day throughout the healing period, usually 6 to 8 weeks (6 to 12 months for ear cartilage, hand web, navel, and penis or clitoris piercings).
- Wash hands with antibacterial soap. Do not touch the healing piercing unless hands are clean.
- Apply cleaning solution to the piercing and jewelry.
- After the first several cleanings, rotate the jewelry to make sure the solution reaches all areas of the piercing.
- Allow cleaning solution to remain on the piercing for 1 minute.
- Rinse the area under running water and rotate jewelry.
- Pat dry with disposable paper products.

Oral Piercings

- Rinse the mouth for 30 to 60 seconds with saline solution (¼ tsp salt with 1 cup water) after meals, but no >4 to 5 times a day.
- If the tongue begins to turn yellow-white, reduce the number of cleansings per day.
- Use a new, soft-bristle brush to gently clean the mouth and around the piercing.
- Keep the mouth as hygienic as possible throughout the healing period. Remember the piercing is an open wound similar to a cut and should be treated properly to prevent infection.

P

Additional Instructions

Report the Following Problems to Your PCP/Clinic/ED

- No improvement or condition worsens after home care measures
- Increased pain or swelling
- Increased redness or red streaks extending from inflamed area
- Thick white, yellow, or green foul-smelling drainage
- Temperature >100.4°F (38°C)
- Warmth over the area
- Darkened hard and painful area around the piercing

If the caller agrees with the advice given, document the call and encourage the caller to call back or see PCP if the problem worsens. If the caller does not agree with the advice given, reevaluate and advise the caller to follow up with PCP, Clinic, or ED.

Pinkeye

>> **Key Questions** Name, Age, Onset, Cause, Eye Appears Pink or Red, History, Medications, Pain Scale

>> **Other Protocols to Consider** Contact Lens Problem (163); Eye Injury (225); Eye Problems (228); Foreign Body, Eye (269); Vision Problems (639).

> *Nurse Alert:* Use this protocol if previously diagnosed with pinkeye, known or suspected exposure to someone with pinkeye, and eye appears pink or red. Pinkeye is highly contagious.

Reminder: Document caller response to advice, home care instructions, and when to call back.

ASSESSMENT	ACTION
A. Are any of the following present?	
• Injury to the eye • Foreign body in the eye	**YES** Go to Eye Injury protocol (225) or Foreign Body, Eye protocol (269)
	NO Go to B
B. Are any of the following present?	
• History of glaucoma • Abdominal pain or nausea • Unable to move eye • Partial loss of field of vision	**YES** "Seek emergency care now" **NO** Go to C
C. Are any of the following present?	
• Red swollen eyelids • Ulcer or gray-white sore on eyeball • Severe pain • Flashes of light • Age younger than 5 years and severe redness or swelling around eye	**YES** "Seek medical care within 2 to 4 hours" **NO** Go to D

P

449

D. Are any of the following present?

- Persistent blinking, tearing with pain
- Yellow/green eye discharge
- Eyelids slightly puffy with red rims
- Blurred vision
- Sensitivity to light
- History of previous eye infections
- Eyelids stuck together upon awakening
- Redness >7 days
- Exposure to welders or ultraviolet light
- Earache on same side as pinkeye

YES "Seek medical care within 24 hours"

NO Go to E

E. Are any of the following present?

- Blood in the white part of the eye with no change in vision
- Cold symptoms: congestion, earache, sore throat, or cough
- Exposure to environmental irritants: smog, smoke, pool water, shampoo, onions, household cleaning products, or jalapeño peppers
- History of hay fever or allergies, and eye itching
- Clear eye discharge

YES "Call back or call PCP for appointment if no improvement" and Follow **Home Care Instructions**

NO Follow **Home Care Instructions**

Home Care Instructions
Pinkeye

- Rinse eyes frequently with warm water, every 1 to 2 hours when awake. Use a soft warm moist cloth to remove crusting and drainage.
- If exposed to chemical irritants, rinse eyes with warm water for 5 minutes.
- Apply alternating warm and cold compresses to eyes for 10 minutes every 2 hours for 24 hours.
- Do not share towels or linens with other household members.
- To control itching, try Benadryl for 24 to 48 hours. Follow instructions on the label.
- Encourage children to avoid touching eyes and to wash hands frequently.

Additional Instructions

Report the Following Problems to Your PCP/Clinic/ED

- Red swollen eyelids
- Ulcer or gray-white sore on eyeball
- Severe pain
- Flashes of light
- Persistent blinking, tearing, or pain
- Persistent eye drainage

Seek Emergency Care Immediately If Any of the Following Occur

- Unable to move eye
- Abdominal pain or nausea

If the caller agrees with the advice given, document the call and encourage the caller to call back or see PCP if the problem worsens. If the caller does not agree with the advice given, reevaluate and advise the caller to follow up with PCP, Clinic, or ED.

P

Pinworms

 Key Questions Name, Age, Onset, Known or Suspected Pinworms, Medications, History

 Other Protocols to Consider Bedbug Exposure or Concerns (67); Itching (382); Rectal Problems (513).

Reminder: Document caller response to advice, home care instructions, and when to call back.

ASSESSMENT		ACTION
A. Are any of the following present?		
• Signs of infection (pain, swelling, redness, drainage, warmth, or fever) in rectal area	**YES**	"Seek medical care within 24 hours"
• Severe rectal itching worsening at night and early morning	**NO**	Go to B
• ¼ to ½ inch white, thread-like worms in rectal or vaginal area		
• Worms visible in stool		
B. Are any of the following present?		
• Mild redness, itching, or tenderness in rectal area	**YES**	"Call back or call PCP for appointment if no improvement" and Follow **Home Care Instructions**
• Child has difficulty sleeping, irritability, or vaginal irritation		
• Exposed to bedclothes or bed linens of child with pinworms	**NO**	Follow **Home Care Instructions**
• Rectal symptoms persist >1 week after treatment		
• Family member diagnosed with pinworms and concerned about transmission		

Home Care Instructions
Pinworms

- To detect pinworms in a child, shine a light on the child's anus in a darkened room several hours after bedtime. If present, the worms will move back into the anus.
- Trim nails closely and encourage good handwashing.
- Discourage nail biting or thumb sucking.
- Wash linen and underwear in hot soapy water until pinworms are gone.
- Vacuum or mop bedroom daily for 2 weeks after treatment.
- Bathe every morning and clean the affected area. Showers are preferable.
- Wear shorts or panties under pajamas.
- To reduce itching:
  - Apply zinc oxide or 1% hydrocortisone cream ointment to affected area.
  - Take a warm bath with Epsom salts or table salt.
- A prescription medication may be necessary to eliminate the pinworms. Take medication completely and as directed.
- Try OTC pinworm medication (Reese's) and follow instructions on the label.

Additional Instructions

Report the Following Problems to Your PCP/Clinic/ED

- Signs of infection: pain, swelling, redness, drainage, or warmth
- Condition persists >3 weeks after treatment

If the caller agrees with the advice given, document the call and encourage the caller to call back or see PCP if the problem worsens. If the caller does not agree with the advice given, reevaluate and advise the caller to follow up with PCP, Clinic, or ED.

Poisoning, Suspected

 Key Questions Name, Age, Onset, Cause, History, Associated Symptoms, Medications

 Other Protocols to Consider Depression (184); Diarrhea, Adult (192), Child (195); Food Poisoning, Suspected (262); Overdose (438); Substance Abuse, Use, or Exposure (582); Suicide Attempt, Threat (585); Vomiting, Adult (642), Child (645).

Nurse Alert: Use this protocol if known or suspected poisoning. Ask what was swallowed, how much, when, and any associated symptoms. Ask about other children who might have also been exposed who might not readily volunteer the information if they think they might be in trouble.

Reminder: Document caller response to advice, home care instructions, and when to call back.

ASSESSMENT	ACTION
A. Are any of the following present?	
<ul><li>Altered mental status, unresponsive</li><li>Severe difficulty breathing or respirations <10 breaths per minute</li><li>Chest pain</li><li>Suicide attempt</li><li>Seizure activity</li><li>Change in level of consciousness</li></ul>	**YES** "Call ambulance and take container and substance with you to hospital." Instruct to start CPR or rescue breathing if no pulse or respirations **NO** Go to B
B. Are any of the following present?	
<ul><li>Excessive sweating or saliva</li><li>Wheezing or shortness of breath</li><li>Blue lips, mouth, or nail beds</li></ul>	**YES** "Seek emergency care now and take container and substance with you to hospital" **NO** Go to C

C. Are any of the following present?

- Nausea, vomiting, diarrhea
- Abdominal pain
- Burns on lips, tongue, or skin
- Palpitations
- Headache, irritability, or fever
- History of psychiatric problems

YES "Seek medical care now" and Follow **Home Care Instructions**

NO Go to D

D. Are any of the following present and no symptoms?

- Children with open spilled containers, pill bottles, or substance on face, skin, or clothes
- Smell of product on breath or clothes
- Suspected ingestion of aspirin, acetaminophen, or other OTC medication, hallucinogen, or unknown mushroom

YES "Call Poison Control" (Telephone number: 1-800-222-1222) and Follow **Home Care Instructions**

NO "Call back or call PCP for appointment if no improvement" and Follow **Home Care Instructions**

P

Home Care Instructions
Poisoning, Suspected

- Follow instructions as directed by the Poison Control Center. Provide the Center with the following information:
  - Identify the substance ingested. Read the exact name from the container label.
  - Describe how much was ingested or is missing from the container.
  - Indicate the time the substance was ingested.
- Read the instructions on the container for accidental ingestion.
- Take the container, remaining contents, plant, or mushroom with you to the hospital.
- If the Poison Control Center is not readily available, call an ambulance.
- Do not induce vomiting if the person has an altered level of consciousness or has difficulty swallowing. Do not induce vomiting until directed to do so by the Poison Control Center. Do not induce vomiting if any of the following have been ingested: acid, alkalis, or petroleum products; battery, sulfuric or hydrochloric acid; bleach; drain or oven cleaners; gasoline; furniture polish; kerosene; or lighter fluid.
- All overdoses should be evaluated by a physician unless the Poison Control Center indicates there is no reason for concern.
- Do not try to arouse the victim by placing in the shower or forcing the ingestion of coffee.
- Do not give anything to eat or drink unless instructed to do so by the Poison Control Center.

Additional Instructions

Report the Following Problems to Poison Control

- Persistent problems or illness after initial treatment
- Unsure whether or not substance was ingested and nausea or vomiting occurs

Seek Emergency Care Immediately If Any of the Following Occur

- Excessive swallowing or saliva
- Wheezing or breathing problems
- Blue lips, mouth, or nail beds

If the caller agrees with the advice given, document the call and encourage the caller to call back or see PCP if the problem worsens. If the caller does not agree with the advice given, reevaluate and advise the caller to follow up with PCP, Clinic, or ED.

Postoperative Problems

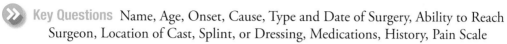 **Key Questions** Name, Age, Onset, Cause, Type and Date of Surgery, Ability to Reach Surgeon, Location of Cast, Splint, or Dressing, Medications, History, Pain Scale

Other Protocols to Consider Bleeding, Severe (90); Breathing Problems (106); Cast/Splint Problems (121); Chest Pain (123); Constipation (160); Fever, Adult (250), Child (253); Leg Pain/Swelling (398); Vomiting, Adult (642), Child (645); Swelling (597); Weakness (649); Wound Care: Sutures or Staples (660); Wound Healing and Infection (664).

Reminder: Document caller response to advice, home care instructions, and when to call back.

ASSESSMENT	ACTION
A. Are any of the following present?	
• Sudden onset of severe pain	**YES** "Call ambulance" or "Seek emergency care now"
• Surgical wound split or gaping and large amount of fluid drainage or material protruding from the wound	
• If cast, splint, or orthopedic surgery:	**NO** Go to B
• fingers or toes cold, blue, or numb	
• severe pain, swelling, or tightness unresponsive to elevation or home care measures	
• Chest pain	
• Coughing up blood or pink frothy sputum	
• Leg swelling and no pulse in foot of affected leg, numbness, or tingling	
• Shortness of breath	

P

457

B. Are any of the following present?

- Surgical wound split or gaping
- Signs of infection (pain, swelling, drainage, warmth, or red streaks extending from the wound)
- Swelling and pain in thigh, calf, ankle, or toes
- Dressing, splint, or cast feels too tight
- Large amount of bleeding from incision and unresponsive to home care measures
- Area over ankle, calf, shin, or thigh is warm to the touch or red
- Sudden swelling in one leg or ankle
- Temperature >100.4°F (38°C)

YES "Seek medical care within hours"

NO Go to C

C. Are any of the following present?

- History of diabetes, HIV infection, chronic disease, use of steroids, blood thinners, or chemotherapy and wound is not healing well
- Pain gradually worsens
- Pain unrelieved by prescribed medication
- Cracked or unstable cast, splint, or appliance
- Persistent oozing or bleeding at the incision site
- Persistent nausea and vomiting

YES "Seek medical care within 24 hours"

NO Go to D

D. Are any of the following present?

- Itching around wound edges
- Persistent swelling or tightness within cast or splint but improves with home care measures
- Small amount of bloody drainage on dressing
- Constipation
- Has questions about activity or diet
- Wound vacuum-assisted closure (VAC) device in place and
  - leaking
  - container full
  - turned off for 8 hours or more

YES "Call back or call PCP for appointment if no improvement" and Follow **Home Care Instructions**

NO Follow **Home Care Instructions**

Home Care Instructions
Postoperative Problems

- Take pain medications at regular intervals.
- Follow home care plan as directed by PCP, including antibiotics, wound checks, exercise, diet, bowel care, and elevation.
- Keep wound clean and dry as directed by PCP.
- Remember that itching along the edges of the wound is a sign of healing.
- If dressing is loose or there is a small amount of drainage, reinforce dressing. Remember that some drainage usually is expected.
- After orthopedic surgery, apply ice pack over the dressing for the first 48 hours.
- If there is a moderate to severe amount of bleeding, reinforce dressing and apply pressure over the wound for 10 minutes. If no improvement, contact PCP.
- Monitor temperature daily.
- Consider alternative methods for pain control: deep breathing, relaxation, ice, heat, elevation, positioning, or distraction.
- For wound VAC problems:
  - If wound VAC is off for >8 hours, replace dressing with wet-to-dry dressing, and contact HH nurse to replace dressing.
  - If VAC is leaking around the tube or at dressing edges, reinforce VAC dressing, and notify HH nurse.
  - If canister is full, discard it in the garbage and replace it with a new canister.

Additional Instructions

Report the Following Problems to Your PCP/Clinic/ED

- Pain persists or worsens
- Signs of infection: redness, swelling, pain, foul-smelling drainage, warmth, or red streaks extending from the wound
- Signs of circulation problems; fingers or toes become cold, blue, or numb
- Temperature >100.4°F (38°C)
- Headache, muscle aches, general ill feeling, and fever
- Persistent nausea and vomiting

P

Seek Emergency Care Immediately If Any of the Following Occur

- Sudden onset of severe pain
- Surgical wound split or gaping and large amount of fluid drainage or material protruding from the wound
- If cast, splint, or orthopedic surgery:
  - fingers or toes cold, blue, or numb
  - severe pain, swelling, or tightness unresponsive to elevation or home care measures
- Chest pain
- Coughing up blood or pink frothy sputum
- Leg swelling and no pulse in foot of affected leg, numbness, or tingling
- Shortness of breath

If the caller agrees with the advice given, document the call and encourage the caller to call back or see PCP if the problem worsens. If the caller does not agree with the advice given, reevaluate and advise the caller to follow up with PCP, Clinic, or ED.

Postpartum Problems

 Key Questions Name, Age, Onset, Date of Delivery, Medications, History

 Other Protocols to Consider Abdominal Pain, Adult (9); Breastfeeding Problems (98); Constipation (160); Depression (184); Vaginal Discharge/Pain/Itching (636); Wound Healing and Infection (664).

> *Nurse Alert:* There are many conditions that can occur following a delivery. When there are multiple associated symptoms, focus on the primary concern that has the highest probability of a referral to a higher level of care.

Reminder: Document caller response to advice, home care instructions, and when to call back.

ASSESSMENT	ACTION

A. Are any of the following present?

<ul><li>Shortness of breath or difficulty breathing</li><li>Vaginal bleeding requiring use of more than one full-size pad per hour and weakness, dizziness</li><li>Altered mental status</li><li>Skin pale, moist, and cool</li><li>Severe lower abdominal pain <48 hours after delivery</li><li>Thoughts of harming infant or self</li><li>Cesarean section and incision is separating</li></ul>	**YES** "Call ambulance" or "Seek emergency care now" **NO** Go to B

P

461

B. Are any of the following present?

- Temperature >100°F (37.8°C) 4 to 10 days after delivery
- Bleeding with fever or abdominal pain
- Increased bleeding and abdominal cramping first week after delivery (saturating one pad with bright red bleeding in <1 hour)
- Abnormal vaginal discharge with bleeding, fever, or pain or discharge is foul smelling
- Vomiting, diarrhea, fever, or rash
- Calf swelling, pain, or redness
- Clots of blood larger than a lemon
- Headache unrelieved by home care measures
- Muscle aches, fever, and painful red area on breast
- Chills or fever and headache
- Vaginal bleeding requiring use of more than one full-size pad per hour

YES "Seek medical care within 2 to 4 hours"

NO Go to C

C. Are any of the following present?

- Persistent depression >2 to 3 weeks
- Urgency, frequency, or pain with urination
- Abnormal vaginal discharge without fever
- Increased pain at episiotomy incision site
- Increased pain, swelling, foul-smelling drainage, redness, or warmth at cesarean section incision site

YES "Seek medical care within 24 hours"

NO Go to D

D. Are any of the following present?

- Engorged, tender, hard breasts
- Cramping
- Constipation
- Stretching or pulling sensation at episiotomy site

YES "Call back or call PCP for appointment if no improvement" and Follow **Home Care Instructions**

NO Follow **Home Care Instructions**

Home Care Instructions
Postpartum Problems

- Balance activity and rest for first 2 weeks after delivery.
- Can usually return to work after 6-week checkup if cleared by physician (8 weeks for cesarean section).
- Remember that contractions 3 to 4 days after delivery are normal and are stimulated by breastfeeding.
- Bowel movements may not occur 1 to 2 days after delivery. Drink 6 to 8 glasses of water and juices a day and increase intake of fruits, vegetables, and bran. Laxatives (Metamucil) may help. Follow instructions on the label.
- Sit in a warm bath or sitz bath to relieve discomfort.
- Apply dry heat to perineum after bath for 10 minutes. May try exposing perineum a foot away from a 25-watt light bulb or using a hair dryer on the low setting.
- After toileting or changing pad, clean area using soap and warm water in a squirt bottle or antiseptic wipes, cleaning from front to back.
- Change pad after toileting.
- Remember that blood and mucus vaginal discharge may persist for several weeks after delivery, and the discharge increases with activity.
- Vaginal bleeding 4 to 8 weeks after delivery is not a cause for alarm and usually is the return of menstruation.
- Discomfort and dryness during intercourse after delivery can be reduced with use of K-Y Jelly. Avoid intercourse until discharge has stopped and stitches are healed. Discuss contraception options with PCP. If breastfeeding, milk letdown may occur.
- Wear a good supportive bra 24 hours a day for 10 days. If breasts become tender and hard, take a warm bath or apply warm compresses to breasts.
- Remember that depression after delivery is not unusual and should subside. Discuss depression with PCP.

Cesarean Section Delivery

- Expect vaginal bleeding for as long as 6 weeks.
- Do not insert anything into the vagina for 6 weeks.
- Avoid stairs and lifting anything heavier than 10 lb.
- Do not soak in tub.
- Get plenty of rest.
- Change dressing daily until drainage has stopped.
- Remove sterile strips after 7 to 10 days.

Postpartum Depression (Blues)

- Get as much rest as possible, nap while infant naps.
- Exercise, such as walking.
- Eat a well-balanced diet.
- Encourage family and friends to help with meal preparation, chores, infant care, and housework.
- Talk about your feelings.

P

Additional Instructions

Report the Following Problems to Your PCP/Clinic/ED

- No improvement with home care measures or condition worsens
- Fever, abdominal pain, or unusual vaginal discharge
- Signs of infection: increased redness, pain, red streaks from the wound, warmth, foul-smelling or thick green drainage, or fever
- Persistent depression

Seek Emergency Care Immediately If Any of the Following Occur

- Shortness of breath or difficulty breathing
- Vaginal bleeding requiring use of more than one full-size pad per hour and weakness or dizziness
- Altered mental status
- Skin pale and moist

If the caller agrees with the advice given, document the call and encourage the caller to call back or see PCP if the problem worsens. If the caller does not agree with the advice given, reevaluate and advise the caller to follow up with PCP, Clinic, or ED.

Pregnancy, Cold Symptoms

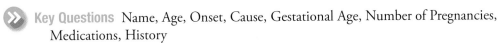 **Key Questions** Name, Age, Onset, Cause, Gestational Age, Number of Pregnancies, Medications, History

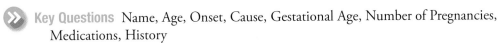 **Other Protocols to Consider** Breathing Problems (106); Congestion (153); Cough (170); Earache, Drainage (206); Fever, Adult (250); Pregnancy Problems (481); Sore Throat (564).

Reminder: Document caller response to advice, home care instructions, and when to call back.

ASSESSMENT		ACTION

A. Are any of the following present?

- Shortness of breath, difficulty talking, or inability to talk
- Chest pain
- Temperature >103°F (39.5°C)
- Difficulty breathing for reasons other than nasal congestion

YES "Seek emergency care now"

NO Go to B

B. Is the following present at 24 weeks of pregnancy?

- No fetal movement

YES "Seek medical care immediately"

NO Go to C

C. Are any of the following present?

- Strong, regular contractions
- Temperature >101°F (38.4°C)
- >20 respirations per minute
- Decreased fetal movement
- Wheezing and unresponsive to home care measures
- Fewer than 10 fetal movements in 1 hour

YES "Seek medical care within 2 to 4 hours"

NO Go to D

P

D. Are any of the following present?

- Green or brown sputum or nasal discharge
- Severe sore throat
- History of asthma, diabetes, heart disease, or immunosuppression
- Ear pain or drainage

YES "Seek medical care within 24 hours"

NO Go to E

E. Are any of the following present?

- Nasal congestion
- Cough
- Sore throat
- Temperature <101°F (38.4°C)
- Malaise
- Headache

YES "Call back or call PCP for appointment if no improvement" and Follow **Home Care Instructions**

NO Follow **Home Care Instructions**

Home Care Instructions
Pregnancy, Cold Symptoms

- Monitor temperature every 4 hours.
- Increase oral fluids to 6 to 8 glasses daily.
- Use a warm moist vaporizer and change the water daily.
- Gargle with salt water; sip warm chicken broth or suck on frozen hard candy for additional relief.
- Limit activity; rest.
- Monitor fetal movement; if fewer than 10 fetal movements in 1 hour, seek medical care.
- Monitor contractions.
- Apply petroleum jelly to nasal opening to protect from infection.
- Use saline nose drops as needed for nasal congestion.

Additional Instructions

Report the Following Problems to Your PCP/Clinic/ED

- Sputum or nasal discharge green or brown
- Severe sore throat
- Temperature >101°F (38.4°C)
- Condition worsens or no improvement with home care measures
- No or decreased fetal movement

Seek Emergency Care Immediately If Any of the Following Occur

- Shortness of breath, difficulty talking, or inability to talk
- Chest pain
- Significant vaginal bleeding
- Temperature >103°F (39.5°C)

P

If the caller agrees with the advice given, document the call and encourage the caller to call back or see PCP if the problem worsens. If the caller does not agree with the advice given, reevaluate and advise the caller to follow up with PCP, Clinic, or ED.

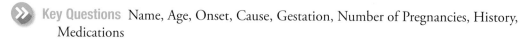

Pregnancy, Fetal Movement Problems

>> **Key Questions** Name, Age, Onset, Cause, Gestation, Number of Pregnancies, History, Medications

>> **Other Protocols to Consider** Pregnancy, Hypertension (471); Pregnancy, Leaking Vaginal Fluid (474); Pregnancy Problems (481); Pregnancy, Suspected Labor (485); Pregnancy, Suspected Labor <36 Weeks (488); Pregnancy, Vaginal Bleeding (493).

Reminder: Document caller response to advice, home care instructions, and when to call back.

ASSESSMENT	ACTION

A. Is there significant vaginal bleeding and pregnancy is >20 weeks?

YES	"Call ambulance" or "Seek emergency care now"
NO	Go to B

B. Are any of the following present and pregnancy is >24 weeks?

- Severe abdominal pain
- No fetal movement
- Severe headache
- Recent trauma to abdomen
- Rupture of membrane with green-, brown-, or red-stained fluid

YES	"Seek medical care immediately"
NO	Go to C

C. Are any of the following present?

- Fewer than 10 fetal movements in 1 hour
- Leakage of clear vaginal fluid
- Strong, regular contractions
- Headache not relieved by home care measures
- Epigastric pain (right upper quadrant pain)
- Vomiting and inability to keep fluids down
- Small amount of bright red blood on pad, underwear, bed, or clothes
- Visual disturbances

YES	"Seek medical care within 2 to 4 hours"
NO	Go to D

D. Is the following present?

- Decreased fetal movement, less than normal daily activity

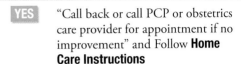 "Call back or call PCP or obstetrics care provider for appointment if no improvement" and Follow **Home Care Instructions**

NO Follow **Home Care Instructions**

P

Home Care Instructions
Pregnancy, Fetal Movement Problems

- Empty the bladder.
- Drink a glass of juice.
- Lie down on left side and place hand on abdomen. Count any fetal movement (kick, jab, or roll). If fewer than 10 fetal movements in 1 hour, seek medical care.

Additional Instructions

Report the Following Problems to Your PCP/Clinic/ED

- Decreased fetal movement, less than normal daily pattern
- Condition persists or worsens

Seek Emergency Care Immediately If Any of the Following Occur

- Severe abdominal pain
- Significant vaginal bleeding

If the caller agrees with the advice given, document the call and encourage the caller to call back or see PCP if the problem worsens. If the caller does not agree with the advice given, reevaluate and advise the caller to follow up with PCP, Clinic, or ED.

Pregnancy, Hypertension

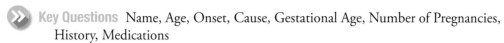

Key Questions Name, Age, Onset, Cause, Gestational Age, Number of Pregnancies, History, Medications

Other Protocols to Consider Pregnancy, Fetal Movement Problems (468); Pregnancy Problems (481); Pregnancy, Suspected Labor (485); Pregnancy, Suspected Labor <36 Weeks (488).

Nurse Alert: Use this protocol if pregnant and under treatment for known pregnancy-induced hypertension.

Reminder: Document caller response to advice, home care instructions, and when to call back.

ASSESSMENT	ACTION
A. Are any of the following present?	

• Seizure activity
 • Convulsions
 • Unresponsiveness
 • >20 weeks' gestation and:
  • severe abdominal pain
  • significant vaginal bleeding
  • imminent delivery, with fetal head crowning
	YES "Call ambulance" or "Seek emergency care now"
	
	 NO Go to B

B. Are any of the following present?	
• Bright red vaginal bleeding • Severe headache • No fetal movement • Sudden increase in swelling of hands, face, legs, or lower back • Epigastric pain (right upper quadrant) • Visual disturbances (blurred or double vision, spots before eyes, or seeing stars or halo around objects)	**YES** "Seek medical care immediately" **NO** Go to C

P

C. Are any of the following present?

- Headache unrelieved by home care measures
- Fewer than 10 fetal movements in 1 hour
- Regular, strong contractions
- Abdominal pain
- Blood pressure elevated (if monitoring at home after resting)
- Vomiting and inability to keep fluids down

YES "Seek medical care within 2 to 4 hours"

NO Go to D

D. Are any of the following present?

- Gradual swelling of the feet or legs
- Headache relieved by home care measures
- Weight gain >2 lb per week
- Nausea

YES "Call back or call PCP or obstetrics care provider for appointment if no improvement" and Follow **Home Care Instructions**

NO Follow **Home Care Instructions**

Home Care Instructions
Pregnancy, Hypertension

- Rest on left side.
- Monitor fetal movement; if fewer than 10 fetal movements in 1 hour, seek medical care.

Additional Instructions

_____

_____

_____

Report the Following Problems to Your PCP/Clinic/ED

- Headache not relieved by home care measures
- Weight gain >2 lb per week
- Bright red vaginal bleeding
- Fewer than 10 fetal movements in 1 hour
- Sudden increase in swelling of hands, face, legs, or lower back
- Epigastric pain (right upper quadrant)
- Visual disturbances (blurred or double vision, spots before eyes, or seeing stars or halo around objects)

Seek Emergency Care Immediately If Any of the Following Occur

- Seizure activity
- Unresponsiveness
- Convulsions
- Significant vaginal bleeding
- Severe abdominal pain
- Imminent delivery with fetal head crowning

If the caller agrees with the advice given, document the call and encourage the caller to call back or see PCP if the problem worsens. If the caller does not agree with the advice given, reevaluate and advise the caller to follow up with PCP, Clinic, or ED.

Pregnancy, Leaking Vaginal Fluid

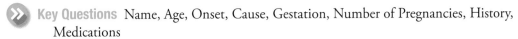

>> **Key Questions** Name, Age, Onset, Cause, Gestation, Number of Pregnancies, History, Medications

>> **Other Protocols to Consider** Pregnancy Problems (481); Pregnancy, Suspected Labor (485); Pregnancy, Suspected Labor <36 Weeks (488); Pregnancy, Vaginal Bleeding (493).

Reminder: Document caller response to advice, home care instructions, and when to call back.

ASSESSMENT	ACTION

A. Are any of the following present and pregnancy is >20 weeks?

- Rupture of membrane with prolapsed umbilical cord
- Imminent delivery, with fetal head crowning
- Significant vaginal bleeding (soaking >1 pad per hour in >2 hours or 6 pads in 12 hours)

YES "Call ambulance" and Follow **Emergency Instructions**

NO Go to B

B. Are any of the following present?

- Severe abdominal pain
- No fetal movement
- Green-, brown-, or red-stained fluid
- Known breech or transverse position of fetus
- <37 weeks' pregnant
- Current herpes outbreak with regular, strong contractions or leaking of fluid

YES "Seek medical care immediately"

NO Go to C

C. Are any of the following present?

- Clear fluid leaking from vagina
- Strong, regular contractions
- Fever or chills
- Fewer than 10 fetal movements in 1 hour

YES "Seek medical care within 2 hours"

NO Go to D

D. Are any of the following present?

- Lost mucus plug
- Irregular contractions
- Increase of mucus-like vaginal discharge

YES   "Call back or call PCP or obstetrics care provider for appointment if no improvement" and Follow **Home Care Instructions**

NO   Follow **Home Care Instructions**

P

Emergency Instructions
Pregnancy, Leaking Vaginal Fluid

- If leaking vaginal fluid and umbilical cord is prolapsed, calmly tell the patient to:
  - hand telephone to someone else to call ambulance
  - get on hands and knees in the knee–chest position, with head down and buttocks up

Home Care Instructions
Pregnancy, Leaking Vaginal Fluid

- Remember it is not unusual to lose the mucus plug in the weeks before true labor.
- Monitor fetal movement; if fewer than 10 fetal movements in 1 hour, seek medical care.
- Monitor contractions; if contractions are strong, last 45 to 60 seconds, and occur in a regular pattern every 5 minutes for 1 to 2 hours, or if contractions are increasing in intensity or strength, go to the delivering facility.
- Empty the bladder.
- Put on a clean, dry sanitary pad. Reevaluate in 1 hour. If the pad is wet, there is continued leakage of vaginal fluid, or if you are unsure, seek medical care.

Additional Instructions

Report the Following Problems to Your PCP/Clinic/ED

- Spotting
- Fewer than 10 fetal movements in 1 hour
- Strong regular contractions
- Fever or chills
- Clear fluid leaking from vagina

Seek Emergency Care Immediately If Any of the Following Occur

- Rupture of membranes with prolapsed umbilical cord
- Imminent delivery, with fetal head crowning
- Severe abdominal pain
- Green- or brown-stained fluid
- Significant vaginal bleeding
- No fetal movement

If the caller agrees with the advice given, document the call and encourage the caller to call back or see PCP if the problem worsens. If the caller does not agree with the advice given, reevaluate and advise the caller to follow up with PCP, Clinic, or ED.

Pregnancy, Nausea and Vomiting

>> **Key Questions** Name, Age, Onset, Cause, Frequency, Gestation, Number of Pregnancies, History, Medications

>> **Other Protocols to Consider** Dehydration (180); Dizziness (199); Diarrhea, Adult (192); Headache (308); Head Injury (311); Pregnancy, Hypertension (471); Pregnancy Problems (481).

Reminder: Document caller response to advice, home care instructions, and when to call back.

ASSESSMENT	ACTION

A. Are any of the following present?

- Chest pain
- Difficulty breathing
- Altered mental status
- Pregnancy >20 weeks and any of the following are present:
  - vomiting bright red blood or dark coffee grounds–like emesis
  - recent head injury
  - fainting
  - sweating or palpitations

YES "Call ambulance" or "Seek emergency care now"

NO Go to B

B. Is the following present?

- No fetal movement and gestational age >24 weeks

YES "Seek medical care now"

NO Go to C

C. Are any of the following present?

- Diarrhea
- Temperature >100.4°F (38.9°C)
- Dehydration symptoms
- Diabetes
- Cramps or regular, strong contractions
- Inability to keep down fluids for >24 hours
- Dark amber urine
- Epigastric pain (right upper quadrant pain)
- Fewer than 10 fetal movements <1 hour

YES "Seek medical care within 2 to 4 hours"

NO Go to D

D. Are any of the following present?

- Nausea and vomiting or heartburn unrelieved by home care measures
- Nausea but able to keep down some fluids or food

YES   "Seek medical care within 24 hours"

NO   Go to E

E. Are any of the following present?

- Urine yellow
- Heartburn

YES   "Call back or call PCP or obstetrics care provider for appointment if no improvement" and Follow **Home Care Instructions**

NO   Follow **Home Care Instructions**

P

Home Care Instructions
Pregnancy, Nausea and Vomiting

- Do not drink or eat for 1 hour after last emesis.
- Take small sips of clear fluid for first 12 hours after vomiting.
- Increase fluids as tolerated.
- After 12 hours of no vomiting, try bland foods (crackers, dry toast, bananas).
- Resume normal diet after 12 hours if no emesis.
- Morning sickness:
  - Eat dry bread, cereal, or crackers upon rising in the morning.
  - Get up slowly.
  - Open window for fresh air while sleeping or cooking.
  - Eat several meals during the day; avoid fluids with meals.
  - Drink ginger ale or orange or grape juice between meals.
  - Avoid fatty or highly seasoned foods.
  - Avoid lying down immediately after a meal.
  - Eat crackers, cheese, or pretzels if nauseated.

Additional Instructions

Report the Following Problems to Your PCP/Clinic/ED

- Nausea and vomiting or heartburn unrelieved by home care measures
- Continuous nausea but able to keep down food
- Condition worsens
- No or decreased fetal movements

Seek Emergency Care Immediately If Any of the Following Occur

- Fainting
- Altered mental status
- Vomiting bright red blood or dark coffee grounds–like emesis
- Chest pain or difficulty breathing

If the caller agrees with the advice given, document the call and encourage the caller to call back or see PCP if the problem worsens. If the caller does not agree with the advice given, reevaluate and advise the caller to follow up with PCP, Clinic, or ED.

Pregnancy Problems

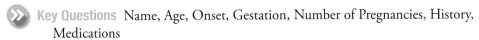 **Key Questions** Name, Age, Onset, Gestation, Number of Pregnancies, History, Medications

Other Protocols to Consider Back Pain (62); Breast Problems (103); Constipation (160); Diarrhea, Adult (192); Foot Problems (265); Headache (308); Heartburn (316); Hemorrhoids (327); Pregnancy, Hypertension (471); Pregnancy, Leaking Vaginal Fluid (474); Pregnancy, Nausea and Vomiting (478); Pregnancy, Suspected Labor (485); Pregnancy, Suspected Labor <36 Weeks (488); Pregnancy, Urination Problems (491); Pregnancy, Vaginal Bleeding (493); Swelling (597).

Nurse Alert: There are many conditions that can occur during pregnancy. When there are multiple associated symptoms, focus on the primary concern that has the highest probability of a referral to a higher level of care.

Reminder: Document caller response to advice, home care instructions, and when to call back.

ASSESSMENT	ACTION

A. Pregnancy of >20 weeks, and are any of the following present?

- Imminent delivery with fetal head crowning
- Severe headache, double or blurred vision, disorientation, dizziness, or irritability
- Previous trauma to mitral valve area, fall, blunt injury to abdomen, etc.
- Passing large clots
- Seizure
- Severe abdominal pain
- Leaking fluid with prolapsed umbilical cord
- Diagnosed preeclampsia with new symptoms

 "Call ambulance" or "Seek emergency care now"

NO Go to B

B. Are any of the following present?

- No fetal movement
- Sudden swelling in face, hands, legs, or lower back
- Headache, spots in front of eyes, dizziness, fainting, or vomiting
- Regular contractions or leaking vaginal fluid

 "Seek medical care immediately"

 NO Go to C

P

481

C. Are any of the following present?

- Known hypertension and blood pressure is increasing
- Leg pain, swelling, redness, or warmth that worsens with weight bearing
- Pain, vaginal bleeding, or fever
- Persistent headache unresponsive to pain relievers
- Persistent vomiting of all foods and fluids and/or abdominal pain
- Fewer than 10 fetal movements in 1 hour

YES "Seek medical care within 2 hours"

NO Go to D

D. Are any of the following present?

- Urgent, frequent, or painful urination
- Sudden weight gain >3 lb per week during the second trimester or >1 lb per week during the third trimester
- Cough with pain, shortness of breath, or yellow, green, or bloody sputum
- Fever >101°F (38.3°C) for >2 days
- Earache or sore throat >2 days
- Generalized rash of unknown cause and itching
- Diarrhea and fever, bloody stools, >10 stools a day, severe abdominal pain, vomiting

YES "Seek medical care within 24 hours"

NO Go to E

E. Are any of the following present?

- Nausea and vomiting (morning sickness) during first trimester
- Dizziness, light-headedness, or fainting
- Heartburn
- Hemorrhoids
- Swelling of hands, fingers, feet, or legs
- Aches and pain in back, legs, feet, or groin

YES "Call back or call PCP for appointment if no improvement" and Follow **Home Care Instructions**

NO Follow **Home Care Instructions**

Home Care Instructions
Pregnancy Problems

- If diagnosed with preeclampsia or preterm labor, rest while lying on left side.

Nausea and Vomiting
- Do not eat or drink for 1 hour after last emesis.
- Take small sips of clear fluid for first 12 hours after vomiting.
- Increase fluids as tolerated.
- After 12 hours of no vomiting, try bland foods (crackers, dry toast, bananas).
- Resume normal diet after 12 hours if no emesis.
- Morning sickness:
  - Eat dry bread, cereal, or crackers upon rising in the morning.
  - Get up slowly.
  - Open window for fresh air while sleeping or cooking.
  - Eat several small meals during the day. Avoid fluids with meals.
  - Drink ginger ale or orange or grape juice between meals.
  - Avoid fatty or highly seasoned foods.
  - Avoid lying down immediately after a meal.
  - Eat crackers, cheese, or pretzels if nauseated.

Light-Headedness and Dizziness
- Get up slowly; avoid sudden changes in posture.
- Avoid lying flat on back or standing for prolonged periods of time.
- Avoid hot, stuffy rooms.
- Do not skip meals.

Heartburn
- Sleep with several pillows or elevate the head of the bed on several blocks.
- Eat frequent small meals.
- Change position frequently.
- Suck on hard candy or sip hot tea.
- Antacids (Maalox, Tums) may help reduce discomfort. Follow instructions on the label.

Hemorrhoids
- Avoid straining with bowel movements.
- Drink 10 to 12 glasses of water a day.
- Eat lots of fresh fruits, whole grains, and vegetables.
- Take warm baths.
- Use hemorrhoidal creams, suppositories, or medicated pads (Preparation H) as needed for discomfort. Follow instructions on the label.

P

Swelling
- Minimize salt in diet.
- Massage feet.
- Elevate legs above the heart.
- Wear supportive hose.
- Avoid tight-fitting clothing or bands around the abdomen.
- Sleep on left side.

Aches and Pains
- Massage affected areas.
- Apply moist heat to area.
- Lie on affected side and draw leg up to chest.
- Crawl on all fours and rock pelvis forward several times a day.
- Take acetaminophen for discomfort if desired, and follow instructions on the label. Do not take aspirin.

Additional Instructions

Report the Following Problems to Your PCP/Clinic/ED
- Conditions persist or worsen after home care measures
- Less than 10 movements in <1 hour

Seek Emergency Care Immediately If Any of the Following Occur
- Imminent delivery
- Severe headache, double or blurred vision, disorientation, dizziness
- Passing large clots
- Severe abdominal pain
- Leaking vaginal fluid with prolapsed umbilical cord
- Sudden swelling in face, hands, legs, or lower back
- Headache, spots in front of eyes
- Regular contractions or leaking vaginal fluid
- No fetal movement

If the caller agrees with the advice given, document the call and encourage the caller to call back or see PCP if the problem worsens. If the caller does not agree with the advice given, reevaluate and advise the caller to follow up with PCP, Clinic, or ED.

Pregnancy, Suspected Labor

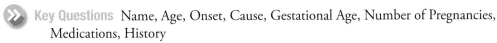 **Key Questions** Name, Age, Onset, Cause, Gestational Age, Number of Pregnancies, Medications, History

Other Protocols to Consider Abdominal Pain, Adult (9); Pregnancy, Fetal Movement Problems (468); Pregnancy, Leaking Vaginal Fluid (474); Pregnancy Problems (481); Pregnancy, Suspected Labor <36 Weeks (488); Pregnancy, Urination Problems (491); Pregnancy, Vaginal Bleeding (493).

Reminder: Document caller response to advice, home care instructions, and when to call back.

ASSESSMENT	ACTION

A. More than 20 weeks pregnant, and are any of the following present?

- Imminent delivery with fetal head crowning
- Significant vaginal bleeding
- Seizure or convulsions
- Severe abdominal pain
- Rupture of membranes with prolapsed umbilical cord

YES "Call ambulance" or "Seek emergency care now"

NO Go to B

B. Are any of the following present?

- Severe headache
- Known breech or transverse position of fetus at first sign of contractions or leaking of fluid
- Leaking brown or green vaginal fluid
- Current herpes outbreak with regular, strong contractions
- Contractions and <37 weeks' gestation
- No fetal movement

YES "Seek medical care immediately"

NO Go to C

P

485

C. Are any of the following present?

- First pregnancy and strong, regular contractions (every 5 minutes, lasting 45 to 60 seconds, for 1 to 2 hours)
- Pregnancy other than first and strong, regular contractions (every 5 to 10 minutes, lasting 45 to 60 seconds, for 1 to 2 hours)
- Leaking clear vaginal fluid
- History of known hypertension, diabetes, or other pregnancy complications
- History of rapid labor
- Long driving distance to delivering facility
- Fewer than 10 fetal movements in 1 hour
- Contractions increasing in intensity or strength
- Pelvic pressure

YES   "Seek medical care within 2 hours"

NO   Go to D

D. Are any of the following present?

- Irregular contractions
- Spotting
- Aches and pain in back, feet, or groin
- Urgency, frequency, or pain with urination

YES   "Call back or call PCP or obstetrics care provider for appointment if no improvement" and Follow **Home Care Instructions**

NO   Follow **Home Care Instructions**

Home Care Instructions
Pregnancy, Suspected Labor

- Walk, shower, massage, apply warm or cold packs to back for comfort, change positions, or use pelvic rocking to help with early labor.
- Eat light meals.
- Monitor contractions: frequency = start of one contraction to the start of the next contraction (i.e., 5 minutes); duration = how long the contraction lasts (i.e., 30 to 45 seconds).
- Monitor fetal movement; if fewer than 10 fetal movements in 1 hour, seek medical care.
- If leaking vaginal fluid and umbilical cord is prolapsed:
  - hand telephone to someone else to call ambulance
  - get on hands and knees in the knee–chest position, with head down and buttocks up
- Increase fluid intake; avoid caffeine. If contracting, drink 32 ounces of fluid, lie on left side, and monitor contractions. If >4 contractions in 1 hour, call back. Keep bladder empty.

Additional Instructions

Report the Following Problems to Your PCP/Clinic/ED
- Conditions persist or worsen after home care measures
- Leaking clear, brown, or green vaginal fluid
- Fewer than 10 fetal movements in 1 hour

Seek Emergency Care Immediately If Any of the Following Occur
- Imminent delivery with fetal head crowning
- Seizure
- Significant vaginal bleeding
- Severe abdominal pain
- Rupture of membranes with prolapsed umbilical cord

P

If the caller agrees with the advice given, document the call and encourage the caller to call back or see PCP if the problem worsens. If the caller does not agree with the advice given, reevaluate and advise the caller to follow up with PCP, Clinic, or ED.

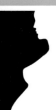

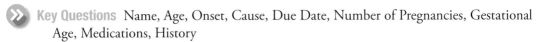

Pregnancy, Suspected Labor <36 Weeks

>> **Key Questions** Name, Age, Onset, Cause, Due Date, Number of Pregnancies, Gestational Age, Medications, History

>> **Other Protocols to Consider** Pregnancy, Fetal Movement Problems (468); Pregnancy, Leaking Vaginal Fluid (474); Pregnancy, Suspected Labor (485); Pregnancy, Urination Problems (491); Pregnancy, Vaginal Bleeding (493).

Reminder: Document caller response to advice, home care instructions, and when to call back.

ASSESSMENT	ACTION

A. Are any of the following present and pregnancy between 20 and 36 weeks?

- Severe abdominal pain
- Leaking fluid and prolapsed umbilical cord
- Significant bright red vaginal bleeding
- Imminent delivery with fetal head crowning

YES "Call ambulance" or "Seek emergency care now"

NO Go to B

B. Are any of the following present?

- No fetal movement
- History of cervical cerclage
- Six or more contractions in 1 hour
- Leaking of vaginal fluid
- Multiple gestation and four or more contractions in 1 hour
- Any contractions with known placenta previa or partial abruption

YES "Seek medical care immediately"

NO Go to C

C. Are any of the following present?

- Four to five contractions in 1 hour
- Fever/chills
- Painful, frequent, or urgent urination
- Current herpes outbreak with first sign of contractions
- Any contractions with known breech or transverse lie of fetus
- Fewer than 10 fetal movements in 1 hour
- Menstrual-like cramps
- Pelvic pressure
- New-onset lower backache
- Any rhythmic pain
- Increasing vaginal discharge
- Groin pain
- History of preterm labor medications

YES "Seek medical care within 2 hours"

NO Go to D

D. Are any of the following present?

- Lost mucus plug
- Fewer than four painless contractions in 1 hour

YES "Call back or call PCP or obstetrics care provider for appointment if no improvement" and Follow **Home Care Instructions**

NO Follow **Home Care Instructions**

P

Home Care Instructions
Pregnancy, Suspected Labor <36 Weeks

- Rest on left side, and monitor contractions.
- Drink fluids.
- Monitor fetal movement.
- Empty the bladder.
- Avoid nipple stimulation and intercourse.

Additional Instructions

Report the Following Problems to Your PCP/Clinic/ED

- No fetal movement or fewer than 10 movements in 1 hour
- More than four contractions in 1 hour
- Increasing vaginal discharge
- Any contractions with known placenta previa or partial abruption
- Urgent, frequent, or painful urination
- Fever or chills

Seek Emergency Care Immediately If Any of the Following Occur

- Imminent delivery, with fetal head crowning
- Leaking vaginal fluid and prolapsed umbilical cord
- Significant vaginal bleeding
- Severe abdominal pain

If the caller agrees with the advice given, document the call and encourage the caller to call back or see PCP if the problem worsens. If the caller does not agree with the advice given, reevaluate and advise the caller to follow up with PCP, Clinic, or ED.

Pregnancy, Urination Problems

 Key Questions Name, Age, Onset, Cause, Gestational Age, Number of Pregnancies, Medications, History

 Other Protocols to Consider Pregnancy, Leaking Vaginal Fluid (474); Pregnancy Problems (481); Pregnancy, Suspected Labor (485); Pregnancy, Suspected Labor <36 Weeks (488); Pregnancy, Vaginal Bleeding (493).

Reminder: Document caller response to advice, home care instructions, and when to call back.

ASSESSMENT	ACTION

A. Are any of the following present and pregnancy of >20 weeks?

- Temperature >100°F (37.8°C)
- Chills or headache
- Flank pain
- Hematuria (blood in urine)
- Symptoms of preterm labor (<37 weeks' gestation):
  - pelvic pressure
  - lower backache
  - any rhythmic pain
  - groin pain
  - menstrual-like cramps
  - pink discharge
  - bloody show
- Decreased fetal movement
- Strong, regular contractions

YES "Seek medical care within 2 hours"

NO Go to B

B. Are any of the following present?

- Pain or burning with urination
- Cloudy or dark urine
- Difficulty starting a stream
- Frequent, urgent, or painful urination

YES "Seek medical care within 24 hours"

NO Go to C

C. Is the following present?

- Difficulty urinating after sexual activity

YES "Call back or call PCP for appointment if no improvement" and Follow **Home Care Instructions**

NO Follow **Home Care Instructions**

P

491

492   Pregnancy, Urination Problems

Home Care Instructions
Pregnancy, Urination Problems

- Drink lots of fluids.
- Drink cranberry juice 3 times a day or take 500 mg of vitamin C 3 times a day.
- Urinate before and after intercourse.
- Wipe from front to back after using the bathroom.
- Wash hands after using the bathroom.
- Wear cotton underwear.
- Monitor temperature, fetal movements, and contractions.
- For difficulty starting to urinate, turn on water faucet (sound of running water can help to stimulate urination) and pour warm water over perineum while sitting on the toilet.

Additional Instructions

Report the Following Problem to Your PCP/Clinic/ED

- Condition worsens or no improvement

If the caller agrees with the advice given, document the call and encourage the caller to call back or see PCP if the problem worsens. If the caller does not agree with the advice given, reevaluate and advise the caller to follow up with PCP, Clinic, or ED.

Pregnancy, Vaginal Bleeding

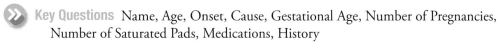 **Key Questions** Name, Age, Onset, Cause, Gestational Age, Number of Pregnancies, Number of Saturated Pads, Medications, History

Other Protocols to Consider Pregnancy Problems (481); Pregnancy, Suspected Labor <36 Weeks (488); Pregnancy, Urination Problems (491).

Reminder: Document caller response to advice, home care instructions, and when to call back.

ASSESSMENT	ACTION

A. Pregnancy >20 weeks, and are any of the following present?

- Severe abdominal pain
- Imminent delivery with fetal head crowning
- Rupture of membranes with suspected prolapsed umbilical cord
- Decreased level of consciousness
- Fainting
- Soaking more than one full-size pad in <1 hour and weakness
- Soaking more than one full-size pad per hour for >2 hours or more than six pads in 12 hours

YES "Call ambulance" or "Seek emergency care now"

NO Go to B

B. Are any of the following present?

- No fetal movement and >20 weeks pregnant
- Moderate vaginal bleeding (need to wear a sanitary pad but not saturating)
- Bright red bleeding, trickling down leg
- Known placenta previa or abruption with any bleeding
- Any recent trauma
- Abdominal pain

YES "Seek medical care immediately"

NO Go to C

P

C. Are any of the following present?

- Fewer than 10 fetal movements in 1 hour
- Strong, regular contractions
- Leaking of clear amniotic fluid
- Small amount of bright red blood on pad, underwear, bed, or clothes

YES "Seek medical care within 2 hours"

NO Go to D

D. Is the following present?

- Spotting; dark brown or pink blood seen when wiping or a small amount on underwear

YES "Call back or call PCP or obstetrics care provider for appointment if no improvement" and Follow **Home Care Instructions**

NO Follow **Home Care Instructions**

Home Care Instructions
Pregnancy, Vaginal Bleeding

- Dark brown or pink spotting can occur after recent intercourse or recent vaginal examination.
- Monitor fetal movements; if fewer than 10 fetal movements in 1 hour, seek medical care.
- Monitor contractions.

Additional Instructions

Report the Following Problems to Your PCP/Clinic/ED

- Spotting is dark brown or pink when wiping or on underwear
- No improvement or condition worsen

Seek Emergency Care Immediately If Any of the Following Occur

- Significant vaginal bleeding
- Fainting or decreased level of consciousness
- Severe abdominal pain
- Imminent delivery with fetal head crowning
- Leaking fluid and prolapsed umbilical cord

If the caller agrees with the advice given, document the call and encourage the caller to call back or see PCP if the problem worsens. If the caller does not agree with the advice given, reevaluate and advise the caller to follow up with PCP, Clinic, or ED.

P

Puncture Wound

 Key Questions Name, Age, Onset, Cause, Location, Medications, Tetanus Immunization Status, Pain Scale, History

 Other Protocols to Consider Bites, Animal/Human (76); Bruising (109); Foreign Body, Skin (278); Immunization, Tetanus (355); Laceration (395); Piercing Problems (445); Tattoo Problems (604); Wound Healing and Infection (664).

Nurse Alert: Puncture wounds are at high risk for infection when foreign debris and bacteria are pushed deep into the tissue. Puncture wounds to the hand such as a cat bite have the highest rate of infection due to the relatively poor blood supply of many structures in the hand. Local infections and cellulitis are the leading cause of morbidity from bite wounds and can potentially lead to sepsis, particularly in immunocompromised individuals.

Reminder: Document caller response to advice, home care instructions, and when to call back.

ASSESSMENT	ACTION

A. Is there a deep wound to the head, chest, neck, scrotum, abdomen, or are any of the following present?

- Inability to control bleeding with pressure or spurting blood
- Decreased level of consciousness
- No pulse distal to injury
- Difficulty breathing
- Pale skin, sweating, or rapid heartbeat
- Skin cold, blue, and numb distal to the wound
- High-pressure injection injury
- Contaminated needle-stick

 "Call ambulance" or "Seek emergency care now" and Follow **Emergency Instructions**

 Go to B

B. Are any of the following present?

- Numbness or tingling
- Difficulty moving affected part
- Puncture wound into a joint
- Visible debris in the wound and unable to remove
- Puncture wound through shoe sole
- Fever, drainage, or red streaks
- Severe pain
- Increasing swelling or bruising around wound and injured person takes blood-thinning medication
- Persistent foreign body sensation
- Foot wound and history of diabetes

 YES "Seek medical care within 2 to 4 hours"

 NO Go to C

C. Are any of the following present?

- Unable to remove large splinter
- History of diabetes
- No tetanus immunization, immunization status unknown, or last tetanus immunization >5 years ago

YES "Seek medical care within 24 hours"

 NO Go to D

D. Are any of the following present?

- Persistent pain or swelling >5 days
- Minor puncture wound
- Unable to remove small splinter
- Gradual swelling
- Gradual bruising
- No improvement in pain or swelling >3 days and unresponsive to home care measures

YES "Call back or call PCP for appointment if no improvement" and Follow **Home Care Instructions**

NO Follow **Home Care Instructions**

Emergency Instructions
Puncture Wound

- If bleeding is profuse or spurting, apply pressure with a clean bandage or cloth directly over the wound and call an ambulance. Do not check to see if the bleeding has stopped. Do not try to remove embedded material from the wound. Seek medical care.

Home Care Instructions
Puncture Wound

- Clean well with soap and water.
- Soak the affected area for 10 to 15 minutes several times a day using warm water or Epsom salts in warm water. This will help to prevent infection and promote healing.
- Apply a bandage to the wound for a few days after the injury to help keep the wound clean.
- Watch for signs of infection: increased redness, pain, swelling, drainage, streaks, or fever.
- If no tetanus immunization within 5 years for a dirty or contaminated wound, contact PCP or clinic for tetanus immunization within 24 hours of injury.
- If no tetanus immunization within 10 years for a clean wound, contact PCP or clinic for tetanus immunization within 72 hours of injury.
- Apply antibiotic ointment 2 to 3 times a day. Soak affected area before applying ointment.
- DO NOT soak a splinter area in water or solution, which will cause the wood to swell and hinder removal.

Additional Instructions

Report the Following Problems to Your PCP/Clinic/ED

- Signs of infection: increased redness, pain, swelling, drainage, streaks, or fever
- Numbness, tingling, or increased pain
- Wound does not heal within 2 weeks
- Persistent foreign body sensation

Seek Emergency Care Immediately If Any of the Following Occur

- Difficulty breathing
- Pale skin, sweating, or rapid heartbeat
- Pulses absent distal to wound
- Skin cyanotic distal to wound

If the caller agrees with the advice given, document the call and encourage the caller to call back or see PCP if the problem worsens. If the caller does not agree with the advice given, reevaluate and advise the caller to follow up with PCP, Clinic, or ED.

P

Rash, Adult

>> **Key Questions** Name, Age, Onset, Cause, Location, History, Associated Symptoms, Medications

>> **Other Protocols to Consider** Allergic Reaction (25); Bedbug Exposure or Concerns (67); Bee Stings (72); Bites, Insect (79); Heat Exposure Problems (323); Hives (337); Itching (382); Scabies (527); Shingles, Suspected or Exposure (544); Skin Lesions: Lumps, Bumps, and Sores (556); Tattoo Problems (604).

Nurse Alert:

- There are many conditions that cause a rash. When a rash is associated with several other symptoms, use the protocol that is the primary concern and has the highest probability of a referral to a higher level of care.
- Communicable Disease Table in Appendix M (696) is provided to help the nurse gain a better understanding of many communicable diseases that can cause a rash. It is NOT to be used to try and diagnose a caller's condition.

Reminder: Document caller response to advice, home care instructions, and when to call back.

ASSESSMENT	ACTION

A. Is the following present?

- Sudden onset of severe hives or rash, and difficulty breathing, chest tightness, swelling in back of throat or tongue, or change in mental status

YES "Call ambulance"

NO Go to B

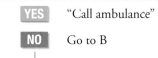

B. Are any of the following present?

- Sudden onset of illness and rapid progression of widespread redness, scaliness, fever, and enlarged lymph nodes
- Purple- or blood-colored flat spots or dots, headache, stiff neck, vomiting, confusion, or fever
- Severe facial or eye swelling
- Fever, headache, or respiratory infection followed by blistering rash
- Blistering rash and painful urination or swallowing

YES "Seek emergency care now"

NO Go to C

C. Are any of the following present?

- Rash around eyes, vision changes, or weeping lesions
- Open sores with signs of infection: redness, swelling, pain, red streaks, drainage, warmth
- Fever in a menstruating woman who uses tampons
- Fever, sore throat, and joint pain
- Fever and painful rash
- Red rash that peels off in sheets of skin
- Tick bite in past 24 days and fever, headache, red or purple rash on wrists, ankles, palms, or soles of feet

YES "Seek medical care within 2 to 4 hours"

NO Go to D

D. Are any of the following present?

- New antibiotic or medication and new onset of rash or hives
- New onset in pregnant woman

YES "Call PCP now"

NO Go to E

E. Are any of the following present?

- Persistent rash for >48 hours that is unresponsive to home care measures
- Persistent hives after taking antihistamine for >24 hours
- Extensive rash, cause unknown
- Painful rash or blisters
- Rash and itching interfere with sleep
- Multiple grouping of painful blisters
- Rash or flu-like symptoms; fever, chills, sore throat, headache 2 to 4 weeks after a tick bite
- Bull's-eye rash

YES "Seek medical care within 24 hours"

NO Go to F

F. Are any of the following present?

- Prolonged exposure to heat
- Exposure to poison oak, ivy, or sumac
- Change in laundry detergent and contact areas affected
- Exposure to chemicals
- Recent immunization
- Other household members have similar rash
- Raised, red, itchy rash followed by blisters
- Dull red spots, runny nose, cough, sore throat, fever, red eyes (suspicion of rubella)
- Pink rash, swollen glands at back of neck, fever, and no prior immunization or history of measles infection
- Circular, raised, rough pink patch with clear center ½ to 1 inch and itchy
- Tender, moist red area in folds of skin
- Tick bite and expanding rash
- No other symptoms but person concerned

YES "Call back or call PCP for appointment if no improvement" and Follow **Home Care Instructions**

NO Follow **Home Care Instructions**

Home Care Instructions
Rash, Adult

- Try to identify the cause and avoid the irritant.
- Initially cleanse the area with soap and water to remove the irritant, then use only water to cleanse the area.
- Apply compresses soaked in water and Domeboro.

To Control Itching

- Take a cool bath with baking soda, Aveeno, or oatmeal (1 cup in a tub of cool water) several times a day, or apply cold packs to localized rashes for 20 minutes every 3 to 4 hours.
- For severe itching, apply 1% hydrocortisone cream and follow the instructions on the label. Refrigerate it for optimal cooling relief. Avoid using it when jock itch, athlete's foot, impetigo, or ringworm is suspected.
- Apply a baking soda paste mixed with white vinegar, or apply OTC preparations such as calamine lotion or Aveeno, to the affected area.
- Take your usual antihistamine (Benadryl, Chlor-Trimeton) and follow the instructions on the label.
- Avoid scratching.
- Apply wet dressings soaked in Burow's solution, 1 part solution to 10 to 40 parts water. Change frequently, as often as 8 times in 2 hours.

For Possible Allergic Reaction

- If the rash is related to a new medication, stop taking the medication. Call PCP if it is a prescription medication.
- Take an antihistamine (Benadryl, Claritin, Alavert, Chlor-Trimeton) as directed on the container until the rash and itching are gone. Do not take an antihistamine if the prostate is enlarged.
- Watch for signs of worsening reaction (swelling or difficulty swallowing or breathing) and see PCP.

For Possible Heat Rash

- Apply calamine lotion or hydrocortisone cream.
- Take a cool bath or shower without soap every 2 to 3 hours as needed for relief, and air-dry.
- Apply baby powder to the affected area.

For Poison Oak, Ivy, or Sumac Exposure

- Wash the exposed area within 1 hour of exposure, if possible.
- Soak the area with cool water or rub it with ice for 20 minutes, as needed.
- Wash all clothes and any animal exposed to the plants.

For Suspected Measles/Chickenpox/Rubella

- If pregnant, contact PCP.
- Stay home until rash is gone to avoid exposing others to the disease.

For Painful Rash Under Pannus or Folds of Skin

- Apply antiperspirant, OTC antifungal cream or Gold Bond Medicated powder to affected area.
- Gently wash area with soap and water then pat dry or use a hairdryer to dry area.

R

Additional Instructions

Report the Following Problems to Your PCP/Clinic/ED

- No improvement in 24 to 48 hours with home care measures or condition worsens
- Fever, sore throat, or joint pain
- Signs of infection

Seek Emergency Care Immediately If Any of the Following Occur

- Difficulty breathing, chest tightness, or swelling in the back of the throat
- Purple- or blood-colored flat spots or dots, headache, stiff neck, vomiting, confusion, or fever
- Severe facial or eye swelling
- Sudden onset of illness and rapid progression of widespread redness, scaliness, fever, and enlarged lymph nodes

If the caller agrees with the advice given, document the call and encourage the caller to call back or see PCP if the problem worsens. If the caller does not agree with the advice given, reevaluate and advise the caller to follow up with PCP, Clinic, or ED.

Rash, Child

» **Key Questions** Name, Age, Onset, Cause, Location, Medications, History, Immunization Status, Associated Symptoms

» **Other Protocols to Consider** Allergic Reaction (25); Bedbug Exposure or Concerns (67); Bee Stings (72); Bites, Insect (79); Chickenpox (129); Diaper Rash (190); Heat Exposure Problem (323); Hives (337); Itching (382); Rubella (German Measles) (520); Rubeola (Measles) (523); Scabies (527); Skin Lesions: Lumps, Bumps, and Sores (556); Tattoo Problems (604); Appendix M (696).

Nurse Alert:

- There are many conditions that cause a rash. When a rash is associated with several other symptoms, use the protocol that is the primary concern and has the highest probability of a referral to a higher level of care.
- Communicable Disease Table in Appendix M (696) is provided to help the nurse gain a better understanding of several communicable diseases that can cause a rash. It is NOT to be used to try and diagnose a caller's condition.

Reminder: Document caller response to advice, home care instructions, and when to call back.

ASSESSMENT	ACTION

A. Is the following present?

• Sudden onset of severe hives and rash, and difficulty breathing, chest tightness, or swelling in back of throat or tongue	**YES**	"Call ambulance"
	NO	Go to B

R

505

B. Are any of the following present?

- Purple- or blood-colored flat spots or dots, headache, pain bending head forward, vomiting, or fever
- Unusual drowsiness, refusal to drink, and noisy or fast breathing
- Rash, fever, red tongue, and enlarged lymph nodes
- Sudden onset of illness and rapid progression of widespread redness, scaliness, fever, and enlarged lymph nodes
- Red peeling rash in rectal area
- Rapidly spreading red or purple rash that develops into blisters on mucous membranes (lips, mouth, eyes, genitals)
- Fever, headache, or respiratory infection followed by blistering rash

YES "Seek emergency care now"

NO Go to C

C. Are any of the following present?

- Severe facial or eye swelling
- Rash around eyes, vision changes, or weeping lesions
- Open sores with signs of infection: redness, swelling, pain, red streaks, drainage, warmth
- Fever in a menstruating child who uses tampons
- Bright-red painful area
- Fever and painful rash
- Red rash peels off in sheets of skin
- Purple- or blood-colored spots or dots
- Age <1 month and grouping of small water blisters
- Rash or flu-like symptoms; fever, chills, sore throat, headache 2 to 4 weeks after a tick bite

YES "Seek medical care within 2 to 4 hours"

NO Go to D

D. Is the following present?

- New antibiotic or medication and new onset of rash or hives

YES "Call PCP now"

NO Go to E

E. Are any of the following present?

- Persistent rash for >48 hours that is unresponsive to home care measures
- Persistent hives after taking Benadryl for 24 hours
- Extensive rash, cause unknown
- Rash and itching interfere with sleep
- Multiple grouping of painful blisters

YES "Seek medical care within 24 hours"

NO Go to F

F. Are any of the following present?

- Prolonged exposure to heat
- Rash restricted to diaper and upper leg area
- Exposure to poison oak, ivy, or sumac
- Change in laundry detergent and contact areas affected
- Exposure to chemicals
- Recent immunization
- Other household members have similar rash
- Raised, red, itchy rash followed by blisters
- Blisters form golden crusts
- Scaly or blistery rash on the face or in folds of skin on elbows or knees
- Dull red spots, runny nose, cough, sore throat, fever, red eyes (suspicion of rubella)
- Pink rash, swollen glands at back of the neck, fever, and no prior immunization or history of measles infection
- Circular, raised, rough pink patch with clear center ½ to 1 inch and itchy
- Tick bite and expanding rash

YES "Call back or call PCP for appointment if no improvement" and Follow **Home Care Instructions**

NO Follow **Home Care Instructions**

R

Home Care Instructions
Rash, Child

- Try to identify the cause and avoid the irritant.
- Cleanse the area with soap and water to remove the irritant, then use only water to cleanse the area.
- Apply compresses soaked in water and Domeboro.

To Control Itching

- Take a cool bath with baking soda, Aveeno, or oatmeal (1 cup in a tub of cool water) several times a day, or apply cold packs to localized rashes for 20 minutes every 3 to 4 hours.
- For severe itching, apply 1% hydrocortisone cream and follow the instructions on the label. Refrigerate it for optimal cooling relief. Avoid using it when jock itch, athlete's foot, impetigo, or ringworm is suspected.
- Apply a baking soda paste mixed with white vinegar, or OTC preparations such as calamine lotion or Aveeno, to the affected area.
- Give an antihistamine (Benadryl, Chlor-Trimeton) and follow the instructions on the label.
- Cut the child's fingernails and discourage scratching.
- Cover the infant's hands with socks to discourage scratching.
- Apply wet dressings soaked in Burow's solution, 1 part solution to 10 to 40 parts water. Change frequently, as often as 8 times in 2 hours.

For Possible Allergic Reaction

- If rash is related to a new medication, stop the medication. Call PCP if it is a prescription medication.
- Take antihistamines as directed on the container until rash and itching are gone.
- Watch for signs of worsening reaction (swelling or difficulty swallowing or breathing) and see PCP.

For Possible Heat Rash

- Apply calamine lotion or hydrocortisone cream.
- Take a cool bath or shower without soap every 2 to 3 hours as needed for relief, and air-dry.
- Apply baby powder to the affected area.

For Poison Oak, Ivy, or Sumac Exposure

- Wash the exposed area within 1 hour of exposure, if possible.
- Soak the area with cool water or rub it with ice for 20 minutes, as needed.
- Wash all clothes and any animal exposed to the plants.

For Suspected Measles/Chickenpox/Rubella

- Keep the child home until the rash is gone to avoid exposing others to the disease.
- Avoid spreading infection to others.
- Wash hands well with soap and water after contact with the infected person.
- Keep weeping areas covered when there is the possibility of contact with others.
- Use cotton balls or gauze to apply lotions or ointments to open areas.

Additional Instructions

Report the Following Problems to Your PCP/Clinic/ED

- No improvement in 24 to 48 hours with home care measures or condition worsens
- Fever, sore throat, or joint pain
- Signs of infection
- Unusual drowsiness, refusal to drink, earache, and noisy or fast breathing

Seek Emergency Care Immediately If Any of the Following Occur

- Difficulty breathing, chest tightness, or swelling in the back of the throat
- Purple spots, headache, stiff neck, vomiting, or fever
- Rash, fever, red tongue, and enlarged lymph nodes
- Red peeling rash in rectal area

If the caller agrees with the advice given, document the call and encourage the caller to call back or see PCP if the problem worsens. If the caller does not agree with the advice given, reevaluate and advise the caller to follow up with PCP, Clinic, or ED.

R

Rectal Bleeding

 Key Questions Name, Age, Onset, Medications, History

 Other Protocols to Consider Abdominal Pain, Adult (9), Child (13); Constipation (160); Diarrhea, Adult (192), Child (195); Foreign Body, Rectum (276); Hemorrhoids (327); Vomiting, Adult (642), Child (645); Stools, Abnormal (573).

Nurse Alert: Rectal bleeding includes black, maroon, or tarry stools, bright-red blood on toilet tissue, on the surface of stool, mixed in with formed or diarrheal stool or passed separately.

Reminder: Document caller response to advice, home care instructions, and when to call back.

ASSESSMENT	ACTION
A. Is abdominal pain present?	
	YES Go to Abdominal Pain protocol (9)
	NO Go to B
B. Are any of the following present?	
• Light-headedness or fainting • Vomiting blood or coffee grounds–like emesis • Intermittent abdominal pain • Frequent black tarry stools • Large amount of bright-red blood mixed in the stool or passing of blood clots	**YES** "Seek emergency care now" **NO** Go to C
C. Is the following present?	
• Use of blood thinners, steroids, nonsteroidal anti-inflammatory medications, or large doses of aspirin	**YES** "Seek medical care within 2 to 4 hours" **NO** Go to D

D. Are any of the following present?

- Recent history of cancer
- Temperature >100°F (37.7°C)

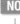 **YES** "Seek medical care within 24 hours"

 NO Go to E

E. Are any of the following present?

- Stool streaked with red blood
- Blood on toilet tissue after wiping
- Constipation or hemorrhoids
- Bleeding persists >2 to 3 days after constipation improves
- Taking iron preparations or bismuth subsalicylate (Pepto-Bismol)
- Recent ingestion of beets or spinach

YES "Call back or call PCP for appointment if no improvement" and Follow **Home Care Instructions**

NO Follow **Home Care Instructions**

R

Home Care Instructions
Rectal Bleeding

- Soak in a warm saline bath for 20 minutes a day to cleanse the area and promote healing. (Add 2 tbsp of salt or baking soda to the water.)
- Keep rectal area clean. May use medicated pads (Tucks) to cleanse and soothe area; follow instruction on the label. Ask pharmacist for additional product suggestions.
- If rectal area is irritated, apply OTC hydrocortisone ointment (Anusol-HC, Cortaid) or zinc oxide paste or powder.
- If hemorrhoids persist, try OTC preparations (Anusol, Nupercainal, Preparation H) to help soothe and shrink hemorrhoids. Follow instructions on the label.
- Increase fluid intake and eat a diet high in fiber: fruits, vegetables, bran, grains, and beans. Avoid constipating foods such as cheese. This is particularly important if taking narcotic pain medications for discomfort.
- If taking iron preparations or bismuth subsalicylate (Pepto-Bismol) or eating spinach or beets, follow up with PCP for stool guaiac.
- Exercise 30 minutes a day even if only at 10- or 15-minute intervals.

Additional Instructions

Report the Following Problems to Your PCP/Clinic/ED

- No improvement in 3 days or bleeding worsens
- Abdominal pain
- Constipation or hemorrhoids persist >1 week after home treatment
- Blood mixed with stool or black stools

Seek Emergency Care Immediately If Any of the Following Occur

- Vomiting blood or coffee grounds–like emesis
- Light-headedness or fainting
- Intermittent abdominal pain
- Large amount of bright-red blood mixed with stool or passing of blood clots
- Frequent black tarry stools

If the caller agrees with the advice given, document the call and encourage the caller to call back or see PCP if the problem worsens. If the caller does not agree with the advice given, reevaluate and advise the caller to follow up with PCP, Clinic, or ED.

Rectal Problems

 Key Questions Name, Age, Onset, Allergies, Medications, History, Pain Scale

 Other Protocols to Consider Constipation (160); Diarrhea, Adult (192), Child (195); Foreign Body, Rectum (276); Hemorrhoids (327); Pinworm (452); Rectal Bleeding (510).

Reminder: Document caller response to advice, home care instructions, and when to call back.

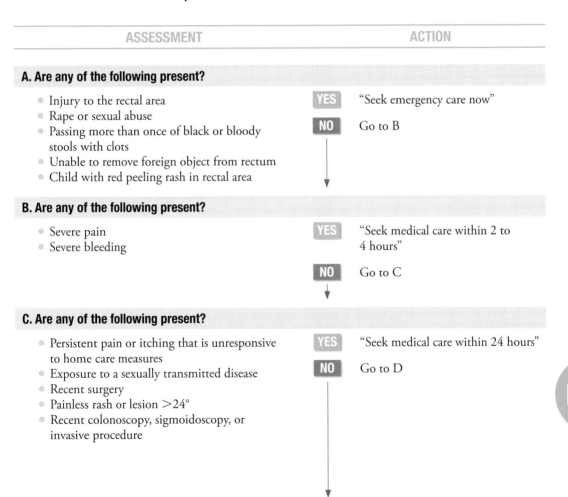

ASSESSMENT	ACTION
A. Are any of the following present?	
• Injury to the rectal area	**YES** "Seek emergency care now"
• Rape or sexual abuse	**NO** Go to B
• Passing more than once of black or bloody stools with clots	
• Unable to remove foreign object from rectum	
• Child with red peeling rash in rectal area	
B. Are any of the following present?	
• Severe pain	**YES** "Seek medical care within 2 to 4 hours"
• Severe bleeding	
	NO Go to C
C. Are any of the following present?	
• Persistent pain or itching that is unresponsive to home care measures	**YES** "Seek medical care within 24 hours"
• Exposure to a sexually transmitted disease	**NO** Go to D
• Recent surgery	
• Painless rash or lesion >24°	
• Recent colonoscopy, sigmoidoscopy, or invasive procedure	

R

D. Are any of the following present?

- Intermittent rectal swelling, pain, itching, or bleeding
- Pain or bleeding for <48 hours
- First episode of rectal bleeding, swelling, pain, or itching
- Rectal itching
- Visible small worms in stools or around rectal area
- Painless rash or growth <24°

YES   "Call back or call PCP for appointment if no improvement" and Follow **Home Care Instructions**

NO   Follow **Home Care Instructions**

Home Care Instructions
Rectal Problems

- Soak in a warm bath for 20 to 30 minutes daily.
- Apply an OTC medication for relief of itching and discomfort.
- Avoid constipating foods (cheese and white flour products). Include fresh fruits, vegetables, and whole grains in the diet. Drink lots of water every day (unless PCP has ordered a restricted fluid intake).
- Try OTC medications for hemorrhoids.

Additional Instructions

Report the Following Problems to Your PCP/Clinic/ED

- Black or bloody stools more than once
- No improvement or condition worsens

Seek Emergency Care Immediately If Any of the Following Occur

- Black or bloody stools with clots more than once
- Child with red peeling rash in rectal area

If the caller agrees with the advice given, document the call and encourage the caller to call back or see PCP if the problem worsens. If the caller does not agree with the advice given, reevaluate and advise the caller to follow up with PCP, Clinic, or ED.

R

Reye Syndrome, Suspected

 Key Questions Name, Age, Onset, Medications, History

 Other Protocols to Consider Chickenpox (129); Confusion (150); Congestion (153); Cough (170); Fever, Child (253).

> *Nurse Alert:* Use this protocol if previously diagnosed with Reye syndrome or caller suspects Reye syndrome in a child or adolescent after a recent illness, taking aspirin during that illness and now has new concerning symptoms.

Reminder: Document caller response to advice, home care instructions, and when to call back.

ASSESSMENT	ACTION
A. Are any of the following present?	
• Recent history of a viral illness such as chickenpox, the flu, or other respiratory illness • History of taking aspirin during the illness and appearance of any of the following symptoms shortly after the viral illness: • headache, incoordination, slurred speech, confusion, lethargy, personality changes • vomiting • weakness in an arm or leg • hearing loss or double vision	**YES** "Seek emergency care now" **NO** "Call back or call PCP for appointment if no improvement" and Follow **Home Care Instructions**

Home Care Instructions
Reye Syndrome, Suspected

- In general, it is not a good idea to give children or adolescents aspirin because symptoms often do not appear until several days after a virus is contracted. Take acetaminophen for fever and discomfort.
- If the child has taken aspirin immediately before or during a viral illness, observe closely for symptoms of Reye syndrome and report to your PCP. Symptoms usually appear shortly after the acute phase of a viral illness and may progress rapidly. Symptoms include the following:
  - headache, incoordination, slurred speech, confusion, lethargy, and personality changes
  - vomiting
  - weakness in an arm or leg
  - hearing loss or double vision

Additional Instructions

Report the Following Problem to Your PCP/Clinic/ED
- Suspected symptoms of Reye syndrome

Seek Emergency Care Immediately If Any of the Following Occur
- Confusion, lethargy, and other mental changes
- Headache, incoordination, slurred speech
- Vomiting
- Weakness in an arm or leg
- Hearing loss or double vision

If the caller agrees with the advice given, document the call and encourage the caller to call back or see PCP if the problem worsens. If the caller does not agree with the advice given, reevaluate and advise the caller to follow up with PCP, Clinic, or ED.

R

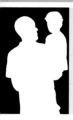

Roseola

>> **Key Questions** Name, Age, Onset, Known Diagnosis or Exposure, Allergies, Medications, History

>> **Other Protocols to Consider** Fever, Child (253); Rubella (German Measles) (520); Itching (382); Rash, Child (505).

Nurse Alert:

- Use this protocol if previously diagnosed with roseola or known exposure and child is now ill with a rash.
- Communicable Disease Table in Appendix M (696) is provided to help the nurse gain a better understanding of many communicable diseases, the mode of disease transmission, incubation period, and contagious period. It is NOT to be used to try and diagnose a caller's condition.

Reminder: Document caller response to advice, home care instructions, and when to call back.

ASSESSMENT		ACTION

A. Diagnosed with roseola, and are any of the following present?

• Purple- or blood-colored rash or spots	**YES**	"Seek emergency care now"
• Child appears very ill		
• Persistent loud crying that is unresponsive to holding and comfort	**NO**	Go to B
• Temperature of >105°F (40.6°C)		

B. Are any of the following present?

• Persistent fever for >4 days	**YES**	"Seek medical care within 24 hours"
• Persistent rash for >3 days	**NO**	Go to C

C. Are any of the following present?

• Known or suspected exposure to roseola and no previous history of the disease	**YES**	"Call back or call PCP for appointment if no improvement" and Follow **Home Care Instructions**
• Fine pink rash on trunk follows 3 to 4 days of fever		
• Irritability	**NO**	Follow **Home Care Instructions**
• Fever		

518

Home Care Instructions
Roseola

- Give acetaminophen for fever. Do not give aspirin to a child. Avoid aspirin-like products if age <20 years. Avoid acetaminophen if liver disease is present. Avoid ibuprofen if kidney disease or stomach problems exist or in the case of pregnancy. Follow the directions on the label.
- Ensure child is taking adequate fluids during fever.

Additional Instructions

Report the Following Problems to Your PCP/Clinic/ED
- Child refuses liquids
- Persistent fever >4 days
- Persistent rash >3 days

Seek Emergency Care Immediately If Any of the Following Occur
- Persistent loud crying that is unresponsive to holding and comfort measures
- Purple- or blood-colored rash or spots
- Child appears very ill
- Temperature >105°F (40.6°C)

If the caller agrees with the advice given, document the call and encourage the caller to call back or see PCP if the problem worsens. If the caller does not agree with the advice given, reevaluate and advise the caller to follow up with PCP, Clinic, or ED.

R

Rubella (German Measles)

Key Questions Name, Age, Onset, Known Diagnosis or Exposure, Allergies, Medications, History, Immunization Status

Other Protocols to Consider Fever, Adult (250), Child (253); Itching (382); Rash, Adult (500), Child (505); Rubeola (Measles) (523).

Nurse Alert:

- Use this protocol if previously diagnosed with rubella or known exposure, now ill, and has a rash.
- Communicable Disease Table in Appendix M (696) is provided to help the nurse gain a better understanding of many communicable diseases, the mode of disease transmission, incubation period, and contagious period. It is NOT to be used to try and diagnose a caller's condition.

Reminder: Document caller response to advice, home care instructions, and when to call back.

ASSESSMENT	ACTION
A. Diagnosed with rubella, and are any of the following present?	
• Purple, flat, nonblanching rash • Child appears very ill • Persistent loud crying that is unresponsive to holding and comfort • Temperature of >105°F (40.6°C)	**YES** "Seek emergency care now" **NO** Go to B
B. Are any of the following present?	
• Persistent fever >3 days • Pain in joints • Pregnant with known or suspected exposure to rubella (contagious period is 7 days before and 5 days after the rash appears)	**YES** "Seek medical care within 24 hours" **NO** Go to C

C. Are any of the following present?

- Known or suspected exposure to rubella and no previous history of the disease or immunization
- Generalized red rash spreading over entire body in 24 hours
- Swollen nodes at the back of the neck
- Fever
- Persistent itching

YES "Call back or call PCP for appointment if no improvement" and Follow **Home Care Instructions**

NO Follow **Home Care Instructions**

R

Home Care Instructions
Rubella (German Measles)

- Avoid exposing pregnant women. Condition is contagious for 5 days after rash initially appears.
- Women of childbearing age should avoid pregnancy for 3 months.
- Take acetaminophen for pain. Do not give aspirin to a child. Avoid aspirin-like products if age <20 years. Avoid acetaminophen if liver disease is present. Avoid ibuprofen if kidney disease or stomach problems exist or in the case of pregnancy. Follow the directions on the label.
- Try soda or oatmeal baths for itching.

Additional Instructions

Report the Following Problems to Your PCP/Clinic/ED

- First trimester of pregnancy and exposed to rubella
- Pain in joints
- Persistent fever >3 days
- Persistent rash >5 days

Seek Emergency Care Immediately If Diagnosed With Rubella and Any of the Following Occur

- Purple, flat, nonblanching rash
- Child appears very ill
- Persistent loud crying that is unresponsive to holding and comfort
- Temperature >105°F (40.6°C)

If the caller agrees with the advice given, document the call and encourage the caller to call back or see PCP if the problem worsens. If the caller does not agree with the advice given, reevaluate and advise the caller to follow up with PCP, Clinic, or ED.

Rubeola (Measles)

 Key Questions Name, Age, Onset, Known Rubeola Diagnosis or Exposure, Allergies, Medications, History, Immunization Status

 Other Protocols to Consider Cough (170); Earache, Drainage (206); Fever, Adult (250), Child (253); Rash, Adult (500), Child (505); Rubella (German Measles) (520); Sore Throat (564).

Nurse Alert:

- Use this protocol if previously diagnosed with rubeola or known exposure and now ill.
- Communicable Disease Table in Appendix M (696) is provided to help the nurse gain a better understanding of many communicable diseases, the mode of disease transmission, incubation period, and contagious period. It is NOT to be used to try and diagnose a caller's condition.

Reminder: Document caller response to advice, home care instructions, and when to call back.

ASSESSMENT	ACTION

A. Known rubeola diagnosis or exposure, and are any of the following present?

- Difficulty breathing
- Severe headache and/or neck pain
- Confusion
- Difficulty awakening
- Decreased level of consciousness
- Seizures

YES "Seek emergency care now"

NO Go to B

B. Are any of the following present?

- Fever >4 days after onset of rash
- Yellow or green nasal discharge >48 hours
- Ill appearance

YES "Seek medical care within 24 hours"

NO Go to C

R

C. Are any of the following present?

- Red, watery or itchy eyes, cough, and runny nose
- Earache
- Eyes crusted closed in the morning or yellow discharge
- Eyes sensitive to light
- Bluish-white spots in mouth
- Blotchy red rash spreads from the face down the body and persists >7 days
- Fever
- Known exposure to measles within past 12 days and no prior vaccination for measles

YES "Call back or call PCP for appointment if no improvement" and Follow **Home Care Instructions**

NO Follow **Home Care Instructions**

Home Care Instructions
Rubeola (Measles)

- Take acetaminophen for fever and discomfort. Do not give aspirin to a child. Avoid aspirin-like products if age <20 years. Avoid acetaminophen if liver disease is present. Avoid ibuprofen if kidney disease or stomach problems exist or in the case of pregnancy. Follow the directions on the label.
- To soothe cough, give ½ to 1 tsp corn syrup to child 4 years old or younger; give cough drops, hard candy, or cough syrup to older children. Warm clear fluids, such as apple juice and herbal teas, are soothing to the throat and can be given to children older than 4 months.
- Remove eye drainage with a wet cotton ball, which should be discarded after use. Use a separate cotton ball for each eye.
- If eyes are sensitive to light, keep the child in a darkened or dimly lit room.
- Enforce rest until fever is gone.
- Call PCP for confirmed diagnosis.
- Keep child away from others who have not had the illness or been immunized until the rash is gone (about 7 days).

Additional Instructions

_____

_____

_____

Report the Following Problems to Your PCP/Clinic/ED

- Earache or sore throat
- Yellow or green nasal discharge for >48 hours
- Fever for >4 days after onset of rash
- Eyes crusted closed in the morning or yellow discharge

R

Seek Emergency Care Immediately If Any of the Following Occur
- Difficulty breathing
- Severe headache
- Confusion
- Difficulty awakening
- Seizures

If the caller agrees with the advice given, document the call and encourage the caller to call back or see PCP if the problem worsens. If the caller does not agree with the advice given, reevaluate and advise the caller to follow up with PCP, Clinic, or ED.

Scabies

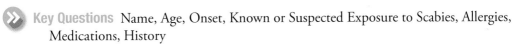

S

>> **Key Questions** Name, Age, Onset, Known or Suspected Exposure to Scabies, Allergies, Medications, History

>> **Other Protocols to Consider** Itching (382); Rash, Adult (500), Child (505).

> *Nurse Alert:* Use this protocol if previously diagnosed with scabies, known or suspected exposure to someone with scabies, and small blisters present. Scabies is highly contagious.

Reminder: Document caller response to advice, home care instructions, and when to call back.

ASSESSMENT	ACTION
A. Are any of the following present?	

• Lines of small itchy blisters:
  • between fingers or toes
  • on wrists, elbows, or armpits
  • on waist, buttock creases, inner thighs, or creases under breasts
• Other household members have same symptoms
• Blisters break easily when scratched
• Increased itching at night
• Signs of infection: increased discomfort, drainage, redness, red streaks from wound, or warmth
• Adult with scabies on face or scalp
	YES "Seek medical care within 48 hours" or "Call back or call PCP for appointment if no improvement" and Follow **Home Care Instructions**
	
	NO Follow **Home Care Instructions**

Home Care Instructions
Scabies

- Scabies is highly contagious, and all members of a household should be treated after exposure to diagnosed scabies. Symptoms can take 30 days to appear after exposure.
- If using crotamiton (Eurax), as prescribed by physician, leave on for 24 hours, then apply a second coat. Do not wash off the first coat. After 48 hours, wash off the second coat. Repeat process in 1 week.
- Take cool baths without soap to help relieve itching.
- Take an antihistamine (Benadryl) to help relieve itching, and follow instructions on the label.
- Wash all clothes, linens, and undergarments in hot soapy water.
- Store blankets for 3 to 4 days. Scabies cannot live if separated from a host body.
- Use OTC or prescribed medications as directed by your PCP or pharmacist.

Additional Instructions

Report the Following Problems to Your PCP/Clinic/ED

- Rash shows signs of infection: redness, swelling, drainage, red streaks, or pain
- Persistent rash after two treatments or 3 weeks
- Condition worsens

If the caller agrees with the advice given, document the call and encourage the caller to call back or see PCP if the problem worsens. If the caller does not agree with the advice given, reevaluate and advise the caller to follow up with PCP, Clinic, or ED.

Scrotal Problems

 Key Questions Name, Age, Onset, Cause, Allergies, Medications, History, Pain Scale

 Other Protocols to Consider Genital Lesions (291); Genital Problems, Male (294); Piercing Problems (445); Sexually Transmitted Disease (542); Urination, Painful (628).

Reminder: Document caller response to advice, home care instructions, and when to call back.

ASSESSMENT	ACTION

A. Severe testicular pain and swelling and are any of the following present?

- Injury to genitals <48 hours ago
- No known injury, sudden onset of pain, swelling, fever, nausea, vomiting
- Scrotum black, blue, or bright red

 YES "Seek emergency care now"

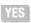 **NO** Go to B

B. Are any of the following present?

- Injury to genitals >48 hours ago with pain and swelling
- Gradual onset of pain, fever, or swelling
- One enlarged testicle
- Unable to reduce scrotal swelling in infant in whom fever, vomiting, and irritability are present

 YES "Seek medical care within 2 to 4 hours"

 NO Go to C

C. Are any of the following present?

- Painless lump or swelling
- Sores or painful red rash on scrotal sac
- Signs of infection: pain, swelling, redness, warmth, red streaks, or drainage
- Scrotal itching, redness, swelling, or discomfort

 YES "Seek medical care within 24 hours"

NO Go to D

D. Is the following present?

- Painless rash <24 hours

 YES "Call back or call PCP for appointment if no improvement" and Follow **Home Care Instructions**

 NO Follow **Home Care Instructions**

529

Home Care Instructions
Scrotal Problems

- While waiting for appointment or visit, support scrotum on rolled towel, apply ice pack to area, and wear supporter. Do not apply ice directly to the skin; use a washcloth or other cloth barrier between ice and the skin.
- Take your usual pain medication (aspirin, acetaminophen, ibuprofen) for discomfort. Do not give aspirin to a child. Avoid aspirin-like products if age <20 years. Avoid acetaminophen if liver disease is present. Avoid ibuprofen if kidney disease or stomach problems exist or in the case of pregnancy. Follow the directions on the label.

Additional Instructions

Report the Following Problems to Your PCP/Clinic/ED

- Any lump
- No improvement after 48 hours or condition worsens
- Signs of infection: pain, swelling, redness, warmth, red streaks, or drainage
- Pain for >2 weeks
- Pain with urination
- Fever

Seek Emergency Care Immediately If the Following Occurs

- Testicles turn black, blue, or bright red

If the caller agrees with the advice given, document the call and encourage the caller to call back or see PCP if the problem worsens. If the caller does not agree with the advice given, reevaluate and advise the caller to follow up with PCP, Clinic, or ED.

Seizure

 Key Questions Name, Age, Onset, History of Seizures, Allergies, Medications, History

 Other Protocols to Consider Alcohol Problems (21); Altered Mental Status (28); Confusion (150); Fever, Adult (250), Child (253); Head Injury (311); Seizure, Febrile (533).

Reminder: Document caller response to advice, home care instructions, and when to call back.

ASSESSMENT	ACTION

A. Are any of the following present?

- Multiple seizures
- Difficulty breathing
- Seizure lasts >5 minutes
- Severe headache
- Persistent unusual lethargy
- History of recent head injury
- History of recent drug ingestion
- First-time seizure
- Pregnancy

YES "Call ambulance" or "Seek emergency care now"

NO Go to B

B. Are any of the following present?

- Injury during seizure
- History of habitual heavy alcohol or drug use and recently quit drinking or taking drugs
- High fever
- Frequent seizures while on seizure medication

YES "Seek medical care within 2 hours"

NO Go to C

C. Are any of the following present?

- Stopped taking seizure medication
- History of diabetes, cerebrovascular accident, cancer, or cardiovascular or neuromuscular disease

YES "Seek medical care within 24 hours"

NO Go to D

D. Is the following present?

- History of seizures and alert and oriented after waking up from the seizure

YES "Call back or call PCP for appointment if no improvement" and Follow **Home Care Instructions**

NO Follow **Home Care Instructions**

Home Care Instructions
Seizure

Protect the Airway
- Lay the victim on side or stomach with the head turned toward the side to prevent choking on secretions or vomit.
- If there is noisy breathing, pull the jaw and chin forward. Do not put your fingers, medication, or any other object in the seizing person's mouth.
- Loosen tie or other restrictive clothing.

Protect from Injury
- Move the seizing person to a safe area away from objects that could cause injury.
- Protect the head from hitting a hard surface.
- Do not try to hold the person and restrict movement. Allow the seizure to run its course.

Postictal Phase
- Expect the person to sleep approximately 30 minutes after the seizure and slowly awaken.
- Do not allow the person to drive after a seizure.
- Do not give anything by mouth until fully awake.

Reduce High Fever after the Seizure
- Remove clothing and sponge with cool water.
- Apply cool compresses to the forehead, face, and neck.
- Give acetaminophen for fever. Use acetaminophen suppositories if the person is still groggy. Do not give aspirin to a child. Avoid aspirin-like products if age <20 years. Avoid acetaminophen if liver disease is present. Avoid ibuprofen if kidney disease or stomach problems exist or in the case of pregnancy. Follow the directions on the label.

Additional Instructions

Report the Following Problems to Your PCP/Clinic/ED
- Repeated seizure activity
- No improvement or condition worsens
- Fever unresponsive to fever-reducing measures after a seizure

Seek Emergency Care Immediately If Any of the Following Occur
- Difficulty breathing
- Severe headache, stiff or painful neck
- Persistent confusion

If the caller agrees with the advice given, document the call and encourage the caller to call back or see PCP if the problem worsens. If the caller does not agree with the advice given, reevaluate and advise the caller to follow up with PCP, Clinic, or ED.

Seizure, Febrile

>> **Key Questions** Name, Age, Onset, History of Seizures, Temperature (if known), Does Child Feel Hot, Allergies, Medications, History

>> **Other Protocols to Consider** Altered Mental Status (28); Confusion (150); Fever, Adult (250), Child (253); Head Injury (311).

Reminder: Document caller response to advice, home care instructions, and when to call back.

ASSESSMENT	ACTION

A. Are any of the following present?

- Multiple seizures
- Difficulty breathing or breathing stopped >60 seconds
- Seizure lasts >5 minutes

YES → "Call ambulance" and "Begin rescue breathing if child is not breathing"

NO → Go to B

B. Are any of the following present?

- First-time seizure
- Child younger than 6 months or older than 5 years of age
- Severe headache, stiff or painful neck

YES → "Seek emergency care now"

NO → Go to C

C. Is the following present?

- Persistent temperature >102°F (38.9°C) that is unresponsive to fever-reducing measures

YES → "Seek medical care within 24 hours"

NO → Go to D

D. Are any of the following present?

- Alert and oriented after seizure
- Child wants to sleep after seizure but can be aroused without irritability

YES → "Call back or call PCP for appointment if no improvement" and Follow **Home Care Instructions**

NO → Follow **Home Care Instructions**

Seizure, Febrile

Protect the Airway
- Lay the victim on side or stomach with the head turned toward the side to prevent choking on secretions or vomit.
- If there is any noisy breathing, pull the jaw and chin forward. Do not put your fingers, medication, or any other object in the seizing person's mouth.
- Loosen clothing.

Protect from Injury
- Move the seizing person to a safe area away from objects that could cause injury.
- Protect the head from hitting a hard surface.
- Do not try to hold the person and restrict movement. Allow the seizure to run its course.

Postictal Phase
- Expect drowsiness. Allow rest in a cool room. Lightly dress the victim in undergarments.
- Do not give anything by mouth until fully awake.

Reduce High Fever after the Seizure
- Remove clothing and sponge with cool water. Stop the bath if shivering occurs.
- Apply cold compresses to the forehead, face, neck, and underarms.
- Give acetaminophen for fever, and follow instructions on the label. Use acetaminophen suppositories if drowsiness persists. Give every 4 hours if fever persists, even during the night, until fever <100°F (37.8°C). Do not give aspirin to a child. Avoid aspirin-like products if age <20 years. Avoid acetaminophen if liver disease is present. Avoid ibuprofen if kidney disease or stomach problems exist or in the case of pregnancy. Follow the directions on the label.
- Do not bathe with alcohol rubs.

Additional Instructions

Report the Following Problems to Your PCP/Clinic/ED

- Repeated seizure activity
- No improvement or condition worsens
- Fever unresponsive to fever-reducing measures

Seek Emergency Care Immediately If Any of the Following Occur

- Difficulty breathing or breathing stops >60 seconds
- Seizure lasts >5 minutes
- Face, lips, or nails turn blue
- Injury occurs during seizure
- Persistent confusion
- Severe headache, stiff or painful neck

If the caller agrees with the advice given, document the call and encourage the caller to call back or see PCP if the problem worsens. If the caller does not agree with the advice given, reevaluate and advise the caller to follow up with PCP, Clinic, or ED.

Severe Acute Respiratory Syndrome (SARS)

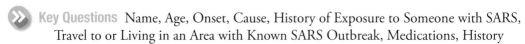 **Key Questions** Name, Age, Onset, Cause, History of Exposure to Someone with SARS, Travel to or Living in an Area with Known SARS Outbreak, Medications, History

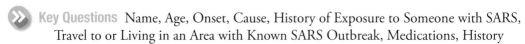 **Other Protocols to Consider** Breathing Problems (106); Common Cold Symptoms (146); Cough (170); Fever, Adult (250), Child (253); Influenza (372).

> *Nurse Alert:* Use this protocol if diagnosed with SARS, known or suspected exposure to SARS, travel to or living in an area with known SARS outbreak.

Reminder: Document caller response to advice, home care instructions, and when to call back.

ASSESSMENT	ACTION
A. Are any of the following present?	
• Altered mental status • Severe difficulty breathing • Chest pain • High fever >104.9°F (40.5°C)	**YES** "Call ambulance" or "Go to Emergency Department now" and Notify health-care workers of potential exposure **NO** Go to B
B. Are any of the following present?	
• Cough and fever within 10 days of SARS exposure • Difficulty breathing within 10 days of SARS exposure	**YES** "Seek medical care immediately" **NO** Go to C

C. Are any of the following present?

- Fever within 10 days of SARS exposure
- Cough within 10 days of SARS exposure
- Exposure to SARS within past 10 days and the development of
  - headache
  - muscle aches
  - diarrhea
  - malaise

YES "Seek medical care within 24 hours"

NO Go to D

D. Is the following present?

- SARS exposure with no signs or symptoms

YES "Call back or call PCP for appointment if no improvement" and
Follow **Home Care Instructions**

NO Follow **Home Care Instructions**

Home Care Instructions
Severe Acute Respiratory Syndrome (SARS)

- Isolation if cough or fever develops within 10 days of SARS exposure. Do not go to work, school, or other public area for 10 days after respiratory symptoms are gone.
- Frequent handwashing with soap and water or alcohol-based hand rubs.
- Good respiratory etiquette: cover mouth and nose with a tissue when coughing or sneezing. Wear a surgical mask during close contact with others to prevent the spread of droplets. Change the mask once a day or if it becomes soiled or moist.
- Use disposable gloves if touching bodily fluids.
- Do not share eating utensils, bedding, towels, etc.
- Frequently disinfect surfaces in kitchen, bathroom, and other areas that the person may have touched.

Additional Instructions

Report the Following Problems to Your PCP/Clinic/ED

- No improvement or condition worsens
- Fever >72 hours
- Productive cough

Seek Emergency Care Immediately If Any of the Following Occur

- Severe difficulty breathing
- Chest pain
- Altered mental status
- High fever >104.9°F (40.5°C)

If the caller agrees with the advice given, document the call and encourage the caller to call back or see PCP if the problem worsens. If the caller does not agree with the advice given, reevaluate and advise the caller to follow up with PCP, Clinic, or ED.

Sexual Assault

 Key Questions Name, Age, Onset, Medications, History

 Other Protocols to Consider Blood/Body Fluid Exposure (93); Child Abuse (132); Domestic Abuse (202); Foreign Body, Rectum (276); Foreign Body, Vagina (282); Rectal Problems (513); Sexually Transmitted Disease (STD) (542); Vaginal Bleeding (633); Vaginal Discharge/Pain/Itching (636).

> *Nurse Alert:* Many sexual assault victims are confused about what to do after an assault. Encourage to go to the ED where a sexual assault examination can be performed by staff specially trained in sexual assault evidence collection, examination, support, and follow-up. Instruct not to shower before going to the ED. In some states the RN sexual assault examiner can examine victims and collect evidence in locations other than the ED. Refer to the services available in your local area.

Reminder: Document caller response to advice, home care instructions, and when to call back.

ASSESSMENT	ACTION

A. Are any of the following present?

- Sexual assault is in process at time of call
- Victim is seriously injured, unconscious, or dead

 "Call ambulance and local police"

 Go to B

B. Sexual assault has occurred and are any of the following present?

- Vaginal or anal tearing or bleeding
- Suspected fractures or dislocations
- Abrasions, lacerations, bruising, discoloration, or swelling
- Difficulty breathing, chest pain, or abdominal pain
- Victim requests an examination and collection of evidence
- Victim is a minor

 "Seek emergency care now"
and
Follow **Home Care Instructions**

 Go to C

C. Sexual assault has occurred and victim requests a medical examination without collection of evidence or has questions and concerns. Ask the following questions:

- Are you in a safe environment now?
- Are you alone?
- Where is the abuser now?
- Do you have family or friends who can help you?
- Have you called the police?
- Have you called a rape crisis center or rape hotline?
- Victim of rape drug (e.g., GHB, Rohypnol, Ketamine) and requesting rape drug blood or urine test

YES "Seek medical care within 24 hours" and
Follow **Home Care Instructions**

NO Follow **Home Care Instructions**

Home Care Instructions
Sexual Assault

- Advise the victim to stay in a safe and supportive environment.
- Encourage the victim to have a medical examination with testing for STDs and pregnancy.
- Encourage the victim to report the incident to the police.
- Encourage the victim to call a rape crisis center or rape hotline.
- Advise caller not to shower or change clothes before the medical examination.

S

Referral Telephone Numbers

_____

_____

_____

Additional Instructions

_____

_____

_____

Report the Following Problems to Your PCP/Clinic/ED

- Pain or bleeding persists or worsens
- Feelings of anger, depression, suicidal thoughts, or uncontrollable crying
- Fever, discharge, or sores develop

If the caller agrees with the advice given, document the call and encourage the caller to call back or see PCP if the problem worsens. If the caller does not agree with the advice given, reevaluate and advise the caller to follow up with PCP, Clinic, or ED.

Sexually Transmitted Disease (STD)

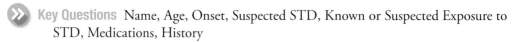 **Key Questions** Name, Age, Onset, Suspected STD, Known or Suspected Exposure to STD, Medications, History

Other Protocols to Consider Blood/Body Fluid Exposure (93); Genital Lesions (291); Genital Problems, Male (294); Sexual Assault (539); Urination, Painful (628); Vaginal Discharge/Pain/Itching (636).

Nurse Alert: Use this protocol if known STD, exposure or suspected exposure to STD. Sexually Transmitted Disease Table: Appendix N (687) is provided to help the nurse gain a better understanding of many STDs, their mode of disease transmission, incubation period, and contagious period. It is NOT to be used to try and diagnose a caller's condition.

Reminder: Document caller response to advice, home care instructions, and when to call back.

ASSESSMENT	ACTION
A. Are any of the following present?	
• Victim of sexual assault • Unprotected sex with known HIV carrier • Unprotected anal, oral, or vaginal sex with suspected HIV carrier	**YES** "Seek medical care now to discuss options" **NO** Go to B
B. Are any of the following present?	
• Suspected or known exposure to STD • Vaginal or penile discharge • Vaginal, penile, or perineal lesions • Pelvic pain with or without fever	**YES** "Seek medical care within 24 hours to discuss options" **NO** Go to C
C. Are any of the following present?	
• Possible vaginal yeast infection • Known genital herpes	**YES** "Call back or call PCP for appointment if no improvement" and Follow **Home Care Instructions** **NO** Follow **Home Care Instructions**

Home Care Instructions
Sexually Transmitted Disease (STD)

S

- A warm bath may ease discomfort of herpes but will not cure it. Avoid sex when open sores are present. Use latex condoms at all times.
- If unprotected sex has occurred with multiple partners or with a person who is known to have or is suspected of having HIV, obtain a laboratory test for HIV infection immediately and then 3 and 6 months after the initial exposure. Avoid the potential of infecting others and yourself by using a condom or abstaining from sex. Contact PCP or Health Department Clinic for testing. Possible medical treatment is available immediately after contact.
- Both partners should be tested and treated for STDs and should avoid unprotected sexual contact.
- Discuss STD and HIV exposure history with a new partner before engaging in sexual intimacy.
- Use latex condoms (unless an allergy to latex exists).

Additional Instructions

Report the Following Problems to Your PCP/Clinic/ED

- At risk for HIV infection and persistent illness, fatigue, weight loss, diarrhea, swollen glands, sores, dry cough, or night sweats
- Suspected exposure to STD
- Unusual vaginal or penile discharge, genital lesions, or genital pain
- Known genital herpes and unable to tolerate persistent discomfort
- Pelvic pain with or without fever

Seek Emergency Care Immediately If Any of the Following Occur

- High fever and known shingles outbreak
- New-onset confusion or delirium
- Pain, redness, or rash in or around the eye

If the caller agrees with the advice given, document the call and encourage the caller to call back or see PCP if the problem worsens. If the caller does not agree with the advice given, reevaluate and advise the caller to follow up with PCP, Clinic, or ED.

Shingles: Suspected or Exposure

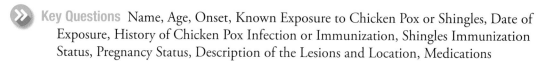

>> **Key Questions** Name, Age, Onset, Known Exposure to Chicken Pox or Shingles, Date of Exposure, History of Chicken Pox Infection or Immunization, Shingles Immunization Status, Pregnancy Status, Description of the Lesions and Location, Medications

>> **Other Protocols to Consider** Breathing Problems (106); Chicken Pox (129); Eye Problems (228); Facial Skin Problems (234); Fever, Adult (250); Itching (382); Rash, Adult (500); Skin Lesions: Lumps, Bumps, and Sores (556).

Nurse Alert: Use this protocol if known or suspected exposure to shingles or chicken pox and have developed a painful skin rash in a band, strip, or small area on one side of the body or face.

- Seek medical attention within 72 hours of developing a rash for possible antiviral medications to reduce the chance of prolonged neuralgia and other complications.
- Greatest risk of contracting shingles if age >50 years, history of chicken pox in the past, and weakened immune system.
- If no history of chicken pox or immunization in the past, exposure to shingles can result in developing chicken pox but not shingles.

Reminder: Document caller response to advice, home care instructions, and when to call back.

ASSESSMENT	ACTION

A. Are any of the following present?

- High fever and known shingles outbreak
- New-onset confusion or delirium
- Pain, redness, or rash in or around the eye

YES "Seek emergency care now"

NO Go to B

B. Are any of the following present?

- Rash with blisters on face
- Blisters rapidly spread to other areas of the body
- Painful rash with blisters and chills, fever, or headache
- New-onset band-like rash or blisters, pain and current/recent steroid treatment, weakened immune system, or age >65 years

YES "Seek medical care within 2 hours"

NO Go to C

C. Are any of the following present?

- Pain followed by rash or blisters in same area in 1 to 3 days
- Rash is widespread and painful
- Shingles exposure, age >50 years, and no history of prior chicken pox, shingles outbreak, or immunization
- Persistent severe itching or pain unresponsive to home care measures

YES "Seek medical care within 24 hours"

NO Go to D

D. Are any of the following present?

- Pus-filled blisters form scabs in 10 to 12 days
- Scabs fall off in 2 to 3 weeks
- Pain persists in same area after rash is gone

YES "Call back or call PCP for appointment if no improvement" and Follow **Home Care Instructions**

NO Follow **Home Care Instructions**

S

Home Care Instructions
Shingles: Suspected or Exposure

- During the first few days of an attack, may apply ice packs to affected area for 10 minutes. Do not place ice directly on the skin; use a washcloth or other cloth barrier between ice and the skin.
- Wash the affected area with cool water and mild soap and apply cool compresses after cleansing.
- Apply cool compresses to open blisters for 20 minutes several times a day to help dry out blisters.
- Practice good handwashing practices. Spreads through direct contact.
- While lesions are open and draining, avoid contact with persons who are steroid dependent, have a weakened immune system, are pregnant, or have not had chicken pox and newborn. Exposed persons with weakened immune systems should be treated within 72 hours.
- Avoid picking or scratching. Allow blisters to dry up and scabs to fall off on their own.
- Apply cornstarch, baking soda, Burow's or Domeboro solution to blistered area to keep them dry and promote healing. Leave the area open to the air as much as possible.
- To control itching, try OTC preparations (Benadryl [oral], Caladryl, Cortaid, Cortizone [topical]) and follow instructions on the label.
- Take your usual medication for pain. Follow instructions on the label.

Additional Instructions

Report the Following Problems to Your PCP/Clinic/ED

- Rash with blisters develops on face
- Blisters spread to other areas of the body
- Painful rash with blisters and chills, fever, or headache
- No improvement or condition worsens

If the caller agrees with the advice given, document the call and encourage the caller to call back or see PCP if the problem worsens. If the caller does not agree with the advice given, reevaluate and advise the caller to follow up with PCP, Clinic, or ED.

Shock, Suspected

 Key Questions Name, Age, Onset, Cause, Medication, History

 Other Protocols to Consider Altered Mental Status (28); Anxiety (36); Bleeding, Severe 90); Breathing Problems (106); Confusion (150); Electric Injury (219); Heart Rate Problems (320); Heat-Exposure Problems (323); Hypotension (352); Weakness (649).

Reminder: Document caller response to advice, home care instructions, and when to call back.

ASSESSMENT	ACTION

A. In addition to the classic signs of shock (pale, sweaty skin, and confusion or drowsiness), are any of the following present?

- Weak, rapid heart rate
- Rapid, shallow breathing
- Anxiety, restlessness
- Thirst
- Faintness, dizziness, weakness, altered mental status, unresponsive

 YES "Call ambulance"
and
Follow **Home Care Instructions**

NO "Seek medical care now"
and
Follow **Home Care Instructions**
and
See Other Protocols to Consider

Home Care Instructions
Shock, Suspected

- Clear the airway and provide CPR as needed.
- Lay the victim down with a pillow under the head and the legs elevated about 12 inches (30 cm).
- If suspected injury to head, neck, back, or chest, keep the legs flat and support neck.
- Control any bleeding by applying firm direct pressure to the area.
- Keep warm; cover with a blanket. In hot climates, keep the victim cool.
- If vomiting occurs, roll the victim to one side, keeping the head, neck, and body in a straight line.
- Do not give anything to drink, even if the victim is thirsty.
- Provide comfort and reassurance to help relieve anxiety.

Additional Instructions

If the caller agrees with the advice given, document the call and encourage the caller to call back or see PCP if the problem worsens. If the caller does not agree with the advice given, reevaluate and advise the caller to follow up with PCP, Clinic, or ED.

Shoulder Pain/Injury

 Key Questions Name, Age, Onset, Cause, Allergies, Medications, History, Pain Scale

 Other Protocols to Consider Abdominal Pain, Adult (9), Child (13); Bone, Joint, and Tissue Injury (95); Chest Pain (123); Extremity Injury (222); Joint Pain/Swelling (390).

Reminder: Document caller response to advice, home care instructions, and when to call back.

ASSESSMENT	ACTION
A. Are any of the following present?	
• Sudden pain in shoulder and neck, jaw, or chest and shortness of breath or sweating • Deformity, bruising, and limited movement in shoulder after an injury • Sudden shoulder and abdominal pain in woman with menses >4 weeks late	**YES** "Call ambulance" or "Seek emergency care now" **NO** Go to B
B. Are any of the following present?	
• Recent history of blunt trauma to shoulder, abdomen, or back • Fever, joint swollen, red, or warm, and recent illness • Unable to raise arm or move shoulder • Abdominal pain radiating to shoulder	**YES** "Seek medical care within 2 to 4 hours" **NO** Go to C
C. Are any of the following present?	
• Sudden onset of pain in other joints • Recent shoulder injury and no improvement in pain after >3 days of ice, heat, and rest	**YES** "Seek medical care within 24 hours" **NO** Go to D
D. Are any of the following present?	
• Progressive soreness in shoulder, increased with movement • Progressive pain and stiffness • Pain worsens by end of day and repetitive use or reaching to the side • Pain in shoulder or upper chest after laparoscopic surgery	**YES** "Call back or call PCP for appointment if no improvement" and Follow **Home Care Instructions** **NO** Follow **Home Care Instructions**

Home Care Instructions
Shoulder Pain/Injury

- After initial injury, apply ice pack every 20 to 30 minutes, 4 to 6 times a day, for 24 to 48 hours, then apply moist heat. Rest shoulder for 24 to 48 hours. Do not apply ice directly on skin. Do not sleep on a heating pad.
- No lifting, pulling, or pushing.
- For pain (no injury), apply moist heat to area every 20 to 30 minutes, 4 to 6 times a day.
- If no known injury, exercise joint with slow, gradual stretching, raising arm as high as tolerated. Reach down, forward, up, and to each side.
- Take your usual pain medication (aspirin, acetaminophen, or ibuprofen) for discomfort, and follow the instructions on the label. Do not give aspirin to a child. Avoid acetaminophen if liver disease is present.
- If working at a computer or other repetitive movement activity, consider having an ergonomic assessment of workstation if shoulder pain consistently worsens at the end of the day.

Additional Instructions

Report the Following Problems to Your PCP/Clinic/ED
- Pain persists or worsens
- New symptoms

Seek Emergency Care Immediately If Any of the Following Occur
- Recurring or sudden pain in shoulder and neck, jaw, or chest and shortness of breath or sweating

If the caller agrees with the advice given, document the call and encourage the caller to call back or see PCP if the problem worsens. If the caller does not agree with the advice given, reevaluate and advise the caller to follow up with PCP, Clinic, or ED.

Sickle Cell Disease Problems

 Key Questions Name, Age, Onset, Medications, Pain Scale, History

 Other Protocols to Consider Abdominal Pain, Adult (9), Child (13); Breathing Problems (106); Chest Pain (123); Jaundice (385); Joint Pain/Swelling (390); Urine, Abnormal Color (631).

Nurse Alert: Use the protocol if known sickle cell disease and problems or questions.

Reminder: Document caller response to advice, home care instructions, and when to call back.

ASSESSMENT	ACTION

A. Are any of the following present?

- Fever >101°F (38.3°C)
- Chest pain with or without cough
- Severe abdominal pain
- Severe joint or bone pain
- Syncope
- Difficulty breathing
- Nonblanching dark red or purple rash
- Severe headache
- Persistent erection of the penis
- Altered mental status
- Transient neurologic symptoms
- Worst-pain crisis

YES "Call ambulance"
or
"Seek emergency care now"

NO Go to B

B. Are any of the following present?

- Moderate pain not responsive to normal pain management
- Blood in urine
- Difficulty walking
- Joint swelling, redness, or warmth
- Pallor
- Vomiting
- Jaundice
- Tachycardia

YES "Seek medical care immediately"

NO Go to C

C. Are any of the following present?

- Fatigue
- Persistent sore unresponsive to treatment

`YES` "Seek medical care within 24 hours"

`NO` Go to D

D. Are any of the following present?

- Fever
- Worsening pain

`YES` "Call back or call PCP for appointment if no improvement" and Follow **Home Care Instructions**

`NO` Follow **Home Care Instructions**

Home Care Instructions
Sickle Cell Disease Problems

- Rest.
- Increase oral hydration. Drink lots of fluids.
- Apply topical heat to affected area for first 24 to 48 hours.
- Do not smoke.
- Take medications as directed.

Additional Instructions

Report the Following Problems to Your PCP/Clinic/ED

- Fever
- Worsening pain
- Decreased range of motion
- Increased swelling
- Blood in urine
- Increased difficulty walking, joint swelling, redness, or warmth
- Increased vomiting or jaundice

Seek Emergency Care Immediately If Any of the Following Occur

- Chest pain with or without cough, syncope, or difficulty breathing
- Severe abdominal pain
- Severe joint or bone pain
- Nonblanching dark red or purple rash
- Severe headache or altered mental status
- Persistent erection of the penis

If the caller agrees with the advice given, document the call and encourage the caller to call back or see PCP if the problem worsens. If the caller does not agree with the advice given, reevaluate and advise the caller to follow up with PCP, Clinic, or ED.

Sinus Problems

 Key Questions Name, Age, Onset, Allergies, Medications, Prior Sinus Problems, History, Pain Scale

 Other Protocols to Consider Breathing Problems (106); Common Cold Symptoms (146); Congestion (153); Cough (170); Earache, Drainage (206); Facial Problems (231); Fever, Adult (250), Child (253); Headache (308); Sore Throat (564).

Nurse Alert: Use the protocol if history of sinus problems or under current treatment for a sinus condition.

Reminder: Document caller response to advice, home care instructions, and when to call back.

ASSESSMENT	ACTION
A. Are any of the following present?	
• Redness and swelling in cheek, forehead, or eyelid • Vision change	**YES** "Seek medical care within 2 to 4 hours" **NO** Go to B
B. Are any of the following present?	
• Persistent fever and sinus congestion or facial pain >2 to 3 days • Yellow or green nasal discharge >3 to 5 days • Persistent dull ache or tenderness around eyes or cheekbones • No improvement after 48 hours of antibiotic therapy • Pain worsens when bending over	**YES** "Seek medical care within 24 hours" **NO** Go to C
C. Are any of the following present?	
• Some sinus discomfort and clear nasal discharge • Recent cold • History of allergies • Postnasal drainage • Chronic cough	**YES** "Call back or call PCP for appointment if no improvement" and Follow **Home Care Instructions** **NO** Follow **Home Care Instructions**

Home Care Instructions
Sinus Problems

- Use a vaporizer or humidifier to keep air moist, especially at night, and change the water daily.
- Breathe steam several times a day to help promote sinus drainage. Sit in a steam-filled bathroom for 10 to 20 minutes or cover head with a towel and breathe steam from a tea kettle or basin filled with hot water.
- Apply hot packs to area around the eyes and cheekbones. Diabetics should use heat with caution.
- Take OTC decongestant of choice, and follow instructions on the label. If hypertensive or pregnant, such medications may not be appropriate. Check label on container before taking such medications.
- For nasal congestion, use saline nose drops or spray.
- For postnasal drainage, may try phenylephrine (Neo-Synephrine) or oxymetazoline (Afrin) nasal drops for as long as 3 days. Then discontinue use. Prolonged use may worsen congestion when use of spray is discontinued. Do not take if cardiac disease, hypertension, or prostate problems are present.
- Take your usual pain medication (aspirin, acetaminophen, ibuprofen) as tolerated for discomfort. Do not give aspirin to a child. Avoid aspirin-like products if age <20 years. Avoid acetaminophen if liver disease is present. Avoid ibuprofen if kidney disease or stomach problems exist or in the case of pregnancy. Follow the directions on the label.
- Avoid dairy products.
- Drink at least six 8-ounce glasses of liquids a day, unless on fluid restriction diet.

Additional Instructions

Report the Following Problems to Your PCP/Clinic/ED

- Yellow or green nasal discharge for >3 to 5 days
- No improvement after 48 hours of antibiotic therapy
- Redness and swelling in cheek, forehead, or eyelid
- No improvement after 5 days or condition worsens

If the caller agrees with the advice given, document the call and encourage the caller to call back or see PCP if the problem worsens. If the caller does not agree with the advice given, reevaluate and advise the caller to follow up with PCP, Clinic, or ED.

Skin Lesions: Lumps, Bumps, and Sores

 Key Questions Name, Age, Onset, Allergies, Medications, History

 Other Protocols to Consider Bedbug Exposure or Concerns (67); Eye Problems (228); Facial Skin Problems (234); Genital Lesions (291); Impetigo (361); Itching (382); Mouth Problems (407); Piercing Problems (445); Rash, Adult (500), Child (505); Scabies (527); Shingles: Suspected or Exposure (544); Tattoo Problems (604); Vaginal Discharge/Pain/Itching (636).

Reminder: Document caller response to advice, home care instructions, and when to call back.

ASSESSMENT	ACTION

A. Are any of the following present?

- New large lesion on the face or near the eyes, rectum, or genitals
- Severe pain
- Painful blisters
- Fever
- Recent use of sulfa drugs
- Diabetic or weakened immune system and signs of infection in the lesion

YES "Seek medical care within 2 to 4 hours"

NO Go to B

B. Are any of the following present?

- Lesion located near upper lip, on tip or opening of nose, on eye or eyelid
- Temperature >100°F (37.8°C)
- Recent rapid change in color, shape, or size of a mole
- Painful or bleeding mole
- Signs of infection: pain, swelling, redness, drainage, red streaks, or warmth
- Lesion on bottom of foot that makes walking painful
- Persistent tender lesion after 48 to 72 hours of home care treatment
- Bumps under armpit
- New lesions develop on other parts of the body
- Pain followed by a rash, then blisters in a band, strip, or small area

YES "Seek medical care within 24 hours"

NO Go to C

C. Are any of the following present?

- Warts or moles that protrude so far they are frequently bumped or in the way
- Request for wart removal
- History of frequently occurring boils, warts, or lesions
- New warts develop after 2 weeks of treatment
- Persistent wart after 8 weeks of treatment
- New onset of pimples
- Circular, raised, rough pink patch with clear center ½ to 1 inch and itchy
- Circular, raised, rough pink patch on scalp with clear center ½ to 1 inch and itchy
- Concern for possible sexually transmitted disease
- Persistent painless lesion after 10 days of home care treatment
- Recurring lesion and person requests prescription to prevent future breakouts

YES "Call back or call PCP for appointment if no improvement" and
Follow **Home Care Instructions**

NO Follow **Home Care Instructions**

S

Home Care Instructions
Skin Lesions

- Do not pick at or irritate the lesion. Do not squeeze boils.
- Apply warm soaks for 10 to 15 minutes, 4 to 6 times a day, to tender lesions or if there are signs of infection. Boils usually drain after a few days of heat treatment. People with diabetes should use heat with caution.
- Examine lesions frequently that are often irritated or rubbed by clothing.
- Take aspirin, acetaminophen, or ibuprofen as tolerated for discomfort. Do not give aspirin to a child. Avoid aspirin-like products if age <20 years. Avoid acetaminophen if liver disease is present. Avoid ibuprofen if kidney disease or stomach problems exist or in the case of pregnancy.
- Wash pimples with antibacterial soap and apply OTC or prescription antibiotic ointment 3 times a day.

For Warts

- Follow instructions on the OTC wart removal preparations. Do not use if the person has diabetes or circulatory problems, or the wart is on the face.
  - Apply an OTC product (salicylic acid preparation) and follow the instructions on the package. Do not apply these products if diabetes or impaired circulation is present. Consult a pharmacist or PCP for product suggestions.
  - Alternative home remedy: Apply clear nail polish to wart daily for a few weeks. The wart will stop growing from lack of oxygen.

For Cold Sores

- Apply OTC cream (i.e., Abreva) 5 times a day until healed. Ask a pharmacist or PCP for product suggestions and follow the instructions on the package. Begin using OTC or prescription cream at first sign of outbreak.
- Sores are contagious until dry. Avoid spreading them to another person's eyes, lips, or genitals or exposing a person with a weakened immune system.

For Abscesses

- Lanced or unlanced abscesses are highly resistant to antibiotics and susceptible to MRSA infections.
  - Wash hands with microbial cleanser >3 times per day or more often when soiled.
  - Shower immediately with hot water as tolerated after activity.
  - Advise others in close contact to wash their hands with microbial cleanser.
  - Keep wounds covered with clean, dry bandages particularly if drainage is present.
  - Disinfect all towels, sheets, and surfaces in contact with wound with a solution of 1:100 of household bleach to water.
  - Wash and dry clothes, linens, and towels in a setting as hot as possible. Make sure all items are dry before removing them from the dryer.
  - Avoid participating in contact sports or skin-to-skin contact with others until the infection has healed.
  - Use a skin antiseptic to treat MRSA on the skin in combination with antibiotics prescribed by PCP.
  - Avoid hot tubs.
  - Do not share bars of soap, razors, towels, or athletic gear.
  - Call PCP if the condition worsens or fails to improve with home care and treatment.

Additional Instructions

Report the Following Problems to Your PCP/Clinic/ED

- Persistent growth, change, bleeding, color change, pain, or poor healing after 72 hours of home care treatment
- Signs of infection: pain, swelling, redness, drainage, red streaks, or warmth
- Requests for skin tag, mole, or wart removal

If the caller agrees with the advice given, document the call and encourage the caller to call back or see PCP if the problem worsens. If the caller does not agree with the advice given, reevaluate and advise the caller to follow up with PCP, Clinic, or ED.

S

Sleep Apnea, Adult

 Key Questions Name, Age, Onset, Medications, History

 Other Protocols to Consider Breathing Problems (106).

Reminder: Document caller response to advice, home care instructions, and when to call back.

ASSESSMENT	ACTION
A. Are any of the following present?	
• Person not breathing • Skin turning blue	**YES** "Call ambulance" and "Start CPR" **NO** Go to B
B. While sleeping, did the following occur?	
• Lapse in breathing for several minutes • Skin turned gray or blue and is normal color now • Abnormal breathing after the episode • Rescue breathing was necessary	**YES** "Seek medical care within 2 hours" **NO** Go to C
C. While sleeping, did the following occur?	
• Lapse in breathing <2 minutes • No change in skin color • Breathing normally after the episode • Rescue breathing was not necessary • Cycles of sleep, choking, sudden awakening, drowsiness, and sleep • Persistent drowsiness and episodes of falling asleep during the day • Decreased ability to function or depression caused by lack of sleep	**YES** "Call back or call PCP for appointment if no improvement" and Follow **Home Care Instructions** **NO** Follow **Home Care Instructions**

Home Care Instructions
Sleep Apnea, Adult

S

- Try to remain calm.
- Eliminate as many contributing risk factors as possible: stress, anxiety, depression, obesity, smoking, and drug or alcohol abuse.
- Obtain CPR training. Rapid identification of prolonged apnea and prompt CPR can help to prevent death or serious problems related to a lack of oxygen to the brain.
- If apnea occurs only when sleeping on the back, sleep on the side or stomach. Use pillows for support. Consider attaching an object to the back of sleepwear to encourage other sleep positions.

Additional Instructions

Report the Following Problem to Your PCP/Clinic/ED

- Persistent episodes of apnea

Call Ambulance Immediately If Any of the Following Occur

- Prolonged period of not breathing
- Skin turning blue
- CPR in progress

If the caller agrees with the advice given, document the call and encourage the caller to call back or see PCP if the problem worsens. If the caller does not agree with the advice given, reevaluate and advise the caller to follow up with PCP, Clinic, or ED.

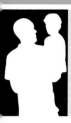

Sleep Apnea, Infant

 Key Questions Name, Age, Onset, Medications, History

 Other Protocols to Consider Newborn Problems (421); Spitting Up, Infant (570).

Reminder: Document caller response to advice, home care instructions, and when to call back.

ASSESSMENT	ACTION

A. Are any of the following present?

- Infant not breathing
- Skin turning blue

YES "Call ambulance"
and
"Start CPR"

NO Go to B

B. While infant was sleeping, did the following occur?

- Lapse in breathing for 1 minute
- Skin turned gray or blue but is normal color now
- Abnormal breathing after the episode
- Rescue breathing was necessary

YES "Seek medical care immediately"

NO Go to C

C. While infant was sleeping, did the following occur?

- Lapse in breathing <1 minute
- No change in skin color
- Infant breathing normally after episode
- Rescue breathing was not necessary

YES "Seek medical care within 24 hours"

NO Follow **Home Care Instructions**

Home Care Instructions
Sleep Apnea, Infant

- Provide reassurance. Some infants have a pause in breathing of <15 seconds after several rapid respirations.
- Reinforce importance of placing child on back for sleep.
- Discuss use of a respiration monitor with PCP.
- Obtain CPR training. Rapid identification of apnea and prompt CPR can successfully revive an infant without serious problems.

S

Additional Instructions

Report the Following Problem to Your PCP/Clinic/ED

- Persistent episodes of apnea

Call Ambulance Immediately If Any of the Following Occur

- Infant not breathing
- Skin turning blue
- CPR in progress

If the caller agrees with the advice given, document the call and encourage the caller to call back or see PCP if the problem worsens. If the caller does not agree with the advice given, reevaluate and advise the caller to follow up with PCP, Clinic, or ED.

Sore Throat

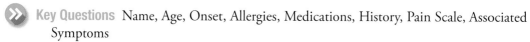

>> **Key Questions** Name, Age, Onset, Allergies, Medications, History, Pain Scale, Associated Symptoms

>> **Other Protocols to Consider** Allergic Reaction (25); Congestion (153); Cough (170); Earache, Drainage (206); Fever, Adult (250), Child (253); Hoarseness (342); Mouth Problems (407); Pregnancy, Cold Symptoms (465); Swallowing Difficulty (591).

Reminder: Document caller response to advice, home care instructions, and when to call back.

ASSESSMENT	ACTION

A. Are any of the following present?

- Difficulty breathing (for reasons other than nasal congestion)
- Excessive drooling by a small child
- Stridor
- Inability to swallow own saliva
- Inability to open mouth fully

YES "Seek emergency care now"

NO Go to B

B. Are any of the following present?

- Significant difficulty swallowing because of pain
- Temperature >104°F (40°C)
- Temperature >101°F (38.3°C) in the elderly or immunosuppressed
- Signs of dehydration

YES "Seek medical care within 2 to 4 hours"

NO Go to C

C. Are any of the following present?

- History of rheumatic fever, mitral valve prolapse, or other heart valve problem
- Skin rash
- Close contact with someone with strep throat within the past 2 weeks
- Yellow pus or white mucus at back of throat
- Red or enlarged tonsils
- Persistent sore throat >3 days
- Ear pain
- Fever or chills unresponsive to fever-reducing measures
- Diabetes, elderly, or immunosuppressed
- Dizziness/faintness
- Foul-smelling breath

YES "Seek medical care within 24 hours" and
Follow **Home Care Instructions**

NO Go to D

D. Are any of the following present?

- Nasal congestion
- Cough or sneezing
- Feeling of fullness in ear

YES "Call back or call PCP for appointment if no improvement" and
Follow **Home Care Instructions**

NO Follow **Home Care Instructions**

S

Home Care Instructions
Sore Throat

- Take your usual pain medication (acetaminophen, aspirin, ibuprofen) for headache or fever. Do not give aspirin to a child. Avoid aspirin-like products if age <20 years. Avoid acetaminophen if liver disease is present. Avoid ibuprofen if kidney disease or stomach problems exist or in the case of pregnancy. Follow the directions on the label.
- Gargle with salt water several times a day for throat discomfort (¼ tsp regular salt to ½ cup warm water) or sip warm chicken broth. Use frozen cough drops or hard candy for additional relief if age >4 years.
- Increase fluids; try warm tea with lemon and honey, apple juice, gelatin, or sucking on flavored ice. Take frequent small sips if it is painful to swallow.
- If you smoke, decrease or stop smoking.
- Use a vaporizer or humidifier to keep the air moist, especially at night, or put a pot of water near the heat source.
- Take decongestants to help relieve congestion, unless there is a history of hypertension or pregnancy. Discuss with PCP or pharmacist.

Additional Instructions

Report the Following Problems to Your PCP/Clinic/ED

- Fever >101°F (38.3°C) for several days
- Sore throat persists >3 days or worsens
- Earache
- No improvement or condition worsens
- Drooling
- Signs of dehydration

Seek Emergency Care Immediately If Any of the Following Occur

- Unable to swallow own saliva
- Difficulty breathing/stridor
- Chest pain
- Excessive drooling
- Unable to open mouth fully

If the caller agrees with the advice given, document the call and encourage the caller to call back or see PCP if the problem worsens. If the caller does not agree with the advice given, reevaluate and advise the caller to follow up with PCP, Clinic, or ED.

Speaking Difficulty

 Key Questions Name, Age, Onset, Medications, History

 Other Protocols to Consider Anxiety (36); Asthma (52); Breathing Problems (106); Confusion (150); Headache (308); Mouth Problems (407); Neurologic Symptoms (418); Piercing Problems (445); Sore Throat (564); Stroke, Suspected (576); Tongue Problems (610).

> *Nurse Alert:* Sudden changes in vision, speech, or mental status, weakness, and numbness may be signs of a stroke or other serious neurologic disorder. Prompt treatment may prevent extensive damage to the brain or spinal cord and reduce permanent disability. Medications used to break up a clot in the brain need to be administered within 3 hours of symptom onset.
>
> - Ask how current condition is different from normal.

Reminder: Document caller response to advice, home care instructions, and when to call back.

ASSESSMENT	ACTION

A. In addition to difficulty speaking, are any of the following present?

- Weakness on one side of body
- Difficulty breathing
- Difficulty swallowing
- Severe headache
- Confusion/disorientation
- New onset and history of blood clots or heart problems
- Words or ideas are mixed up
- Trauma to the neck

YES "Call ambulance"

NO Go to B

B. Are any of the following present?

- Numbness or weakness
- Frequent or intermittent episodes of difficulty speaking
- Inability to move muscles on one side of face
- History of recent injury or trauma
- Dizziness or light-headedness
- Blurred vision
- New onset and unable to start sentences without repeating first word or unable to start a sentence when ready to speak

YES "Seek emergency care now"

NO Go to C

567

C. Is the following present?

- Pain in mouth or face

 YES "Seek medical care within 24 hours"

NO Go to D

D. Are any of the following present?

- Under medical care for problem and condition is worsening
- Increased stress level
- Taking a new OTC or prescribed medication
- Poor attention span
- New onset of stuttering in child
- Parent concerned

YES "Call back or call PCP for appointment if no improvement" and
Follow **Home Care Instructions**

NO Follow **Home Care Instructions**

Home Care Instructions
Speaking Difficulty

- Speak slowly while facing the person and give short, simple directions.
- Do not rush the person; allow ample time for a response.
- Use paper and pencil to communicate as necessary.
- The person with a diagnosed speech problem may show frustration through swearing, yelling, or acting out. Be patient, positive, and nonjudgmental. Do not take the person's actions personally.
- Encourage and allow for as much independent behavior as possible.
- Decrease the stress level through relaxation, exercise, or taking a break from stressors.

Additional Instructions

Report the Following Problems to Your PCP/Clinic/ED

- Condition persists or worsens, and cause of the problem is unknown
- Numbness or weakness
- Dizziness or light-headedness
- Blurred vision

Seek Emergency Care Immediately If Any of the Following Occur

- Weakness on one side of the body
- Difficulty breathing
- Difficulty swallowing
- Confusion or disorientation
- Severe headache

If the caller agrees with the advice given, document the call and encourage the caller to call back or see PCP if the problem worsens. If the caller does not agree with the advice given, reevaluate and advise the caller to follow up with PCP, Clinic, or ED.

Spitting Up, Infant

 Name, Age, Onset, Medications, History

 Other Protocols to Consider Breast-feeding Problems (98); Dehydration (180); Vomiting, Child (645).

Reminder: Document caller response to advice, home care instructions, and when to call back.

ASSESSMENT	ACTION

A. Are any of the following present?

- Difficulty breathing
- Blue or gray face, lips, fingernails, or earlobes
- Lethargy

YES "Call ambulance"
or
"Seek emergency care now"

NO Go to B

B. Are any of the following present?

- Persistent vomiting
- Choking or coughing afterward
- Blood or dark green bile in spit-up material
- Fever >100.4°F (38°C) and age <3 months
- Signs of dehydration:
  - decreased urine
  - sunken eyes
  - poor skin elasticity (does not spring back when pinched)
  - excessive thirst or dry mouth
  - crying without tears
- Sunken soft spot
- No stools in newborn
- Projectile vomiting

YES "Seek medical care within 2 hours"

NO Go to C

C. Are any of the following present?

- Persistent irritability
- Diarrhea
- Parent concerned about infant's lack of weight gain

 YES "Seek medical care within 24 hours"

 NO Go to D

↓

D. Are any of the following present?

- Fever and age >3 months
- Spitting up frequently occurs after infant consumes volumes larger than 1 to 2 mouthfuls
- Weight loss
- Increasing constipation
- Persistent spitting up
- Parent concerned

YES "Call back or call PCP for appointment if no improvement" and Follow **Home Care Instructions**

NO Follow **Home Care Instructions**

S

Home Care Instructions
Spitting Up, Infant

- Remember that nonforceful spitting up of a small amount of stomach contents shortly after feeding is a common condition of infants. The infant should outgrow this after starting to sit up.
- Burp the baby several times during the feedings.
- Give small frequent feedings and avoid overfeeding or feeding too quickly.
- Place infant in an upright position in a swing or baby carrier after feeding. Avoid hugging or bouncing the infant after feeding.
- Elevate the head of the bed and position infant on side.
- Avoid tight diapers or binding infant when changing diapers.
- If breastfeeding, try feeding one side at a time and pump the other side. Avoid pacifiers.

Additional Instructions

Report the Following Problems to Your PCP/Clinic/ED

- No improvement with home care measures or condition worsens
- Weight loss or failure to gain weight normally
- Increasing constipation
- Persistent spitting up
- Blood or dark green bile in spit-up material
- Signs of dehydration

Seek Emergency Care Immediately If Any of the Following Occur

- Difficulty breathing
- Lethargy
- Blue or gray face, lips, fingernails, or earlobes

If the caller agrees with the advice given, document the call and encourage the caller to call back or see PCP if the problem worsens. If the caller does not agree with the advice given, reevaluate and advise the caller to follow up with PCP, Clinic, or ED.

Stools, Abnormal

 Key Questions Name, Age, Onset, Recent Dietary Habits, Medications, History

 Other Protocols to Consider Abdominal Pain, Adult (9), Child (13); Constipation (160); Diarrhea, Adult (192), Child (195); Hemorrhoids (327); Rectal Bleeding (510).

Reminder: Document caller response to advice, home care instructions, and when to call back.

ASSESSMENT	ACTION
A. Is there abdominal pain?	
	YES Go to Abdominal Pain, Adult, (11), Child (14) protocols
	NO Go to B
B. Is there diarrhea?	
	YES Go to Diarrhea, Adult (192), Child (195) protocol
	NO Go to C
C. Are any of the following present?	
• Black or dark stools for more than two bowel movements and light-headedness or dizziness • Vomiting blood or dark coffee-ground–like emesis • Passing blood clots	**YES** "Seek emergency care now" **NO** Go to D
D. Are any of the following present?	
• Black tarry stools without recent ingestion of iron pills, beets, bismuth salicylate (Pepto-Bismol), or spinach • Large amount of bright red blood mixed in the stool • Bloody stool, fever, vomiting, ill feeling • Age <12 weeks, fever, and bloody stools	**YES** "Seek medical care within 2 to 4 hours" **NO** Go to E

S

573

E. Are any of the following present?

- Pale stool, yellow skin and eyes
- Pale, foamy, bulky, foul-smelling stool
- Blood mixed in stool or black stools for more than two consecutive bowel movements
- Persistent weight loss and thin, pencil-like stools

 "Seek medical care within 24 hours"

 Go to F

F. Are any of the following present?

- Stool streaked with red blood
- Blood on toilet tissue after wiping
- Discolored stool and recent ingestion of iron pills, beets, Pepto-Bismol, spinach, tomatoes, or peppers, or stool is color of recently ingested food
- Persistent discoloration
- Persistent bleeding >3 days
- Constipation or hemorrhoids

YES "Call back or call PCP for appointment if no improvement" and Follow **Home Care Instructions**

NO Follow **Home Care Instructions**

Home Care Instructions
Stools, Abnormal

- For hemorrhoids, soak in a warm saline bath for 20 minutes a day (add 2 tbsp of salt or baking soda to the water).
- Keep rectal area clean.
- If rectal area is irritated, apply OTC hydrocortisone ointment or zinc oxide paste or powder.
- If hemorrhoids persist, try OTC preparations to help soothe and shrink hemorrhoids.
- Increase fluid intake and eat a diet high in fiber: fruits, vegetables, bran, grains, and beans. Avoid constipating foods such as cheese. Note which foods change the color of the stool.
- Remember the color of the stool should return to normal within 24 hours if the discoloration is caused by a change in diet.
- Use products with witch hazel (Tucks) to reduce discomfort.

S

Additional Instructions

Report the Following Problems to Your PCP/Clinic/ED

- No improvement in 3 days or condition worsens
- Abdominal pain
- Bloody stool, fever, vomiting, ill feeling
- Pale stool, yellow skin and eyes
- Pale, foamy, bulky, foul-smelling stool
- Persistent weight loss and thin, pencil-like stools

Seek Emergency Care Immediately If Any of the Following Occur

- Black or dark stools for more than two consecutive bowel movements and light-headedness or dizziness
- Vomiting blood or dark coffee-ground–like emesis
- Passing bloody stools

If the caller agrees with the advice given, document the call and encourage the caller to call back or see PCP if the problem worsens. If the caller does not agree with the advice given, reevaluate and advise the caller to follow up with PCP, Clinic, or ED.

Stroke, Suspected

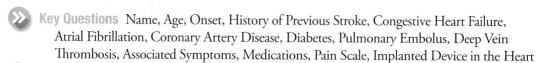

Key Questions Name, Age, Onset, History of Previous Stroke, Congestive Heart Failure, Atrial Fibrillation, Coronary Artery Disease, Diabetes, Pulmonary Embolus, Deep Vein Thrombosis, Associated Symptoms, Medications, Pain Scale, Implanted Device in the Heart

Other Protocols to Consider Alcohol Problems (21); Allergic Reaction (25); Altered Mental Status (28); Diabetes Problems (187); Dizziness (199); Headache (308); Heart Rate Problems (320); Hypertension (347); Neurologic Symptoms (418); Seizure (531); Speaking Difficulty (567); Weakness (649).

> *Nurse Alert:* Use this protocol if known stroke or symptoms sound like a stroke.

- Stroke is the fifth leading cause of death in the United States. A stroke happens when brain cells die from not getting enough oxygen. This is caused by a blocked artery or a blood vessel in the brain that bursts or slowly leaks.
- Think "**FAST**" and act quickly: **F** = face drooping or weak smile on one side, **A** = arm (and/or leg) weakness or numbness on one side, **S** = speech slurred or hard to understand, **T** = time to call 911.
- Sudden changes in vision, weakness, numbness, speech, or mental status may be signs of a stroke or other serious neurologic disorder. Prompt treatment may prevent extensive damage to the brain and reduce permanent disability. Medications used to break up a clot in the brain need to be administered within 3 hours of symptom onset.
- Stroke symptoms are now gone; may be the symptoms of a temporary stroke (or transient ischemic attack [TIA]) and can be the warning signs before an actual stroke.
- Ask how current condition is different from normal.

Reminder: Document caller response to advice, home care instructions, and when to call back.

ASSESSMENT	ACTION
A. Are any of the following present?	
<ul><li>Suddenly one side of the face is drooping, smile is crooked, and when tongue is stuck out it leans to one side</li><li>Sudden arm and/or leg weakness, and/or numbness on one side; if the person is asked to hold arms up, one drops down</li><li>Speech is slurred or hard to understand</li><li>Suddenly becomes confused or disoriented</li><li>Suddenly develops a severe headache</li><li>Suddenly has trouble seeing from one or both eyes or develops involuntary eye movements</li><li>Suddenly has trouble swallowing</li></ul>	**YES** "Call ambulance" **NO** Go to B

B. Are any of the following present?

- Suddenly becomes dizzy or light-headed
- Suddenly has trouble with balance and/or coordination or has trouble walking
- Sudden loss of memory
- Suddenly has muscle stiffness or loss of feeling in any part of the body
- Sudden behavior change
- Rapid or irregular heart beat with dizziness or light-headedness
- Heart palpitations or fluttering
- Recreational street drug or prescription drug abuse within past 24 hours

YES "Seek emergency care now"
"Do not drive yourself. If another driver is not available, call an ambulance"

NO Go to C

C. Are any of the following present and person is concerned about a possible stroke?

- History of blood clots or heart problems
- Slow onset of numbness, tingling, or burning sensation in arm or leg
- Pain spreading to arm or leg
- History of taking cholesterol-lowering medication
- Recent history of frequent falls
  - Increased difficulty with being able to move or walk
  - History of heart disease, heart attack, previous stroke, or diabetes
  - History of CHF, atrial fibrillation, or blood clotting problems
  - Heavy smoker with high blood pressure, high cholesterol, or obesity

YES "Seek medical care within 24 hours"

NO Go to D

D. Are any of the following present?

- History of neuromuscular or nervous system problems that do not respond to medication
- Occasional weakness
- Dizziness that occurs when moving the head, after taking a new medication, or after drinking alcohol

YES "Call back or call PCP for appointment if no improvement" and
Follow **Home Care Instructions**

NO Follow **Home Care Instructions**

S

Home Care Instructions
Stroke, Suspected

- Think "**FAST**" and act quickly if you suspect that the person is having a stroke: **F** = face drooping or weak smile on one side, **A** = arm (and/or leg) weakness or numbness on one side, **S** = speech slurred or hard to understand, **T** = time to call 911.
- If dizziness occurs, stop moving for a few minutes. Reach out and lightly touch something solid and firm, then sit down and stay still.
- If the person has diabetes and experiences a sudden change in level of consciousness, give a fast-acting source of sugar immediately (but only if person is awake enough to eat or drink). Good sources of fast-acting sugar include orange (or other fruit) juice, flavored drink mixes (such as Kool-Aid), regular cola, nonfat or low-fat milk, raisins, a tablespoon of sugar or jelly, or candy (LifeSavers, gummies, etc.).
- If event is alcohol or drug-related, see also Alcohol Problems protocol (21) and Substance Abuse, Use or Exposure protocol (582). For future assistance, contact local resources for assistance: counseling, detoxification programs, inpatient/outpatient treatment programs, AA, or Al-Anon.

Additional Instructions

Report the Following Problems to Your PCP/Clinic/ED

- No improvement or condition worsens

Seek Emergency Care Immediately If Any of the Following Occur

- Suddenly one side of the face is drooping, smile is crooked, and when tongue is stuck out it leans to one side
- Sudden arm and/or leg weakness, and/or numbness on one side; if the person is asked to hold arms up, one drops down
- Speech is slurred or hard to understand
- Suddenly becomes confused or disoriented
- Suddenly becomes dizzy or light-headed
- Sudden trouble with balance and/or coordination or has trouble walking
- Suddenly develops a severe headache
- Suddenly has trouble swallowing
- Sudden loss of memory
- Suddenly has muscle stiffness or loss of feeling in any part of the body
- Suddenly develops involuntary eye movements or has trouble seeing from one or both eyes
- Sudden behavior change
- Rapid or irregular heart beat with dizziness or light-headedness
- Heart palpitations or fluttering
- Recreational street drug or prescription drug abuse within past 24 hours

If the caller agrees with the advice given, document the call and encourage the caller to call back or see PCP if the problem worsens. If the caller does not agree with the advice given, reevaluate and advise the caller to follow up with PCP, Clinic, or ED.

Stye

 Key Questions Name, Age, Onset, Medications, History

 Other Protocols to Consider Eye Injury (225); Eye Problems (228).

Nurse Alert: Use this protocol if previously diagnosed with a stye and has questions or concerns.

Reminder: Document caller response to advice, home care instructions, and when to call back.

ASSESSMENT	ACTION
A. Are any of the following present?	
• Lump interferes with vision • Several lumps suddenly appear at once • Persistent pain unresponsive to home care measures • New onset of red, tender, swollen area on bottom eyelid or near nose • Drainage from lesion and temperature >100.5°F (38.1°C) • Bloody drainage	**YES** "Seek medical care within 24 hours" **NO** Go to B
B. Are any of the following present?	
• Red pimple-like lump persists on upper or lower eyelid or near it >48 hours after home treatment • Lumps frequently appear • Lump breaks open and drains	**YES** "Call back or call PCP for appointment if no improvement" and **NO** Follow **Home Care Instructions** Follow **Home Care Instructions**

Home Care Instructions
Stye

- Avoid rubbing the affected eye.
- Apply warm compresses to the area for 20 minutes, 4 to 6 times a day or more if possible.
- Do not share washcloths and towels with other household members. Sties may be contagious.
- Allow the stye to break open; do not squeeze the lump.
- Avoid eye makeup or contact lenses until the stye heals.
- Apply OTC treatments and follow the instructions on the package (Stye, Bausch & Lomb Eye Wash, Collyrium Eye Wash, OCuSOFT Lid Scrub, and Stygiene, which are available as ointments, solutions, and medicated pads). Ask the pharmacist for other product suggestions.
- If antibiotic ointment is prescribed, apply to the stye at bedtime.
- Do not touch the tip of the applicator with the hand or eye surface.
- To apply eye drops, pull the lower lid down with two fingers. Put drops in the area between the eyelid and eyeball. Close eyes for 30 to 60 seconds.
- Wash hands often and before putting medications into the eye.

Additional Instructions

Report the Following Problems to Your PCP/Clinic/ED

- No improvement in 48 hours or condition worsens
- Several more lumps appear
- Drainage from lesion, and temperature >100.5°F (38.1°C)
- Bloody drainage

If the caller agrees with the advice given, document the call and encourage the caller to call back or see PCP if the problem worsens. If the caller does not agree with the advice given, reevaluate and advise the caller to follow up with PCP, Clinic, or ED.

Substance Abuse, Use, or Exposure

Key Questions Name, Age, Onset, Cause, Drug of Choice and Route, Drug Habits (Amount and Frequency), Hours or Days Since Last Use, Mental Health History, Possible Exposure to Methamphetamine Lab or Chemicals, Medications, History, Medications

Other Protocols to Consider Alcohol Problems (21); Altered Mental Status (28); Chest Pain (123); Diarrhea, Adult (192); Overdose (438); Poisoning, Suspected (262); Suicide Attempt, Threat (585).

Nurse Alert: If overdosed on prescription, nonprescription, recreational drugs, alcohol, or any chemical agent, go to Overdose (438). If suicide attempt/gesture or threat to hurt self or others, go to Suicide Attempt/Threat (585) protocol.

Reminder: Document caller response to advice, home care instructions, and when to call back.

ASSESSMENT	ACTION

A. Are any of the following present?

- Altered mental status
- Apnea or difficulty breathing
- Pale, diaphoretic, and light-headed or weak
- Suicidal or homicidal ideation
- Unresponsive
- Face, lips, or tongue blue or gray
- Seizures

YES "Call ambulance"

NO Go to B

B. Are any of the following present?

- Adolescent with speech slurring, confusion, poor coordination after use of drugs or alcohol
- Chest pain
- Dizziness, difficulty breathing, shakiness
- Possible overdose
- Hallucinations
- Extreme anxiety, agitation, paranoia, or terror
- Signs of withdrawal: rapid or irregular heart rate, tremors, high blood pressure, vomiting, restlessness, diaphoresis
- Exposure to methamphetamine vapors during cooking process (especially children and first responders)

YES "Seek emergency care now" and
See **Home Care Instructions**

NO Go to C

C. Are any of the following present?

- 24 to 48 hours after cessation of substance and hallucinations: auditory (voices, buzzing, clicks), sensory (bug crawling), or visual hallucinations
- Fever
- Difficulty performing simple tasks
- Suicide thoughts but no action
- Suspected ingestion of unknown drug, inability to recall events, possible sexual contact

YES "Seek medical care within 2 to 4 hours"

NO Go to D

D. Are any of the following present?

- Request for addiction services
- History of intermittent use and has concerns
- Ongoing vomiting, diarrhea, heartburn after exposure
- Postexposure eye or skin irritation
- Acute anxiety

YES "Seek medical care within 24 hours"

NO Go to E

E. Are any of the following present?

- No other symptoms or problems but parent or person concerned
- 12 hours after cessation and mild tremors, anxiety, anorexia, nausea or vomiting, weakness, myalgias

YES "Call back or call PCP for appointment if no improvement" and Follow **Home Care Instructions**

NO Follow **Home Care Instructions**

S

Home Care Instructions
Substance Abuse, Use, or Exposure

- For chemical exposure, immediately wash exposed skin surfaces.
- Call Poison Control (1-800-222-1222) for exact care of exposure to methamphetamine processing chemicals.
- Contact local resources for assistance: counseling, detoxification centers, inpatient and outpatient treatment programs, AA, and Al-Anon.
- Take usual pain medication for discomfort. Do not give aspirin to a child. Avoid aspirin-like products if age <20 years. Avoid acetaminophen if liver disease is present. Avoid ibuprofen if kidney disease or stomach problems exist or in the case of pregnancy. Follow the directions on the label.

Additional Instructions

Report the Following Problems to Your PCP/Clinic/ED

- Fever
- Difficulty performing simple tasks
- Dizziness
- Persistent vomiting or diarrhea

Seek Emergency Care Immediately If Any of the Following Occur

- Signs of withdrawal: rapid heart rate, tremors, high blood pressure, vomiting, restlessness, sweating
- Seizures
- Black or tarry stools
- Dark coffee-ground–like emesis
- Suicidal or homicidal ideation
- Chest pain
- Dizziness
- Hallucinations
- Extreme anxiety, agitation, or paranoia
- Exposure to methamphetamine vapors during cooking process

If the caller agrees with the advice given, document the call and encourage the caller to call back or see PCP if the problem worsens. If the caller does not agree with the advice given, reevaluate and advise the caller to follow up with PCP, Clinic, or ED.

Suicide Attempt, Threat

 Key Questions Name, Age, Onset, Cause, Address, Telephone Number, Medications, History

 Other Protocols to Consider Altered Mental Status (28); Alcohol Problems (21); Anxiety (36); Breathing Problems (106); Confusion (150); Depression (184); Laceration (395); Mental Health Challenges in Telephone Triage (App V, 720); Overdose (438); Substance Abuse, Use, or Exposure (582).

Nurse Alert: Assess for suicide risk.

- High Suicide Risk:
  - Specific suicide plan
  - Access to lethal means (weapon)
  - Impaired judgment
  - Chemical dependency
  - Psychosis

- Moderate Suicide Risk:
  - No access to lethal means (weapon)
  - No specific suicide plan
  - Appropriate judgment
  - Supportive family or significant other

- Low Suicide Risk:
  - No specific suicide plan or intent
  - Supportive social circle

Reminder: Document caller response to advice, home care instructions, and when to call back.

ASSESSMENT	ACTION

A. Are any of the following present?

- Unconsciousness
- Severe respiratory distress, chest pain, or abdominal pain
- Suicide attempt, such as physical injury or overdose
- Suicide attempt in progress
- Threat to harm self or others
- Suicidal thoughts with a specific plan (available method such as weapons or pills)
- New onset of confusion or delusional thinking

 "Call ambulance" or "Seek emergency care now"
and
Contact police if necessary

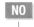 Go to B

B. Are any of the following present?

- Refusal to talk anymore and considered at high risk for suicide
- History of prior suicide attempts
- Depression
- Intoxication
- Suicidal thoughts but no plan or injury
- Recent change in medication

YES "Seek medical care now" and Contact mental health professional now or call police if necessary and Follow **Home Care Instructions**

NO Follow **Home Care Instructions**

S

Home Care Instructions
Suicide Attempt, Threat

- All calls dealing with suicidal thoughts should be referred to an appropriate mental health professional.
- If the caller is alone and high risk, maintain telephone contact as long as possible or transfer the call to a suicide hotline without losing the connection. Trace the call as necessary. Obtain the caller's address and telephone number.
- All calls indicating suicidal thoughts should be considered emergent until cleared by a mental health professional or ED physician.
- Note background noises.

Additional Instructions

Seek Emergency Care or Call Police Immediately If Any of the Following Occur

- Continued suicidal thoughts
- Suicidal thoughts with a specific plan (available method: weapons or pills)
- Suicide attempt (physical injury or overdose)

If the caller agrees with the advice given, document the call and encourage the caller to call back or see PCP if the problem worsens. If the caller does not agree with the advice given, reevaluate and advise the caller to follow up with PCP, Clinic, or ED.

Sunburn

 Key Questions Name, Age, Onset, Allergies, Medications, Tetanus Immunization Status, History

Other Protocols to Consider Dehydration (180); Eye Problems (228); Heat-Exposure Problems (323); Rash, Adult (500), Child (505); Skin Lesions: Lumps, Bumps, and Sores (556).

Reminder: Document caller response to advice, home care instructions, and when to call back.

ASSESSMENT	ACTION

A. Are any of the following present?

- Cool skin, dizziness, faintness
- Dry, hot skin, faintness when temperature >105°F (40.6°C)
- Confusion
- Significant decrease in urine output
- Loss of consciousness or altered mental status

YES "Seek emergency care now"

NO Go to B

B. Are any of the following present?

- Vision changes
- Severe swelling
- Blisters on hands or genitals
- Burn circles around a digit or limb
- Burns on joints

YES "Seek medical care within 2 to 4 hours"

NO Go to C

C. Are any of the following present?

- Multiple blisters
- Open blisters
- Tetanus immunization >10 years ago or no history of immunization
- Signs of infection: pain, swelling, pus, or red streaks extending from blistered area
- Eye pain, decreased vision, light sensitivity

YES "Seek medical care within 24 hours"

NO Go to D

D. Are any of the following present?

- Skin reddened and no blisters
- Pain unresponsive to OTC pain relievers
- Pain >48 hours
- A few blisters

YES "Call back or call PCP for appointment if no improvement" and
Follow **Home Care Instructions**

NO Follow **Home Care Instructions**

S

Home Care Instructions
Sunburn

- Apply cold compresses to burn or take a cool bath for 10 minutes 4 times a day. May add Aveeno or ½ cup baking soda to water. Be careful area does not become numb; frostbite can occur. Do not apply ice to the skin.
- Expect some discomfort for as long as 48 hours. Use your usual pain medication (aspirin, acetaminophen, ibuprofen). Do not give aspirin to a child. Avoid aspirin-like products if age <20 years. Avoid acetaminophen if liver disease is present. Avoid ibuprofen if kidney disease or stomach problems exist or in the case of pregnancy. Follow the directions on the label.
- Do not apply greasy substance or toothpaste to burn area.
- After cooling with water, and if no open blisters are present, apply topical antibiotic, aloe vera, or a mixture of Benadryl elixir and milk of magnesia in equal amounts to burned area for a soothing effect.
- During the drying stage, apply moisturizing lotion to the skin. Peeling usually occurs in 3 to 10 days.
- For painful and swollen eyes, stay in a darkened room, apply cool compresses to the eyes, and rest.
- Increase fluid intake.
- Avoid sun exposure if taking phototoxic medications such as sulfas, tetracycline, phenothiazines, or thiazides. Always read the warning label on medications before taking them.

Additional Instructions

Report the Following Problems to Your PCP/Clinic/ED

- Signs of infection
- Severe swelling
- No improvement or if condition worsens

Seek Emergency Care Immediately If Any of the Following Occur

- Significant decrease in urine output
- Confusion
- Cool skin, dizziness, fainting

If the caller agrees with the advice given, document the call and encourage the caller to call back or see PCP if the problem worsens. If the caller does not agree with the advice given, reevaluate and advise the caller to follow up with PCP, Clinic, or ED.

Swallowing Difficulty

 Key Questions Name, Age, Onset, Cause, Allergies, Medications, History, Pain Scale

 Other Protocols to Consider Foreign Body, Swallowing of (280); Heartburn (316); Mouth Problems (407); Neurologic Symptoms (418); Piercing Problems (445); Sore Throat (564); Stroke, Suspected (576); Weakness (649).

> *Nurse Alert:* Sudden changes in ability to swallow, vision, speech, or mental status; weakness, and numbness may be signs of a stroke or other serious neurologic disorder. Prompt treatment may prevent extensive damage to the brain or reduce permanent disability. Medications used to break up a clot in the brain need to be administered within 3 hours of symptom onset.

Reminder: Document caller response to advice, home care instructions, and when to call back.

ASSESSMENT	ACTION

A. Are any of the following present?

- Weakness of neck, chest, and limbs
- Double or blurred vision, drooling, or drooping eyelids
- Excessive drooling in small child who appears ill
- Sudden swelling in face, tongue, or throat or itching, hives, or wheezing
- Difficulty breathing
- Pain in jaw, throat, neck, shoulders, chest, or arms
- Inability to swallow own saliva

 "Call ambulance"
or
"Seek emergency care now"

NO Go to B

B. Is the following present?

- Sensation that bone or food is stuck in throat or esophagus

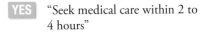 "Seek medical care within 2 to 4 hours"

NO Go to C

C. Is the following present?

- Unexplained weight loss

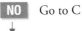 "Seek medical care within 24 hours"

NO Go to D

D. Are any of the following present?

- Difficulty swallowing because of sore throat
- Intermittent chest pain on bending forward or lying down
- Throat feels tight after swallowing
- Recent increase in stress

YES "Call back or call PCP for appointment if no improvement" and
Follow **Home Care Instructions**

NO Follow **Home Care Instructions**

S

Home Care Instructions
Swallowing Difficulty

- Take your usual pain medication (aspirin, acetaminophen, ibuprofen) as tolerated for fever and discomfort. Do not give aspirin to a child. Avoid aspirin-like products if age <20 years. Avoid acetaminophen if liver disease is present. Avoid ibuprofen if kidney disease or stomach problems exist or in the case of pregnancy. Follow the directions on the label.
- Gargle with salt water several times a day for throat discomfort. Suck on hard candy or lozenges.
- Increase fluids. Sip warm tea with lemon and honey.
- Swallow bread or soft foods, as tolerated.
- Try OTC antacids, such as Gelusil, Maalox, Mylanta, Riopan, and Tums, and follow instructions on the label.
- Do not lie down, bend over, or exercise soon after eating.
- Eat small, frequent meals.
- Avoid spicy foods, alcohol, coffee, smoking, chocolate, vinegar, fatty foods, and carbonated beverages.

Additional Instructions

Report the Following Problems to Your PCP/Clinic/ED

- No improvement after 3 days or condition worsens
- Burping or vomiting blood or dark coffee-ground–like emesis
- Excessive drooling
- Persistent fever unresponsive to home care measures

Seek Emergency Care Immediately If Any of the Following Occur

- Weakness of neck, chest, and limbs
- Double or blurred vision, drooling, or drooping eyelids
- Excessive drooling in small child who appears ill
- Sudden swelling in face, tongue, or throat or itching, hives, or wheezing
- Difficulty breathing
- Pain in jaw, throat, neck, shoulders, chest, or arms
- Inability to swallow own saliva

If the caller agrees with the advice given, document the call and encourage the caller to call back or see PCP if the problem worsens. If the caller does not agree with the advice given, reevaluate and advise the caller to follow up with PCP, Clinic, or ED.

Sweating, Excessive

 Key Questions Name, Age, Onset, Cause, Allergies, Medications, History

 Other Protocols to Consider Alcohol Problems (21); Anxiety (36); Breathing Problems (106); Chest Pain (123); Diabetes Problems (187); Fever, Adult (250), Child (253); Heat-Exposure Problems (323); Poisoning, Suspected (454); Substance Use, Abuse, or Exposure (582).

Reminder: Document caller response to advice, home care instructions, and when to call back.

ASSESSMENT	ACTION

A. Are any of the following present?

- Pale, cool skin and rapid pulse
- Pain in chest, throat, neck, jaw, shoulders, or arms
- Difficulty breathing

YES "Call ambulance"
or
"Seek emergency care now"

NO Go to B

B. Are any of the following present?

- Prolonged exposure to heat and fatigue, weakness, dizziness, or nausea
- Signs of dehydration in young children, the elderly, or immunosuppressed individuals:
  - decreased urine for >8 hours
  - sunken eyes
  - crying without tears
  - skin does not bounce back when pinched
  - excessive thirst
  - dry mouth
  - unusual lethargy

YES "Seek medical care within 2 to 4 hours"

NO Go to C

C. Are any of the following present?

- Excessive sweating at night and weight loss, persistent cough, blood in sputum
- Persistent fever and fatigue
- Recent abrupt cessation of drugs (OTC, prescription, or street), alcohol, or caffeine

YES "Seek medical care within 24 hours"

NO Go to D

D. Are any of the following present?

- Weight loss, increased appetite, weakness, difficulty sleeping
- Older than 38 years, sweating without fever, and irregular or absent menstrual periods
- Obesity
- Temperature >100°F (37.8°C)
- Sweating occurs after consuming alcohol or large doses of aspirin
- Sweating occurs when wearing synthetic clothing
- Only the hands and feet sweat
- Recent increase in stress
- Beginning signs of dehydration
- Problems with body odor

YES "Call back or call PCP for appointment if no improvement" and
Follow **Home Care Instructions**

NO Follow **Home Care Instructions**

S

Home Care Instructions
Sweating, Excessive

- Remember that sweating often is a natural response to fever, hormonal changes, exercise, and stress.
- Sweating increases with obesity. Reduction in weight should decrease the amount of sweat.
- Take your usual pain medication (aspirin, acetaminophen, ibuprofen) to reduce fever. Do not give aspirin to a child. Avoid aspirin-like products if age <20 years. Avoid acetaminophen if liver disease is present. Avoid ibuprofen if kidney disease or stomach problems exist or in the case of pregnancy. Follow the directions on the label.
- If sweating is related to heat exposure, cool down with cold compresses, cold bath or shower, and light cotton clothing and drink cool fluids.
- For signs of dehydration, increase fluid intake: give young children Lytren, Pedialyte, or Rehydralyte; older children and adults should consume sports drinks, water, juice, or soft drinks.
- Wash and dry hands and feet frequently for excessive sweating. Wear cotton or other natural-fiber clothing and socks.
- Avoid alcohol and aspirin if consumption is related to sweating.

Additional Instructions

Report the Following Problems to Your PCP/Clinic/ED

- Persistent or worsening of unexplained excessive sweating
- Excessive sweating at night and weight loss, persistent cough, blood in sputum
- Weight loss, increased appetite, weakness, difficulty sleeping
- Persistent fever and fatigue

Seek Emergency Care Immediately If Any of the Following Occur

- Pain in chest, throat, neck, jaw, shoulders, or arms
- Pale, cool skin and rapid pulse
- Difficulty breathing

If the caller agrees with the advice given, document the call and encourage the caller to call back or see PCP if the problem worsens. If the caller does not agree with the advice given, reevaluate and advise the caller to follow up with PCP, Clinic, or ED.

Swelling

Key Questions Name, Age, Onset, No Known Injury, Medications, History

Other Protocols to Consider Abdominal Pain, Adult (9), Child (13); Abdominal Swelling (16); Ankle Problems (33); Breast Problems (103); Bruising (109); Cast/Splint Problems (121); Congestive Heart Failure (157); Finger and Toe Problems (257); Glands, Swollen or Tender (297); Pregnancy Problems (481); Wound Healing and Infection (664).

Reminder: Document caller response to advice, home care instructions, and when to call back.

ASSESSMENT	ACTION

A. In addition to swelling in the face, ankles, or hands, are any of the following present?

- Severe respiratory difficulty, wheezing, or cough
- Swollen tongue or swelling at back of throat
- Rapid progression of swelling
- Coughing up frothy pink-tinged sputum

YES "Seek emergency care now"

NO Go to B

B. Are any of the following present?

- Area warm, red, or tender
- Area cold or blue
- Rings cutting into skin because of increased swelling
- Vomiting or diarrhea
- Persistent painful swelling in groin or abdomen that does not disappear with pressure
- Swelling in groin or abdomen and nausea or vomiting present

YES "Seek medical care within 2 to 4 hours"

NO Go to C

C. Are any of the following present?

- Recent trauma and unexpected swelling
- History of kidney disease
- Persistent water retention that is unresponsive to prescribed diuretic
- Swelling and fever with no other related symptoms
- Swelling in child <3 months old
- Ankle swelling and increased difficulty breathing at night when lying flat
- History of heart disease
- Persistent swelling
- Swelling in groin or abdomen disappears with pressure or enlarges with coughing
- Persistent swelling in armpit, neck, or groin

YES "Seek medical care within 24 hours"

NO Go to D

D. Are any of the following present?

- Intermittent recurring swelling of ankles and fingers
- Swelling interferes with activity
- Recent weight gain >5 lb and no change in dietary or activity habits
- Swelling occurs 1 to 2 weeks before menstruation or at end of the day
- Swelling goes down after removing restrictive clothing
- High intake of salty foods or soda

YES "Call back or call PCP for appointment if no improvement" and
Follow **Home Care Instructions**

NO Follow **Home Care Instructions**

S

Home Care Instructions
Swelling

- Reduce salt in the diet.
- Increase exercise, and avoid prolonged sitting or standing.
- Elevate legs at end of the day.
- Avoid restrictive clothing.
- Avoid crossing legs when sitting.
- Avoid wearing rings if fingers frequently swell.
- Sleep on two pillows or raise head of bed if having difficulty breathing at night.

Additional Instructions

Report the Following Problem to Your PCP/Clinic/ED

- Condition persists or worsens

Seek Emergency Care Immediately If Any of the Following Occur

- Severe respiratory difficulty, wheezing, or cough
- Swollen tongue or swelling at back of throat
- Rapid progression of swelling
- Coughing up frothy, pink-tinged sputum

If the caller agrees with the advice given, document the call and encourage the caller to call back or see PCP if the problem worsens. If the caller does not agree with the advice given, reevaluate and advise the caller to follow up with PCP, Clinic, or ED.

Swine Flu (H1N1 Virus) Exposure

>> **Key Questions** Name, Age, Onset, Symptoms, Known or Suspected Exposure to Swine Flu (H1N1) Virus within Past 7 Days, Medications, History, Health-Care Worker, Public Health-Care Worker, or First Responder

>> **Other Protocols to Consider** Breathing Problems (106); Common Cold Symptoms (146); Congestion (153); Cough (170); Dehydration (180); Fever, Adult (250), Child (253); Headache (308); Influenza (372); Rash, Adult (500), Child (505); Sore Throat (564).

Nurse Alert: Use this protocol if diagnosed with swine flu, known or suspected exposure to swine flu (H1N1) virus within past 7 days.

Reminder: Document caller response to advice, home care instructions, and when to call back.

ASSESSMENT	ACTION

A. Are any of the following present?

- Confusion, delirium, or difficulty arousing
- Severe difficulty breathing for reasons other than congestion
- Flat purple or dark red spots on the face or trunk, fever, stiff or painful neck, or headache
- Severe headache
- Skin or lips turn blue or gray
- Profuse sweating and light-headedness or weakness

YES "Call ambulance"
or
"Seek emergency care now"

NO Go to B

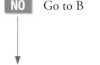

B. Are any of the following present?

- Age >60 years, weakened immune system, diabetes, or bedridden and fever >101°F (38.3°C)
- Infant <3 months old and fever >100.4°F (38°C)
- Fever in an older adult or child who appears very ill, lethargic, or irritable
- Signs of dehydration in the elderly, young child, or persons who have a weakened immune system
- Age <6 weeks

YES "Seek medical care immediately"
NO Go to C

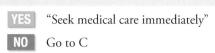

C. Known exposure and are any of the following present?

- Fatigue, fever <103.1°F (39.5°C), dry cough, sore throat, GI symptoms, runny nose or congestion, muscle aches
- Child with fever >104.9°F (40.5°C)
- History of CHF, weakened immune system, age 6 weeks to 23 months, age >65 years, pregnant, long-term-care resident, asthma, COPD, or metabolic disorders
- Caretaker of person with known swine flu and no flu symptoms
- Exposure within the past 7 days in a health-care or public health-care worker or first responder
- Green, brown, or yellow sputum or nasal discharge >72 hours
- Persistent signs of dehydration after home care
- Sinus pain or pressure
- Persistent earache

YES "Seek medical care within 24 hours"

NO Go to D

D. Are any of the following present?

- Green, brown, or yellow sputum or nasal discharge >72 hours
- Cough >3 weeks
- Mild symptoms
- No symptoms but parent or person concerned about exposure to the swine flu virus
- Exposure to swine flu >7 days and no respiratory symptoms

YES "Call back or call PCP for appointment if no improvement" and
Follow **Home Care Instructions**

NO Follow **Home Care Instructions**

Home Care Instructions
Swine Flu (H1N1 Virus) Exposure

- Wash hands frequently with soap and water or alcohol-based hand rubs.
- Reinforce that swine flu virus is highly contagious. Maintain good respiratory etiquette; cover the mouth and nose with a tissue when coughing or sneezing.
- Avoid contact with sick individuals.
- If sick, avoid contact with other people. Stay home for 24 hours after last fever (except for doctor appointments). If coughing and sneezing, wear a surgical mask during close contact with others to prevent the spread of droplets. Change the mask if it becomes soiled or moist.
- Get a lot of rest and drink plenty of fluids.
- Take your usual pain reliever for fever or discomfort. Do not give aspirin to a child. Avoid aspirin-like products if age <20 years. Avoid acetaminophen if liver disease is present. Avoid ibuprofen if kidney disease or stomach problems exist or in the case of pregnancy. Follow the directions on the label.
- Consider antiviral medications to prevent or treat swine flu virus: oseltamivir (Tamiflu) and zanamivir (Relenza).
- Remember that the virus enters the body through the mouth and nose and can be contracted anywhere. Prevent the growth and spread of the virus whether or not you have symptoms by:
  - Resisting touching of the face as much as possible except for bathing and eating
  - Practicing frequent handwashing
  - Gargling twice a day with warm salt water or Listerine to help prevent the growth of the virus in the mouth
  - Cleaning the nostrils once a day with warm salt water. Blow the nose, then swab both nostrils with warm salt water
  - Boosting immunity by consuming foods rich in vitamin C (such as citrus fruits). If taking vitamin C supplements, choose those with zinc to increase absorption
  - Drinking plenty of warm fluids to help flush the virus from the throat into the stomach where the virus cannot survive

Additional Instructions

Report the Following Problems to Your PCP/Clinic/ED

- Persistent fever >103.1°F (39.5°C) and unresponsive to home care measures
- Fever in an older adult or child who appears very ill, lethargic, or irritable
- Signs of dehydration

Seek Emergency Care If Any of the Following Occur

- Flat purple or dark red spots on the face or trunk, fever, headache, or stiff or painful neck
- Skin or lips turn blue or gray
- Profuse sweating and light-headedness or weakness
- Confusion, delirium, or difficulty arousing person
- Severe difficulty breathing for reasons other than congestion

If the caller agrees with the advice given, document the call and encourage the caller to call back or see PCP if the problem worsens. If the caller does not agree with the advice given, reevaluate and advise the caller to follow up with PCP, Clinic, or ED.

S

Tattoo Problems

>> **Key Questions** Name, Age, Date of Recent Tattoo, Location of Tattoo, Medications, History, Pain Scale, Tetanus Immunization Status

>> **Other Protocols to Consider** Abrasions (19); Laceration (395); Piercing Problems (445); Wound Healing and Infection (664).

Reminder: Document caller response to advice, home care instructions, and when to call back.

ASSESSMENT	ACTION

A. Are any of the following present?

- Rapid swelling of tongue or throat
- Difficulty swallowing or breathing
- Inability to speak

YES "Call ambulance"

NO Go to B

B. Are any of the following present?

- Swelling and area below tattoo is cool, clammy, or painful
- Faintness or dizziness
- Rapid joint swelling near site of tattoo
- Diabetic or weakened immune system and signs of infection: pain, swelling, drainage, warmth, or red streaks extending from the tattoo
- Sudden onset of hoarseness
- Recent tattoo and pain at wound site, muscle spasms, stiff jaw and neck, or difficulty swallowing or opening mouth

YES "Seek emergency care now"

NO Go to C

C. Are any of the following present?

- New tattoo and chills, feeling ill, or headache
- No improvement with home care measures
- Wound <24 hours old and tetanus immunization >10 years
- Signs of infection
- Persistent bleeding after 24 hours and unresponsive to home care measures
- Swollen lymph nodes near the tattoo: neck, armpit, or groin
- Blistering around the tattoo
- Temperature >100.4°F (38°C)

 YES "Seek medical care within 24 hours"

NO Go to D

D. Are any of the following present?

- Itching around the tattoo edges
- Painless bumps around the tattoo
- Desire to have tattoo removed and requests referral to a health-care provider

YES "Call back or call PCP for appointment if no improvement" and Follow **Home Care Instructions**

NO Follow **Home Care Instructions**

Home Care Instructions
Tattoo Problems

- Stop bleeding by applying direct pressure to the area.
- Apply a cold pack to reduce swelling, bruising, or itching. Do not put ice directly on the skin; place a cloth barrier between ice and the skin.
- Remove the bandage after 24 hours and apply antibiotic ointment (Triple Antibiotic Ointment or bacitracin). Replace with a nonstick bandage if the wound becomes dirty or irritated by clothing. Replace with a clean bandage daily and change it if it gets wet.
- If the bandage sticks to the tattoo, hold it under running water and gently remove the bandage.
- Keep the skin clean. Do not rub. Avoid strong soaps, detergents, or other chemicals. Pat dry after cleaning. Check the tattoo daily during the healing period for signs of infection.
- Some clear, yellow, or blood-tinged drainage is normal. Report signs of infection: redness, swelling, foul drainage, red streaks, warm to touch, or increased pain.
- Leave the tattoo open to the air whenever possible during the healing period.
- Apply moisturizer several times a day and avoid sun exposure.
- Avoid hot tubs or pools for 14 days.
- Take an antihistamine (Benadryl or Chlor-Trimeton) if hives or itching is present. Follow the instructions on the label.
- Take your usual pain medication. Do not give aspirin to a child. Avoid aspirin-like products if age <20 years. Avoid acetaminophen if liver disease is present. Avoid ibuprofen if kidney disease or stomach problems exist or in the case of pregnancy. Follow the directions on the label.
- Allow up to 2 weeks for healing.
- If you are scheduled for an MRI, inform the radiologist or technician that you have a tattoo and indicate the location and colors. Some tattoos can distort imaging or react to the MRI.

Additional Instructions

Report the Following Problems to Your PCP/Clinic/ED

- Headache, muscle aches, general ill feeling, or fever
- No improvement or condition worsens
- Temperature >100.4°F (38°C)
- Signs of infection

Seek Emergency Care Immediately If Any of the Following Occur

- Swelling and area below tattoo is cool, clammy, or painful
- Rapid joint swelling near the site of the tattoo
- Painful site, muscle spasms, stiff jaw and neck, or difficulty swallowing or opening mouth

If the caller agrees with the advice given, document the call and encourage the caller to call back or see PCP if the problem worsens. If the caller does not agree with the advice given, reevaluate and advise the caller to follow up with PCP, Clinic, or ED.

T

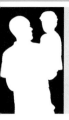

Teething

 Key Questions Name, Age, Onset, Medications, History

 Other Protocols to Consider Crying, Excessive, in Infants (176); Earache, Drainage (206); Fever, Child (253).

Reminder: Document caller response to advice, home care instructions, and when to call back.

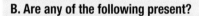

ASSESSMENT	ACTION

A. In addition to drooling, chewing, swollen and bruised gums, are any of the following present?

- Excessive irritability, intermittent lethargy, and high fever
- Constant crying >2 hours and unrelated to colic
- Persistent high fever
- Child appears ill

YES "Seek medical care within 2 to 4 hours"

NO Go to B

B. Are any of the following present?

- Fussiness >2 days
- Crying interferes with child's sleep
- Child pulling on ears

YES "Seek medical care within 24 hours"

NO Go to C

C. Are any of the following present?

- Teething, gums are red and swollen, and child is 4 to 8 months old
- Temperature <101°F (38.3°C)
- Poor appetite

YES "Call back or call PCP for appointment if no improvement" and Follow **Home Care Instructions**

NO Follow **Home Care Instructions**

Home Care Instructions
Teething

- Massage the swollen or irritated gum with finger for 2 minutes.
- Give acetaminophen for discomfort. Do not give aspirin to a child. Avoid aspirin-like products if age <20 years. Avoid acetaminophen if liver disease is present. Avoid ibuprofen if kidney disease or stomach problems exist or in the case of pregnancy. Follow the directions on the label.
- Provide a cold teething ring, flavored ice, frozen banana, or frozen bagel for infant to chew.
- Avoid salty or acidic foods.
- Avoid teething gels with benzocaine, which may numb the throat and cause choking or a drug reaction.
- Remember that infants 3 to 8 months of age may have symptoms of teething (drooling, chewing) when not actually teething.
- Discuss teething remedies with PCP if no tooth or gum swelling is observed.

Additional Instructions

Report the Following Problems to Your PCP/Clinic/ED

- Excessive irritability, intermittent lethargy, and high fever
- Constant crying >2 hours
- Persistent high fever
- Infant stops eating

If the caller agrees with the advice given, document the call and encourage the caller to call back or see PCP if the problem worsens. If the caller does not agree with the advice given, reevaluate and advise the caller to follow up with PCP, Clinic, or ED.

Tongue Problems

 Key Questions Name, Age, Onset, Cause, Allergies, Medications, History, Pain Scale

 Other Protocols to Consider Allergic Reaction (25); Mouth Problems (407); Piercing Problems (445); Sore Throat (564); Swallowing Difficulty (591); Toothache (613).

Reminder: Document caller response to advice, home care instructions, and when to call back.

ASSESSMENT	ACTION

A. Is the following present?

- Sudden onset of tongue swelling and difficulty breathing

YES "Call ambulance"

NO Go to B

B. Are any of the following present?

- Sudden onset of tongue swelling and no difficulty breathing
- Pain, swelling, drainage around piercing
- Gaping laceration from torn piercing

YES "Seek medical care within 2 to 4 hours"

NO Go to C

C. Are any of the following present?

- Pain after taking a new medication
- Pain on one side of face
- Persistent hard lump on tongue or mouth
- Persistent pain and diarrhea with loose, foul-smelling, bulky stools
- Ulcers, cracks, redness, and persistent pain unresponsive to >3 days of home care measures
- Minor tear from piercing and last tetanus shot >10 years

YES "Seek medical care within 24 hours"

NO Go to D

D. Are any of the following present?

- Tongue bright red and swollen
- Red tip and edges
- Tongue appears hairy
- Ulcers
- Sore on one area of tongue
- Tongue appears black from Pepto-Bismol
- Irritation from dentures, rough tooth, or braces

YES "Call back or call PCP for appointment if no improvement" and
Follow **Home Care Instructions**

NO Follow **Home Care Instructions**

T

Home Care Instructions
Tongue Problems

- Drink through a straw to minimize discomfort.
- Note relationship between certain foods and tongue pain and avoid those foods in the diet. Alcohol, hot food or spices, tobacco, chocolate, citrus foods, vinegar, pickles, salted nuts, and chips may irritate the tongue. Milk, gelatin, yogurt, ice cream, and custard are soothing to the tongue.
- Rinse mouth 4 times a day with a salt or baking soda solution. Add ½ tsp salt or baking soda to 8 ounces of water.
- If irritation is caused by a rough tooth or braces, contact your dentist.
- If swelling is related to medication, discontinue use and contact PCP if it is a prescription medication.
- Increase fluid intake.
- If irritation is caused by dentures, remove dentures and contact dentist.

Additional Instructions

_____

_____

_____

Report the Following Problems to Your PCP/Clinic/ED

- No improvement or condition worsens after 3 days of home care measures
- Pain becomes intolerable
- Fever, rash, facial swelling

Seek Emergency Care Immediately If Any of the Following Occur

- Difficulty breathing
- Swelling of the back of the mouth

If the caller agrees with the advice given, document the call and encourage the caller to call back or see PCP if the problem worsens. If the caller does not agree with the advice given, reevaluate and advise the caller to follow up with PCP, Clinic, or ED.

Toothache

T

Key Questions Name, Age, Onset, Cause, Allergies, Medications, History (If injury occurred, see Tooth Injury protocol (616))

Other Protocols to Consider Chest Pain (123); Facial Problems (231); Jaw Pain (387); Mouth Problems (407); Tooth Injury (616).

Reminder: Document caller response to advice, home care instructions, and when to call back.

ASSESSMENT	ACTION

A. Is the following present?

- Gnawing pain in lower teeth and neck, chest, shoulder, or arms

YES "Seek emergency care now"

NO Go to B

B. Are any of the following present?

- History of cardiovascular disease or diabetes and jaw pain (no known injury or dental problem)
- Temperature >100.4°F (38.0°C)

YES "Seek medical care within 2 hours"

NO Go to C

C. Are any of the following present?

- Persistent pain and swelling over upper or lower jaw
- Drainage from dental abscess
- Broken tooth (nontraumatic)

YES "Seek dental care within 24 hours"

NO Go to D

D. Are any of the following present?

- Pain interferes with daily activities
- Red, swollen, bleeding gums
- Pain when biting food for several days
- Recent filling and pain for several days
- History of problems with same tooth (previous break or crack, hot or cold sensitivity)
- Pain without trauma, fracture, fever, or facial swelling
- Sores in mouth
- Tooth loose, chipped, or decayed
- Pain during or just after eating

YES "Call back or call dentist for appointment if no improvement" and Follow **Home Care Instructions**

NO Follow **Home Care Instructions**

Home Care Instructions
Toothache

- Apply ice pack for 20 minutes, 4 times a day, to reduce swelling.
- Do not put ice directly on the skin; place a cloth barrier between ice and the skin.
- Take your usual pain medication (aspirin, acetaminophen, ibuprofen) for discomfort. Do not give aspirin to a child. Avoid aspirin-like products if age <20 years. Avoid acetaminophen if liver disease is present. Avoid ibuprofen if kidney disease or stomach problems exist or in the case of pregnancy. Follow the directions on the label.
- Rinse mouth with ½ tsp baking soda or salt in a cup of warm water several times a day if sores are present.
- Brush teeth at least twice a day.
- Call a dentist for an appointment.

Additional Instructions

Report the Following Problems to Your Dentist/PCP/Clinic

- Persistent pain unresponsive to pain medication
- Facial swelling
- Fever
- Drainage from dental abscess

Seek Emergency Care Immediately If Any of the Following Occur

- Pain in chest, shoulder, or arms
- Gnawing pain in lower teeth and neck

If the caller agrees with the advice given, document the call and encourage the caller to call back or see PCP if the problem worsens. If the caller does not agree with the advice given, reevaluate and advise the caller to follow up with PCP, Clinic, or ED.

Tooth Injury

 Key Questions Name, Age, Onset, Cause, Allergies, Medications, History

 Other Protocols to Consider Back/Neck Injury (59); Jaw Pain (387); Mouth Problems (407); Toothache (613).

> *Nurse Alert:* If the tooth has been knocked out, timing is critical since the success rate of reimplantation decreases significantly after 60 minutes. See home care instructions (618) for specific directions to help save the tooth.

Reminder: Document caller response to advice, home care instructions, and when to call back.

ASSESSMENT	ACTION
A. Are any of the following present?	
• Altered mental status • Severe neck pain • Numbness or tingling in arms or legs	**YES** "Call ambulance" **NO** Go to B
B. Are any of the following present?	
• Tooth (or teeth) knocked out • Tooth or teeth loose and about to fall out • Tooth repositioned • Unable to stop bleeding with pressure	**YES** "Seek dental or emergency care now" and Follow **Home Care Instructions** **NO** Go to C
C. After a traumatic injury to teeth, are any of the following present?	
• Severe pain and swelling over affected area • Loose tooth or teeth • Tooth fractured through crown or to gum line • Painful cracked or chipped tooth • Frenum tear or laceration • Severe jaw pain	**YES** "Seek dental or medical care within 2 to 4 hours" **NO** Go to D

D. Are any of the following present?

- Lacerated gum, cheek, or lip
- Painless cracked or chipped tooth

YES   "Call back or call dentist for appointment if no improvement" and
Follow **Home Care Instructions**

NO   Follow **Home Care Instructions**

T

Home Care Instructions
Tooth Injury

- Find tooth; rinse gently with saliva, milk, or nonchlorinated bottle water; and replace in socket as quickly as possible. Do not remove material adhered to tooth. Do not scrub tooth. Bite down on gauze pad or other material to help keep tooth in place.
- If unable to replace tooth in socket, place tooth in a cup with ¼ tsp salt and 1 cup of milk. May place tooth under tongue if victim is alert and not a young child. Patient must be able to comprehend why it is important to keep tooth segment under the tongue so that there is no chance of swallowing tooth.
- Bite down on a folded gauze dressing or a moistened black tea bag for 20 minutes to control bleeding.
- Call dentist.
- Take your usual pain medication (acetaminophen, ibuprofen) for discomfort. Do not give aspirin to a child. Avoid aspirin-like products if age <20 years. Avoid acetaminophen if liver disease is present. Avoid ibuprofen if kidney disease or stomach problems exist or in the case of pregnancy. Follow the directions on the label.
- Apply ice to injured gum as tolerated to help control pain.

Additional Instructions

Report the Following Problem to Your Dentist/PCP/Clinic

- Persistent bleeding, swelling, or pain

If the caller agrees with the advice given, document the call and encourage the caller to call back or see PCP if the problem worsens. If the caller does not agree with the advice given, reevaluate and advise the caller to follow up with PCP, Clinic, or ED.

Umbilical Cord Care

 Key Questions Name, Age, History

 Other Protocols to Consider Newborn Problems (421); Wound Healing and Infection (664).

Reminder: Document caller response to advice, home care instructions, and when to call back.

ASSESSMENT		ACTION
A. Are any of the following present?		
• Temperature <97.5°F (36.4°C) or >100.4°F (38°C)	YES	"Seek medical care within 2 to 4 hours"
• Signs of infection around the umbilicus: redness, pain, swelling, foul-smelling drainage, red streaks, or warmth	NO	Go to B
• Pain, vomiting, and bulging umbilicus		
B. Are any of the following present?		
• Tissue in navel looks abnormal	YES	"Seek medical care within 24 hours"
• Bleeding longer than 3 days after cord detachment	NO	Go to C
• Moist navel after 2 days of treatment		
C. Are any of the following present?		
• Newly discovered bulging umbilicus when infant cries	YES	"Call back or call PCP for appointment if no improvement" and Follow **Home Care Instructions**
• Small amount of bleeding (a few drops) or discharge after cord detachment		
• Cord has not fallen off within 1 month	NO	Follow **Home Care Instructions**

U

Home Care Instructions
Umbilical Cord Care

- Until the cord dries: Clean stump once a day with alcohol. Only sponge bathe until the cord falls off.
- Keep diapers and plastic pants below umbilicus.
- Remember that the cord usually falls off in 1 to 3 weeks and a small amount of oozing blood is to be expected.
- Remember that it is common for the umbilicus to bulge when the infant cries or strains. This type of hernia will resolve with time.
- If the cord appears infected, wash with antibacterial soap, rinse, wash again with peroxide, and rinse; follow this procedure twice a day. Rub the cord with a cotton swab saturated in 70% rubbing alcohol 6 times a day.
- Leave the cord open to air as much as possible.
- Do not use ointments or powders on the cord.

Additional Instructions

Report the Following Problems to Your PCP/Clinic/ED

- Bleeding longer than 3 days after cord detachment
- Moist navel after 2 days of treatment
- Cord still attached after 3 weeks
- Condition persists or worsens
- Signs of infection inside the umbilicus

If the caller agrees with the advice given, document the call and encourage the caller to call back or see PCP if the problem worsens. If the caller does not agree with the advice given, reevaluate and advise the caller to follow up with PCP, Clinic, or ED.

Urinary Catheter/Nephrostomy Tube Problems

 Key Questions Name, Age, Onset, Cause, Type of Urinary Device, Length of Time in Place, Name of Surgeon or Urologist, Medications, History

 Other Protocols to Consider Dehydration (180); Urination, Difficult (624), Excessive (626), Painful (628); Urine, Abnormal Color (631); Wound Healing and Infection (664).

Reminder: Document caller response to advice, home care instructions, and when to call back.

U

ASSESSMENT	ACTION
A. Are any of the following present?	
• Severe pain • Severe bleeding • Catheter in place and no urine flow for >8 hours	**YES** "Seek emergency care now" **NO** Go to B
B. Are any of the following present?	
• No drainage from catheter for >4 hours and no improvement with home care measures • Taking blood-thinning medication and urine is pink or red • Recent urinary tract surgery and unexpected pain • Temperature >100.4°F (38°C) • Surgically placed catheter or tube dislodged • Large amount of blood in urine • Persistent back, low abdominal, or flank pain	**YES** "Seek medical care within 2 to 4 hours" **NO** Go to C
C. Are any of the following present?	
• Painful, red, and irritated skin surrounding the insertion point of the device or perineal area • Cloudy or foul-smelling urine • Catheter or tube in place but no urine outflow • Urine leaking around the appliance	**YES** "Seek medical care within 24 hours" and Follow **Home Care Instructions** **NO** Go to D

D. Are any of the following present?

- Leaking catheter or tube
- Mild discomfort

YES "Call back or call PCP for appointment if no improvement" and
Follow **Home Care Instructions**

NO Follow **Home Care Instructions**

Home Care Instructions
Urinary Catheter/Nephrostomy Tube Problems

- Check for kinks in tubing.
- Make sure collection bag is lower than the pelvis.
- Make sure person is not lying on the catheter and catheter is in place.
- Check and secure all connections.
- Make sure nephrostomy (if present) stopcock is in the correct position.
- Change position of the person.
- Clean the catheter with soap and water, then advance ½ inch or rotate 90°.
- If individual has received instruction in the irrigation procedure, he or she may irrigate the catheter.
- Drink at least 8 to 10 glasses of fluid daily unless on a fluid-restricted regimen.
- Call back if no improvement after home care measures.
- Keep genital area and catheter clean. Wash away from the insertion site and front to back in female patients. Wash with soap and rinse with warm water.

Additional Instructions

Report the Following Problems to Your PCP/Clinic/ED

- No drainage from catheter for >4 hours and no improvement with home care measures
- Large amount of blood in urine
- Persistent back, low abdominal, or flank pain
- Temperature >100.4°F (38°C)
- Urine leaking around the appliance

Seek Emergency Care Immediately If Any of the Following Occur

- Severe pain
- Severe bleeding

If the caller agrees with the advice given, document the call and encourage the caller to call back or see PCP if the problem worsens. If the caller does not agree with the advice given, reevaluate and advise the caller to follow up with PCP, Clinic, or ED.

Urination, Difficult

 Key Questions Name, Age, Onset, Cause, Medications, History, Pain Scale

 Other Protocols to Consider Abdominal Pain, Adult (9), Child (13); Genital Lesions (291); Urinary Catheter/Nephrostomy Tube Problems (621); Urination, Painful (628); Urine, Abnormal Color (631).

Reminder: Document caller response to advice, home care instructions, and when to call back.

ASSESSMENT	ACTION

A. Are any of the following present?

- Severe abdominal pain and inability to void >8 hours
- Catheter in place but no urine flow >8 hours
- Severe abdominal pain and temperature >102°F (39°C)

YES "Seek emergency care"

NO Go to B

B. Are any of the following present?

- Full bladder and inability to urinate >4 hours
- Persistent flank or low abdominal pain
- History of renal disease or prostatitis
- Recent urinary tract or abdominal surgery
- Large amount of blood in urine
- Recent trauma
- Catheter in place but no urine outflow >4 hours
- Recent back injury

YES "Seek medical care within 2 to 4 hours"

NO Go to C

C. Are any of the following present?

- Nausea, vomiting, diarrhea
- Genital herpes
- Painful, red, and irritated perineal area
- Difficulty urinating after sexual activity
- Decreased fluid intake, excessive sweating, dark yellow or orange urine
- Mild discomfort
- New-onset incontinence
- Fever >102°F (39°C)
- Difficulty starting urination

YES "Call back or call PCP for appointment if no improvement" and Follow **Home Care Instructions**

NO Follow **Home Care Instructions**

Home Care Instructions
Urination, Difficult

- Drink at least six to eight-ounce glasses of water a day (unless physician has ordered a fluid-restricted regimen).
- Avoid caffeine and alcohol.
- For retention problems, try urinating in a warm bath.
- For genital herpes, apply cold compresses to perineal area.
- For difficulty starting to urinate, turn on water faucet (sound of running water can help to stimulate urination), and pour warm water over perineum while sitting on toilet.

Additional Instructions

U

Report the Following Problems to Your PCP/Clinic/ED

- Severe flank or abdominal pain
- Persistent inability to empty bladder for >12 hours
- Signs of dehydration: sunken eyes, loss of skin elasticity, excessive thirst, dry mouth or mucous membranes, infant crying without tears
- Severe nausea, vomiting, or diarrhea
- Blood in urine

Seek Emergency Care Immediately If Any of the Following Occur

- Severe abdominal pain and inability to void for >8 hours, or temperature >102°F (39°C)
- Catheter in place but no urine flow for >8 hours

If the caller agrees with the advice given, document the call and encourage the caller to call back or see PCP if the problem worsens. If the caller does not agree with the advice given, reevaluate and advise the caller to follow up with PCP, Clinic, or ED.

Urination, Excessive

 Key Questions Name, Age, Onset, Cause, Medications, History

 Other Protocols to Consider Abdominal Pain, Adult (9), Child (13); Back Pain (62); Dehydration (180); Diabetes Problems (187); Incontinence, Urine (366).

Reminder: Document caller response to advice, home care instructions, and when to call back.

ASSESSMENT	ACTION
A. Are any of the following present?	

• Diabetes
• Signs of dehydration in a child, elderly adult, or immunosuppressed adult:
  • sunken eyes
  • loose, dry skin that does not spring back when pinched
  • excessive thirst, dry mouth, or dry mucous membranes
  • crying without tears
• Excessive thirst
• History of breast cancer, lung cancer, or multiple myeloma
	YES "Seek medical care within 2 to 4 hours"
	
	NO Go to B

B. Are any of the following present?	
• History of kidney disorder • Flank or back pain • Abdominal pain • History of parathyroid tumor or disorder • Muscle cramps or weakness • Signs of dehydration in normally healthy adult	**YES** "Seek medical care within 24 hours" **NO** Go to C
C. Are any of the following present?	
• Recent change in diuretic therapy • Increased fluid intake, especially tea, coffee, alcohol • Increased stress • Taking a diuretic medication (prescribed, OTC, or herbal)	**YES** "Call back or call PCP for appointment if no improvement" and Follow **Home Care Instructions** **NO** Follow **Home Care Instructions**

Home Care Instructions
Urination, Excessive

- Observe for signs of dehydration.
- Drink fluids such as sports drinks or sodas without caffeine.
- If no other physical symptoms, observe for worsening of condition or new symptoms.
- If diabetic, closely monitor blood glucose levels.

Additional Instructions

U

Report the Following Problems to Your PCP/Clinic/ED

- No improvement in 3 days or condition worsens
- Persistent fever unresponsive to fever-reducing measures
- Vomiting, diarrhea, fatigue, lethargy, or stiff neck
- Fever or swelling

If the caller agrees with the advice given, document the call and encourage the caller to call back or see PCP if the problem worsens. If the caller does not agree with the advice given, reevaluate and advise the caller to follow up with PCP, Clinic, or ED.

Urination, Painful

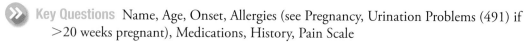

>> **Key Questions** Name, Age, Onset, Allergies (see Pregnancy, Urination Problems (491) if >20 weeks pregnant), Medications, History, Pain Scale

>> **Other Protocols to Consider** Abdominal Pain, Adult (9), Child (13); Pregnancy, Urination Problems (491); Urination, Difficult (624); Urine, Abnormal Color (631).

Reminder: Document caller response to advice, home care instructions, and when to call back.

ASSESSMENT	ACTION

A. Are any of the following present?

- Inability to urinate
- Large amount of red blood in urine
- Back, flank, or abdominal pain and inability to urinate for >8 hours

YES "Seek medical care immediately"

NO Go to B

B. Are any of the following present?

- Recent urinary tract surgery and unexpected pain or fever
- Recent trauma to genitalia or abdomen
- Use of blood-thinning medications and urine is pink or red
- Severe discomfort with urination
- Back or flank pain
- Fever >102°F (39°C)
- Severe scrotal pain or swelling
- Pregnancy
- History of lupus, glomerulonephritis, or single kidney
- Perineal or rectal pain
- Back or flank pain and fever >100.5°F (38.1°C)
- Inability to urinate for >4 hours

YES "Seek medical care within 2 to 4 hours"

NO Go to C

C. Are any of the following present?

- Penile discharge
- Cloudy or foul-smelling urine and <2 years old
- Vomiting or poor fluid intake in a child
- Urgency or frequency for >3 days
- Pain over bladder
- Cloudy or foul-smelling urine

YES "Seek medical care within 24 hours"

NO Go to D

D. Are any of the following present?

- Increased pain at end of urination
- Recurrent urinary tract infections
- Painful urination after sexual contact
- Frequent bubble baths or soap residue on genital area (particularly in young girls)
- Urgency or frequency of <3 days

YES "Call back or call PCP for appointment if no improvement" and
Follow **Home Care Instructions**

NO Follow **Home Care Instructions**

U

Home Care Instructions
Urination, Painful

- Drink lots of fluids, especially cranberry juice.
- Avoid caffeine and alcohol.
- Urinate before and after intercourse or sexual contact.
- Wipe the perineal area from front to back.
- Wear cotton underwear.
- Avoid wearing panty hose for long periods of time.
- Young girls should avoid frequent bubble baths and wash the perineum with water only.
- For irritated and sore perineum, add ½ cup white vinegar to bath and soak for 20 minutes. Repeat in 2 hours and again in 12 hours.
- Take your usual pain medication (aspirin, acetaminophen, ibuprofen) for discomfort. Do not give aspirin to a child. Avoid aspirin-like products if age <20 years. Avoid acetaminophen if liver disease is present. Avoid ibuprofen if kidney disease or stomach problems exist or in the case of pregnancy. Follow the directions on the label.
- When having recurrent urinary tract infections and discomfort, discuss OTC products available (such as phenazopyridine HCl [Pyridium]) with your pharmacist.

Additional Instructions

Report the Following Problems to Your PCP/Clinic/ED

- Persistent discomfort or condition worsens after 48 hours of home care or antibiotic therapy
- Fever, back or flank pain
- Increased blood in urine
- Severe scrotal pain or swelling
- Difficulty urinating

If the caller agrees with the advice given, document the call and encourage the caller to call back or see PCP if the problem worsens. If the caller does not agree with the advice given, reevaluate and advise the caller to follow up with PCP, Clinic, or ED.

Urine, Abnormal Color

 Key Questions Name, Age, Onset, Medications, History

 Other Protocols to Consider Abdominal Pain, Adult (9), Child (13); Dehydration (180); Hepatitis (329); Pregnancy, Urination Problems (491); Urinary Catheter/Nephrostomy Tube Problems (621); Urination, Painful (628).

Reminder: Document caller response to advice, home care instructions, and when to call back.

ASSESSMENT	ACTION
A. Are any of the following present?	
• Pink, red, or smoky brown urine and recent trauma to back or abdomen or severe pain	**YES** "Seek medical care within 2 to 4 hours"
• Fever and flank or back pain	
• Urinary stent present and severe pain or large amount of bright red blood	**NO** Go to B
B. Are any of the following present?	
• Recent onset of dark brown urine, pale stools, and yellow skin and eyes	**YES** "Seek medical care within 24 hours"
• Blood in urine with or without pain	**NO** Go to C
C. Are any of the following present?	
• Dark yellow or orange urine and	**YES** "Call back or call PCP for appointment if no improvement" and
• nausea	Follow **Home Care Instructions**
• vomiting	
• diarrhea	**NO** Follow **Home Care Instructions**
• fever	
• exposure to a hot climate	
• decreased fluid intake	
• decreased urine output	
• Use of medications that cause urine color changes: phenazopyridine HCl (Pyridium), phenytoin (Dilantin), phenolphthalein, metronidazole (Flagyl), or nitrofurantoin (Furadantin)	
• Recent ingestion of rhubarb, beets, blackberries, or other red food	
• New prescription	

U

Home Care Instructions
Urine, Abnormal Color

- Increase fluid intake.
- Avoid foods that may be causing a change in urine color (rhubarb, beets, blackberries, or other red foods) and observe for change in color of urine. Urine should return to normal color within 24 hours.
- If currently taking phenazopyridine HCl (Pyridium) for a urinary tract infection, expect the urine to be red or orange.
- Blue or green urine usually is related to food or medication ingestion.

Additional Instructions

Report the Following Problems to Your PCP/Clinic/ED

- Fever, pain with urination, or back pain
- Condition persists >24 hours or worsens after home care measures
- Unexpected color changes after taking a new medication
- Persistent nausea, vomiting, diarrhea, and decreased fluid intake

Seek Emergency Care Immediately If Any of the Following Occur

- Gross bloody urine and increased abdominal pain after a traumatic blow to the back, side, or abdomen, or a fall or an accident

If the caller agrees with the advice given, document the call and encourage the caller to call back or see PCP if the problem worsens. If the caller does not agree with the advice given, reevaluate and advise the caller to follow up with PCP, Clinic, or ED.

Vaginal Bleeding

 Key Questions Name, Age, Onset (see Pregnancy, Vaginal Bleeding (493) if pregnant), Number of Saturated Pads or Tampons and Size, Medications, History

 Other Protocols to Consider Abdominal Pain, Adult (9), Child (13); Pregnancy Problems (481); Pregnancy, Vaginal Bleeding (493); Sexual Assault (539); Vaginal Discharge/Pain/ Itching (636).

Reminder: Document caller response to advice, home care instructions, and when to call back.

ASSESSMENT	ACTION

A. Are any of the following present?

- Recent rape or trauma
- Pregnancy >20 weeks and sudden bleeding
- Soaking more than one full-size pad in <1 hour and weakness
- Decreased level of consciousness
- Skin pale and moist
- Sudden unexpected bright red bleeding
- Soaking more than two pads or tampons per hour >2 hours or more than one pad or tampon per hour >6 hours

YES "Seek emergency care now"

NO Go to B

B. Are any of the following present?

- Pelvic pain with bleeding (different from usual menstrual discomfort)
- Unusually heavy bleeding
- Postmenopause and sudden bleeding or spotting (not taking medroxyprogesterone [Provera])
- Dizziness or light-headedness when sitting up
- Recent abortion and increased bleeding, pain, or fever

YES "Seek medical care within 2 to 4 hours"

NO Go to C

C. Is the following present?

- Pregnancy and bleeding

YES Go to Pregnancy, Vaginal Bleeding (493) protocol

NO Go to D

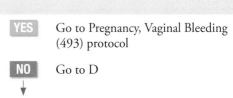

D. Are any of the following present?

- Small amount of bleeding:
  - after intercourse
  - during first 3 months of taking birth control pills
  - missed birth control pill mid-cycle
  - postmenopause and use of Provera
- Bleeding >10 days

YES   "Call back or call PCP for appointment if no improvement" and
Follow **Home Care Instructions**

NO   Follow **Home Care Instructions**

Home Care Instructions
Vaginal Bleeding

- Remember that breakthrough bleeding is not unusual at the time of ovulation, during the first 3 months of a regimen of birth control pills, while taking Provera, or with emotional crisis.
- Change tampons frequently.
- If fever, chills, or muscle aches occur while using tampons, discontinue use and notify PCP if condition persists or worsens.
- If miscarriage is suspected, do not flush toilet; save tissue and clots for physician to examine.

Additional Instructions

Report the Following Problems to Your PCP/Clinic/ED
- Bleeding persists or worsens
- Severe abdominal pain
- Fever, chills, or muscle aches
- Passing tissue or large clots

Seek Emergency Care Immediately If Any of the Following Occur
- Severe pain interferes with activity
- Soaking more than one full-size pad in <1 hour and weakness
- Decreased level of consciousness
- Skin pale and moist
- Soaking more than two pads or tampons per hour for >2 hours or one pad or tampon per hour for >6 hours

If the caller agrees with the advice given, document the call and encourage the caller to call back or see PCP if the problem worsens. If the caller does not agree with the advice given, reevaluate and advise the caller to follow up with PCP, Clinic, or ED.

Vaginal Discharge/Pain/Itching

 Key Questions Name, Age, Onset, Allergies, Medications, History, Pain Scale

 Other Protocols to Consider Abdominal Pain, Adult (9), Child (13); Fever, Adult (250), Child (253); Genital Lesions (291); Menstrual Problems (404); Sexually Transmitted Disease (STD) (542); Vaginal Bleeding (633).

Reminder: Document caller response to advice, home care instructions, and when to call back.

ASSESSMENT	ACTION

A. Are any of the following present?

- Severe pelvic pain interferes with activity
- Temperature >102.0°F (38.9°C), increased pain, chills, shakes, or vomiting
- Foul-smelling vaginal discharge, pain, or itching and history of recent trauma, rape, surgery, pregnancy, or abortion
- Last menstrual period >6 weeks ago, abdominal pain, suspicion of pregnancy

YES "Seek medical care within 2 to 4 hours"

NO Go to B

B. Are any of the following present?

- Itching interferes with activity
- Temperature >100.0°F (37.8°C)
- Foul odor and large amount of discharge
- Green, brown, or white cottage cheese–like discharge
- Exposure to venereal disease or other STD and request for an examination
- Painful sores or irritation on labia or vagina
- History of one ovary and of child-bearing age
- Tampon in place and unable to remove

YES "Seek medical care within 24 hours"

NO Go to C

636

C. Are any of the following present?

- Frequent use of scented feminine hygiene products
- Pain during or after intercourse
- Last Papanicolaou smear >1 year ago
- Small amount of clear, white, or yellow discharge
- Recent prolonged sexual activity
- Concerned about possible STD and no known exposure
- Painless sore on labia or vagina
- Onset of symptoms while on antibiotics
- Exposure to chemicals or bubble bath

YES "Call back or call PCP for appointment if no improvement" and
Follow **Home Care Instructions**

NO Follow **Home Care Instructions**

V

Home Care Instructions
Vaginal Discharge/Pain/Itching

- Note how discharge differs from usual discharge and understand that it is important that there might be a need for further investigation.

For Swelling, Itching, or Irritation
- Soak in a tub of warm water (avoid scented bubble baths).
- Wear loose-fitting undergarments and clothing.
- Wear underwear with cotton-lined crotch.
- Avoid scented feminine hygiene products, tampons, sanitary pads, and toilet tissue.
- Apply clotrimazole (Gyne-Lotrimin) cream to the area. Ask your pharmacist for other OTC product suggestions.
- Apply cool compresses to the area.

For Discharge
- Eat yogurt daily to help prevent infection while taking antibiotics.
- Clean the area frequently.

For Known Infection
- Notify partner of infection and the need for treatment.
- Use a condom during sexual activity to help prevent cross-infection.
- Apply heating pad to abdomen for discomfort.
- Avoid sexual intercourse while symptoms are present or until examined by PCP.

Additional Instructions

Report the Following Problems to Your PCP/Clinic/ED
- Temperature >102.0°F (38.9°C), shakes, chills, vomiting, or increased pain
- Symptoms persist >3 days
- Foul odor and large amount of discharge

If the caller agrees with the advice given, document the call and encourage the caller to call back or see PCP if the problem worsens. If the caller does not agree with the advice given, reevaluate and advise the caller to follow up with PCP, Clinic, or ED.

Vision Problems

 Key Questions Name, Age, Onset, Cause, Medications, History

 Other Protocols to Consider Eye Injury (225); Eye Problems (228); Foreign Body, Eye (269); Neurologic Symptoms (418); Stroke, Suspected (576).

> *Nurse Alert:*
> - If eye injury or foreign body to the eye, use Eye Injury (225) or Foreign Body, Eye (269) protocols.
> - Sudden changes in vision, speech, or mental status, weakness, and numbness may be signs of a stroke or other serious neurologic disorder. Prompt treatment may prevent extensive damage to the brain or reduce permanent disability. Medications used to break up a clot in the brain need to be administered within 3 hours of symptom onset.

Reminder: Document caller response to advice, home care instructions, and when to call back.

ASSESSMENT	ACTION
A. Are any of the following present?	
- Sudden onset of severe eye pain - Sudden loss of partial or total vision in one or both eyes - Blood or pus in colored part of eye - Pupils of unequal size - History of recent head injury and vision changes - Sudden or gradual increase in number of floaters, light flashes, or curtain over field of vision	**YES** "Seek emergency care now" **NO** Go to B
B. Are any of the following present?	
- Sudden onset of blurred or double vision and eye pain - Pain increases with pressure to the eye or eye movement - Age >50 years and recent or present temporal pain/ache - Signs of an eye infection: pain, redness, swelling, drainage, or fever	**YES** "Seek medical care within 2 to 4 hours" **NO** Go to C

V

C. Are any of the following present?

- Increased sensitivity to light
- History of flashing lights followed by a headache
- New and sudden onset of flashing lights (has not occurred in the past) preceded by a headache
- Persistent blurred or double vision
- Change in vision after a change in medication

 YES "Seek medical care within 24 hours"

NO Go to D

D. Are any of the following present?

- Progressive blurred vision and older than 50 years
- Intermittent episodes of blurred vision
- Difficulty seeing distant objects
- Difficulty reading
- Eyes dry and itching

YES "Call back or call PCP for appointment if no improvement" and
Follow **Home Care Instructions**

NO Follow **Home Care Instructions**

Home Care Instructions
Vision Problems

- If drainage is present and eye infection is suspected, encourage family members to use separate towels and washcloths.
- Avoid rubbing or touching eyes. Wash hands frequently.
- Clean crusting or discharge with a cotton ball moistened in warm water. Discard cotton ball after use. Do not use the same cotton ball for both eyes.
- Instill saline drops in dry, itchy eyes.
- Make an appointment to have eyes checked for difficulty seeing close or distant objects.

Additional Instructions

V

Report the Following Problems to Your PCP/Clinic/ED

- Sudden changes in vision
- Signs of infection
- Condition persists or worsens

Seek Emergency Care Immediately If Any of the Following Occur

- Sudden onset of severe eye pain
- Sudden loss of partial or total vision in one or both eyes
- Pupils of unequal size
- Sudden or gradual increase in number of floaters, light flashes, or curtain over field of vision

If the caller agrees with the advice given, document the call and encourage the caller to call back or see PCP if the problem worsens. If the caller does not agree with the advice given, reevaluate and advise the caller to follow up with PCP, Clinic, or ED.

Vomiting, Adult

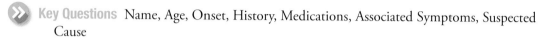 **Key Questions** Name, Age, Onset, History, Medications, Associated Symptoms, Suspected Cause

Other Protocols to Consider Abdominal Pain, Adult (9); Altered Mental Status (28); Chest Pain (123); Dehydration (180); Diabetes Problems (187); Diarrhea, Adult (192); Fever, Adult (250); Food Poisoning, Suspected (262); Headache (308); Head Injury (311); Overdose (438); Postoperative Problems (457); Pregnancy, Nausea and Vomiting (478); Substance Abuse, Use, or Exposure (582).

Nurse Alert: There are many conditions that cause vomiting. When vomiting is associated with several other symptoms, use the protocol that is the primary concern and has the highest probability of a referral to a higher level of care.

Reminder: Document caller response to advice, home care instructions, and when to call back.

ASSESSMENT	ACTION

A. Are any of the following present?

- Altered mental status
- Fainting
- Vomiting bright red blood or dark coffee grounds–like emesis
- Recent injury to head or abdomen and vomiting
- Chest pain or discomfort, difficulty breathing, palpitations, or sweating
- Persistent severe abdominal pain that interferes with activity

YES "Call ambulance" or "Seek emergency care now"

NO Go to B

B. Are any of the following present?

- Signs of dehydration:
  - decreased urine
  - dark yellow urine
  - sunken eyes
  - loose dry skin
  - excessive thirst
  - dry mouth, dry tongue, thick mucous
  - dizziness on standing or rising to sitting position
- Suspicion that recent ingestion of wild mushrooms or plant is causing vomiting
- History of diabetes and unable to control vomiting with home care measures
- Weakness or unusual fatigue

YES "Seek medical care within 2 to 4 hours"

NO Go to C

C. Are any of the following present?

- Persistent vomiting for >24 hours that is unrelieved by home care measures
- Recent surgery, hospitalization, or diagnostic procedure
- New-onset jaundice
- Persistent vomiting and increased use of marijuana or other party/illicit drugs

YES "Seek medical care within 24 hours"

NO Go to D

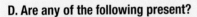

V

D. Are any of the following present?

- Diarrhea or constipation
- Abdominal distension
- History of travel out of the country or a camping trip
- Other household members are ill
- Excessive ingestion of food, alcohol, or fluids
- Recent ingestion of an antibiotic, pain medication, or new medication
- Occasional vomiting and ingestion of party/illicit drugs
- Possible pregnancy

YES "Call back or call PCP for appointment if no improvement" and Follow **Home Care Instructions**

NO Follow **Home Care Instructions**

Home Care Instructions
Vomiting, Adult

- Do not eat or drink anything for 1 hour after last emesis.
- Drink sips of clear fluids for first 12 hours, including gelatin, water, sports drinks, flat soda, clear broth, flavored ice, or apple juice. Do not drink citrus juices.
- Increase fluids as tolerated.
- After 12 hours, try small amounts of bland foods, such as rice, potatoes, soda crackers, pretzels, dry toast, and applesauce.
- After bland food is tolerated, resume normal diet, as tolerated.
- Retake medications if vomiting occurs within 30 minutes of taking usual medication.
- Avoid milk, citrus foods and juices, spicy and fatty foods, alcohol, coffee, and caffeinated beverages.
- Take OTC dimenhydrinate (Dramamine) or phosphorated carbohydrate solution (Emetrol) for nausea, and follow instructions on the package.
- Viruses causing nausea and vomiting are easily spread. Pay special attention to hand washing. Avoid using towels, tableware, and cups used by infected person.

Additional Instructions

Report the Following Problems to Your PCP/Clinic/ED

- Fever, weakness, or abdominal pain
- No improvement in 48 hours or condition worsens
- Signs of dehydration

Seek Emergency Care Immediately If Any of the Following Occur

- Altered mental status
- Vomiting blood or dark coffee grounds–like emesis
- Persistent severe pain that interferes with activity
- Fainting
- Chest pain, difficulty breathing, palpitations, or sweating

If the caller agrees with the advice given, document the call and encourage the caller to call back or see PCP if the problem worsens. If the caller does not agree with the advice given, reevaluate and advise the caller to follow up with PCP, Clinic, or ED.

Vomiting, Child

 Key Questions Name, Age, Onset, Suspected Cause, History, Medications, Associated Symptoms

 Other Protocols to Consider Abdominal Pain, Child (13); Altered Mental Status (28); Constipation (160); Dehydration (180); Diarrhea, Child (195); Fever, Child (253); Food Poisoning, Suspected (262); Headache (308); Head Injury (311); Postoperative Problems (457).

> *Nurse Alert:* There are many conditions that cause vomiting. When vomiting is associated with several other symptoms, use the protocol that is the primary concern and has the highest probability of a referral to a higher level of care.

Reminder: Document caller response to advice, home care instructions, and when to call back.

ASSESSMENT	ACTION

A. Are any of the following present?

- Altered mental status: listless, unusually irritable, confused
- Severe headache, stiff neck, or pain bending head forward
- Vomiting bright red blood or dark coffee grounds–like emesis
- Recent head or abdominal injury
- Exposure to a poisonous substance (such as medications, plants, cleaning agents, pesticides, or wild mushrooms)
- Neonate <1 month of age
- Abdomen is hard or firm when not crying

YES "Seek emergency care now"
If poison ingestion is suspected, go to Poisoning, Suspected (454) protocol

NO Go to B

645

B. Are any of the following present?

- Signs of dehydration:
  - decreased urine
  - sunken eyes or fontanel
  - dry mouth
  - crying without tears
  - unusual listlessness
- Breathing hard or fast
- Persistent abdominal pain interferes with activity
- Child appears very ill
- History of diabetes and unable to control vomiting with home care measures
- Infant <3 months old and has vomited >2 times or has projectile vomiting

YES "Seek medical care within 2 to 4 hours"

NO Go to C

C. Are any of the following present?

- Vomiting >12 hours
- Temperature >101°F (38.3°C) for >24 hours
- Vomited >3 times in the last 6 hours
- Persistent diarrhea
- Infant with forceful vomiting after feeding

YES "Seek medical care within 24 hours"

NO Go to D

D. Are any of the following present?

- Moderate diarrhea or constipation
- History of travel out of the country or a camping trip
- Other household members are ill
- Excessive ingestion of food or fluids
- Recent ingestion of an antibiotic, pain medication, or new medication
- Earache, cold, sore throat, or fever

YES "Call back or call PCP for appointment if no improvement" and Follow **Home Care Instructions**

NO Follow **Home Care Instructions**

Home Care Instructions
Vomiting, Child

Infants
- Introduce 1 tsp Lytren, Pedialyte, Infalyte, or Kao Lectrolyte every 5 minutes and increase as tolerated.
- If infant drinks juice, introduce 1 tsp every 5 minutes, then clear liquids as tolerated. Do not give juice if diarrhea is also present.
- If breastfeeding and infant vomits 3 or more times, offer breast for 4 to 5 minutes every 30 to 60 minutes, and offer rehydration fluids between breastfeeds, 1 tsp every 5 to 15 minutes. It should not be necessary to discontinue breastfeeding.
- If using formula, use small, frequent feedings.

Children
- Avoid eating or drinking for 1 to 2 hours after vomiting.
- Drink 1 tsp every 5 minutes for 4 hours (fruit juice diluted with water, weak tea with sugar, clear broth, gelatin, or flavored ice). After 4 hours without vomiting, the amount of fluids offered may be increased.
- Avoid milk for 12 to 24 hours after vomiting subsides.
- Slowly introduce bland foods, such as rice, potatoes, soda cracker, pretzels, dry toast, applesauce, and bananas, as tolerated 8 hours after last emesis.

Additional Home Care Advice
- Acetaminophen can be given for fever. Do not give aspirin to a child. Avoid aspirin-like products if age <20 years. Avoid acetaminophen if liver disease is present. Avoid ibuprofen if kidney disease or stomach problems exist or in the case of pregnancy. Follow the directions on the label.
- If, after vomiting has subsided, diarrhea is present or continues, follow home care instructions for the treatment of diarrhea. Vomiting should always be treated first.
- Wash hands with soap and water frequently when caring for a child with vomiting and/or diarrhea.

V

Additional Instructions

Report the Following Problems to Your PCP/Clinic/ED

- High fever, weakness, or abdominal pain for >2 hours
- No improvement in 48 hours or condition worsens
- Signs of dehydration

Seek Emergency Care Immediately If Any of the Following Occur

- Altered mental status
- Vomiting blood or dark coffee grounds–like emesis
- Develops a severe headache, stiff neck, or pain bending head forward
- Abdomen becomes hard or firm when not crying

If the caller agrees with the advice given, document the call and encourage the caller to call back or see PCP if the problem worsens. If the caller does not agree with the advice given, reevaluate and advise the caller to follow up with PCP, Clinic, or ED.

Weakness

 Key Questions Name, Age, Onset, Cause, Location (see Back/Neck Injury if suspected back injury caused by trauma), Medications, History, Pain Scale

 Other Protocols to Consider Altered Mental Status (28); Back/Neck Injury (59); Back Pain (62); Extremity Injury (222); Fainting (237); Falls (240); Fatigue (244); Heart Rate Problems (320); Heat-Exposure Problems (323); Leg Pain/Swelling (398); Muscle Cramps (413); Neurologic Symptoms (418); Postoperative Problems (457); Stroke, Suspected (576).

> *Nurse Alert:* There are many conditions that can cause weakness. When weakness is associated with several other symptoms, triage with caution and note signs that may be an indication of a more serious condition.
>
> - Sudden changes in vision, speech, or mental status, weakness, and numbness may be signs of a stroke or other serious neurologic disorder. Prompt treatment may prevent extensive damage to the brain or reduce permanent disability. Medications used to break up a clot in the brain need to be administered within 3 hours of symptom onset.
> - Ask how current condition is different from normal.
> - Use **BEFAST** to remember signs of a stroke:
>   - **Balance**: sudden loss of balance
>   - **Eyes**: sudden loss of vision in one or both eyes
>   - **Face:** one side of the face droops when asked to smile
>   - **Arms**: one arm drifts down when asked to raise both arms
>   - **Speech**: speech is slurred or garbled
>   - **Time**: call 911 if any of these signs are present

Reminder: Document caller response to advice, home care instructions, and when to call back.

W

ASSESSMENT	ACTION
A. Is chest pain present?	
	YES Go to Chest Pain (123) protocol
	NO Go to B

B. Is there difficulty breathing?

YES	Go to Breathing Problems (106) protocol
NO	Go to C

C. Is there an altered mental status?

YES	Go to Altered Mental Status (28) protocol
NO	Go to D

D. Are any of the following present?

- Inability to stand, walk, or bear weight
- Sudden onset of weakness on one side of the body
- Weakness in face, arm, or leg
- Visual disturbances
- Speech and language problems
- Irregular pulse
- Severe headache

YES	"Call ambulance" or "Seek emergency care now"
NO	Go to E

E. Are any of the following present?

- Hand or foot cold or blue
- Pain, swelling, warmth, or redness in affected limb
- Severe pain interferes with normal activity

YES	"Seek medical care within 2 to 4 hours"
NO	Go to F

F. Are any of the following present?

- History of dieting or use of diuretics
- History of blood clots or heart problems
- Gradual onset of numbness, tingling, or burning sensation in extremities
- Pain radiates to arm or leg
- Fever; cough; green, yellow, or brown sputum; body aches for >24 hours and unresponsive to home care measures
- History of taking cholesterol-lowering medication
- Recent history of frequent falls
- Increasing difficulty with mobility

YES	"Seek medical care within 24 hours"
NO	Go to G

G. Are any of the following present?

- Occasional weakness
- History of neuromuscular problems that are unresponsive to medication
- Increased exercise, activity level, or stress
- History of muscular pain
- History of eating disorder

"Call back or call PCP for appointment if no improvement"

and

Follow **Home Care Instructions**

Follow **Home Care Instructions**

W

Home Care Instructions
Weakness

- Rest and eat regular meals.
- Apply moist heat to painful swollen area (if known injury, apply ice during the first 24 hours).
- Do not put ice directly on the skin; place a cloth barrier between ice and the skin.
- Take your usual pain medication (aspirin, acetaminophen, ibuprofen). Do not give aspirin to a child. Avoid aspirin-like products if age <20 years. Avoid acetaminophen if liver disease is present. Avoid ibuprofen if kidney disease or stomach problems exist or in the case of pregnancy. Follow the directions on the label.

Additional Instructions

Report the Following Problem to Your PCP/Clinic/ED

- No improvement or condition worsens

Seek Emergency Care Immediately If Any of the Following Occur

- Limb turns cold, numb, or blue
- Sudden change in ability to walk, stand, bear weight, or move
- Weakness in face, arm, or leg
- Visual disturbances
- Speech and language problems

If the caller agrees with the advice given, document the call and encourage the caller to call back or see PCP if the problem worsens. If the caller does not agree with the advice given, reevaluate and advise the caller to follow up with PCP, Clinic, or ED.

West Nile Virus

>> Key Questions Name, Age, Onset, Cause, Medications, History (Consider this.)

>> Other Protocols to Consider Altered Mental Status (28); Fatigue (244); Fever, Adult (250), Child (253); Headache (308); Neck Pain (415); Neurologic Symptoms (418); Numbness and Tingling (431); Rash, Adult (500), Child (505); Weakness (649).

Nurse Alert: Use this protocol only if diagnosed with West Nile Virus or if caller has concerns about West Nile Virus and signs and symptoms appear 2 to 15 days after known exposure to dead birds or mosquito bites.

Reminder: Document caller response to advice, home care instructions, and when to call back.

ASSESSMENT	ACTION
A. Are any of the following present?	
• Altered mental status • Seizures • Vision loss • Paralysis	**YES** "Call ambulance" **NO** Go to B
B. Are any of the following present?	
• Neck stiffness • High fever >104.9°F (40.5°C) • Nonblanching purple or dark red spots • Shortness of breath	**YES** "Seek emergency care now" **NO** Go to C
C. Are any of the following present?	
• Severe headache • Severe muscle weakness • Numbness • History of immunosuppression	**YES** "Seek medical care immediately" **NO** Go to D

W

D. Are any of the following present?

- Body aches
- Nausea/vomiting
- Raised rash on trunk
- Swollen lymph glands
- Fatigue
- Woman currently pregnant or breast-
  feeding, or baby breastfeeding

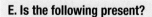

YES   "Seek medical care within 24 hours"

NO   Go to E

E. Is the following present?

- No other symptoms but parent or person
  concerned

YES   "Call back or call PCP for
appointment if no improvement"
and
Follow **Home Care Instructions**

NO   Follow **Home Care Instructions**

Home Care Instructions
West Nile Virus

- Do not touch dead birds with bare hands.
- Call the local health department _____ for directions on how to report and turn over the deceased bird for testing and disposal.
- Reduce risks of West Nile Virus by:
  - applying insect repellent;
  - wearing long-sleeve shirts, long pants, and socks;
  - minimizing exposed skin;
  - wearing light-colored clothing;
  - avoiding being outdoors at peak mosquito-biting times (from dusk to dawn);
  - using screens to cover open doors and windows and repairing or replacing any holes in the screens or ill-fitting screens;
  - avoiding standing water by draining objects or areas on your property;
  - cleaning clogged rain gutters.
- Rest.
- Drink plenty of fluids.
- Take your usual pain medication for discomfort. Do not give aspirin to a child. Avoid aspirin-like products if age <20 years. Avoid acetaminophen if liver disease is present. Avoid ibuprofen if kidney disease or stomach problems exist or in the case of pregnancy. Follow the directions on the label.

Additional Instructions

_____

_____

_____

Report the Following Problems to Your PCP/Clinic/ED

- Severe headache
- Severe muscle weakness
- Numbness
- No improvement or condition worsens

Seek Emergency Care Immediately If Any of the Following Occur

- Altered mental status
- Neck stiffness
- Seizures
- Vision loss
- Paralysis
- High fever >104.9°F (40.5°C)
- Nonblanching dark red or purple rash

If the caller agrees with the advice given, document the call and encourage the caller to call back or see PCP if the problem worsens. If the caller does not agree with the advice given, reevaluate and advise the caller to follow up with PCP, Clinic, or ED.

Wheezing

 Key Questions Name, Age, Onset, Medications, History of Intubation, Hospitalizations, History

 Other Protocols to Consider Allergic Reaction (25); Asthma (52); Breathing Problems (106); Chronic Obstructive Pulmonary Disease (138); Congestion (153); Congestive Heart Failure (157); Cough (170); Croup (173); Hay Fever Problems (305).

> *Nurse Alert:* If known respiratory problems and prescribed inhalers, use O_2 or peak flow meters (to measure how well air is moving out of the lungs). Assess baseline functioning, O_2 saturation level, and % oxygen delivered and method.
>
> Peak flow values are divided into three zones:
> Green: 80% of baseline or higher (mild attack)
> Yellow: 50% to 80% of baseline (moderate attack)
> Red: <50% of baseline (severe attack)

Reminder: Document caller response to advice, home care instructions, and when to call back.

ASSESSMENT	ACTION

A. Are any of the following present?

- Severe respiratory distress
- Inability to speak
- Chest retractions
- Aspiration of foreign body
- Blue lips or face
- Severe chest pain
- Sudden-onset wheezing after medication or exposure to known allergen
- Peak flow rate <50% of baseline (if asthmatic)

YES "Call ambulance"

NO Go to B

B. Are any of the following present?

- Unresponsive to medication treatments
- Unresponsive to home care measures
- Must sit up to breathe
- Wheezing similar to prior episodes that required hospitalization or injections
- History of CHF, cardiac disease, COPD, pulmonary embolus, or blood clot in leg
- Speaking in partial sentences
- Peak flow rate 50% to 80% of baseline (if asthmatic)

YES "Seek medical care within 2 hours"

NO   Go to C

C. Are any of the following present?

- Peak flow rate >80% of baseline (if asthmatic)
- Green, yellow, or rust-colored sputum
- Infant, elderly, or immunosuppressed

YES "Seek medical care within 24 hours"

NO   Go to D

D. Are any of the following present?

- First wheezing episode that resolves in a short period of time
- Fever
- Speaking in full sentences

YES "Call back or call PCP for appointment if no improvement" and
Follow **Home Care Instructions**

NO   Follow **Home Care Instructions**

Home Care Instructions
Wheezing

- Take medication as directed by PCP.
- Use vaporizer with cool mist.
- Identify cause and avoid irritant.

Additional Instructions

Report the Following Problems to Your PCP/Clinic/ED

- Condition worsens
- No improvement with medication

Seek Emergency Care Immediately If Any of the Following Occur

- Lips or face turn blue
- Fighting for air
- Decreased level of consciousness
- Inability to speak or speaking in short words
- Severe chest pain
- Peak flow rate <50% of baseline (if asthmatic)

If the caller agrees with the advice given, document the call and encourage the caller to call back or see PCP if the problem worsens. If the caller does not agree with the advice given, reevaluate and advise the caller to follow up with PCP, Clinic, or ED.

Wound Care: Sutures or Staples

 Key Questions Name, Age, Onset, Date Sutures or Staples Placed, Medications, Pain Scale, History

 Other Protocols to Consider Piercing Problems (445); Postoperative Problems (457); Tattoo Problems (604); Wound Healing and Infection (664).

Reminder: Document caller response to advice, home care instructions, and when to call back.

ASSESSMENT	ACTION
A. Are any of the following present?	
• Altered mental status • Difficulty breathing • Surgical wound split or gaping and large amount of fluid, drainage, or material exposed	**YES** "Call ambulance" or "Seek emergency care now" **NO** Go to B
B. Are any of the following present?	
• Rapidly spreading warmth, swelling, or redness around wound • Recent placement of sutures/staples; headache, muscle aches, general ill feeling, or fever • Fever >101.3°F (38.5°C) • Wound splitting open or gaping • Persistent bleeding after >10 minutes of direct pressure • Numbness or swelling distal to incision • Inability to move the joint distal to the incision • Drain slipped from wound • Loose suture or staple <48 hours since placement • Suture or staple falls out, glue separates, and wound on the face	**YES** "Seek medical care immediately" **NO** Go to C

C. Are any of the following present?

- Persistent incisional pain or discomfort
- Gradual-onset warmth, foul odor, swelling or redness around wound
- Yellow or green drainage and no fever
- History of diabetes, HIV, chronic disease, use of steroids or blood thinners, chemotherapy, and improperly healing wound

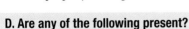 **YES** "Seek medical care within 24 hours"

NO Go to D

D. Are any of the following present?

- Sutures/staples removed and tender to touch
- Questions about sutures/staples/glue
- Missed removal date
- Loose suture or staple and >48 hours since placement
- Itching around the edges of the wound
- Blisters around the wound

YES "Call back or call PCP for appointment if no improvement" and Follow **Home Care Instructions**

NO Follow **Home Care Instructions**

Home Care Instructions
Wound Care: Sutures or Staples

- Keep sutured/stapled/glued area clean and dry for at least 24 hours.
- Clean the wound gently with warm water daily and when soiled.
- Watch for signs of infection: warmth, pain, drainage, redness, or red streaks. Check the wound daily.
- Wash hands with soap and water or alcohol-based hand rub before touching the wound or changing the dressing.
- Apply antibiotic ointment to the wound 3 times a day or as prescribed by surgeon.
- Do not apply lotions, potions, or petroleum-based ointment on abdominal wounds unless prescribed by surgeon or PCP.
- Change dressing when wet or soiled.
- If a suture or staple falls out or glue separates >48 hours after placement, keep the wound closed with tape or a butterfly bandage until ready to have the remaining sutures/staples removed.
- Keep appointment for suture/staple removal.
- Take your usual pain medication for discomfort. Do not give aspirin to a child. Avoid aspirin-like products if age <20 years. Avoid acetaminophen if liver disease is present. Avoid ibuprofen if kidney disease or stomach problems exist or in the case of pregnancy. Follow the directions on the label.
- Avoid bumping or stretching the wound for the first 2 days after suture/staple removal.
- Use sunscreen and avoid direct sun exposure to the healing wound.

Additional Instructions

Report the Following Problems to Your PCP/Clinic/ED

- Signs of infection; pain, warmth, foul odor, swelling, redness, drainage, red streaks extending from the wound
- Fever
- Persistent bleeding
- Increasing pain
- Wound splits open
- Condition worsens or no improvement

Seek Emergency Care Immediately If Any of the Following Occur
- Persistent bleeding with direct pressure >10 minutes
- Difficulty breathing
- Large wound splits open and body tissue is exposed
- Surgical wound opens and surgeon cannot be reached

If the caller agrees with the advice given, document the call and encourage the caller to call back or see PCP if the problem worsens. If the caller does not agree with the advice given, reevaluate and advise the caller to follow up with PCP, Clinic, or ED.

Wound Healing and Infection

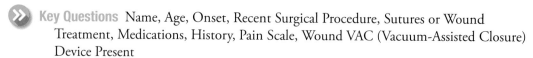

>> **Key Questions** Name, Age, Onset, Recent Surgical Procedure, Sutures or Wound Treatment, Medications, History, Pain Scale, Wound VAC (Vacuum-Assisted Closure) Device Present

>> **Other Protocols to Consider** Abrasions (19); Bites, Animal/Human (76); Piercing Problems (445); Laceration (395); Postoperative Problems (457); Skin Lesions: Lumps, Bumps, and Sores (556); Wound Care: Sutures or Staples (660); Tattoo Problems (604).

Reminder: Document caller response to advice, home care instructions, and when to call back.

ASSESSMENT	ACTION

A. Are any of the following present?

- Gaping, split, jagged, or deep wound
- Surgical wound split or gaping, and large amount of fluid, drainage, or material protruding from wound

YES "Seek emergency care now"

NO Go to B

B. Are any of the following present?

- Surgical wound split or gaping
- Healing wound and headache, muscle aches, general ill feeling, or fever
- Signs of infection: pain, swelling, drainage, warmth, or red streaks extending from wound
- Swollen lymph nodes in neck, armpit, or groin
- Wound caused by a bite
- Temperature > 100.1°F (37°C)
- Dirty wound and no tetanus immunization, immunization status unknown, or last tetanus immunization >5 years ago
- History of diabetes, HIV, chronic disease, use of steroids or blood thinners, chemotherapy, and a wound not healing well

YES "Seek medical care within 2 to 4 hours"

NO Go to C

C. Are any of the following present?

- Chills, ill feeling, or headache
- No improvement with home care measures
- Wound <24 hours old and no tetanus immunization, immunization status unknown, or last tetanus immunization >5 years ago
- Blistering around wound

 YES   "Seek medical care within 24 hours"

NO   Go to D

D. Are any of the following present?

- Itching around wound edges
- Tetanus immunization >5 years ago
- Wound VAC in place and concerns about
  - leaking around the tube or edges of the dressing
  - container is full
  - device has been turned off >8 hours

YES   "Call back or call PCP for appointment if no improvement" and Follow **Home Care Instructions**

NO   Follow **Home Care Instructions**

Home Care Instructions
Wound Healing and Infection

- Keep the wound clean and dry.
- Apply dressing if drainage is present.
- Apply moist hot packs for 20 minutes, 4 times a day.
- Check the wound daily for signs of healing.
- No tetanus immunization, immunization status unknown, or last tetanus immunization >5 years ago. Contact PCP or clinic for tetanus immunization within 72 hours of injury.
- If the wound is bleeding, lie down and apply pressure over the wound for 10 minutes; if no improvement, contact PCP.
- Monitor temperature.
- For wound VAC problems:
  - If the wound VAC is turned off >8 hours, replace the dressing with wet-to-dry dressing and notify home health (HH) nurse.
  - If the VAC is leaking around the tube or edges of the dressing, reinforce the VAC dressing and notify HH nurse.
  - If the canister is full, replace it and discard it in the garbage as directed by HH nurse.

For Abscess

- Lanced or unlanced abscess is highly resistant to antibiotics and susceptible to MRSA infections. Prevent sharing or worsening by using these measures.
  - wash hands >3 times per day or more when soiled with microbial cleanser
  - shower immediately after activity with hot water as tolerated
  - advise others in close contact to wash their hands with microbial cleanser
  - keep wounds covered with clean, dry bandages, particularly if drainage is present
  - disinfect all towels, sheets, and surfaces in contact with the wound with a solution of 1:100 of household bleach to water or white vinegar
  - wash and dry clothes, linens, and towels in a setting as hot as possible; ensure all items are dry before removing them from the dryer
  - avoid participating in contact sports or skin-to-skin contact with others until the infection has healed
  - use a skin antiseptic to treat MRSA on the skin in combination with antibiotics prescribed by PCP
  - avoid hot tubs
  - do not share bars of soap, razors, towels, or athletic gear
  - call PCP if condition worsens or fails to improve with home care and treatment

Additional Instructions

_____

_____

_____

Report the Following Problems to Your PCP/Clinic/ED

- Headache, muscle aches, general ill feeling, or fever
- No improvement or condition worsens
- Temperature >100°F (37.8°C)
- Blisters develop

Seek Emergency Care Immediately If Any of the Following Occur

- Surgical incision opens and surgeon cannot be reached

If the caller agrees with the advice given, document the call and encourage the caller to call back or see PCP if the problem worsens. If the caller does not agree with the advice given, reevaluate and advise the caller to follow up with PCP, Clinic, or ED.

W

Zika Virus

>> **Key Questions** Name, Age, Onset, Cause, Medications, History, Pregnancy Status, Recent travel to area where Zika Virus is spreading, Recent Mosquito Bites

>> **Other Protocols to Consider** Altered Mental Status (28); Fever, Adult (250); Child (253); Headache (308); Numbness and Tingling (431); Rash, Adult (500); Child (505); Weakness (649).

Nurse Alert: Use this protocol only if diagnosed with Zika virus or if caller has concerns about Zika virus and signs and symptoms appear 3 to 14 days after a mosquito bite, and known travel to a Zika-infected area or exposure to an infected person through unprotected sex. Currently, there is no cure for Zika virus, and treatment is directed toward symptom management.

Reminder: Document caller response to advice, home care instructions, and when to call back.

ASSESSMENT	ACTION

A. Are any of the following present?

- Shortness of breath
- Severe muscle weakness
- Severe pain
- Numbness
- Fever >100.0°F (37.8°C) and history of immunosuppression
- Fever >101°F (38.3°C) in the elderly

YES "Seek medical care immediately"

NO Go to B

B. Are any of the following present?

- Muscle pain
- Headache
- Rash
- Joint pain
- Fever
- Red eyes
- Woman currently pregnant and new onset of rash, joint pain, fever, red eyes

YES "Seek medical care within 24 hours"

NO Go to C

C. Are any of the following present?

- No other symptoms but parent or person |concerned
- Pregnant, no symptoms, and recent travel to Zika-infected area or exposed to infected person, person who lives in or recently traveled to Zika-infected area and unprotected sex

YES   "Call back or call PCP for appointment if no improvement" and
Follow **Home Care Instructions**

NO   Follow **Home Care Instructions**

Z

Home Care Instructions
Zika Virus

- Reduce risks of Zika virus by:
  - avoiding coming into contact with an infected person's body fluid, urine, or feces, if pregnant. If contact cannot be avoided, use gloves and bleach.
  - applying insect repellent. Do not use insect repellents on babies younger than 2 months. Mosquito netting can be used to cover babies younger than 2 months in carriers, strollers, or cribs to protect them from mosquito bites. Do not use products containing oil of lemon eucalyptus or para-menthane-diol on children younger than 3 years. Do not apply insect repellent onto a child's hands, eyes, mouth, and any cut or irritated skin. If you are also using sunscreen, apply sunscreen first and insect repellent second.
  - wearing long-sleeve shirts, long pants, and socks.
  - minimizing exposed skin.
  - wearing light-colored clothing.
  - using screens to cover open doors and windows and repairing or replacing any holes in the screens or ill-fitting screens.
  - avoiding standing water by draining objects or areas on your property.
  - cleaning clogged rain gutters.
- Avoid sexual activity with a person known to be or suspected to be infected with the Zika virus. Use condoms (male or female condoms).
- Rest.
- Drink plenty of fluids.
- Take your usual pain medication for discomfort. Avoid aspirin and aspirin-like products (NSAIDs). Avoid acetaminophen if liver disease is present. Follow the directions on the label. Use the dosing device that comes with the medication, a measuring device, or a medication syringe from the pharmacy. Household teaspoons often do not give the correct amount of medication.
- For current information on Zika travel information and areas impacted, see CDC's website: cdc.gov/zika or wwwnc.cdc.gov/travel/page/zika-travel-information

Additional Instructions

Report the Following Problems to Your PCP/Clinic/ED

- Severe pain
- Severe muscle weakness
- Numbness
- No improvement or condition worsens
- Fever >100.0°F (37.8°C) and history of immunosuppression
- Fever >101°F (38.3°C) in the elderly

Seek Emergency Care Immediately If Any of the Following Occur

- Difficulty breathing
- Paralysis
- High fever

If the caller agrees with the advice given, document the call and encourage the caller to call back or see PCP if the problem worsens. If the caller does not agree with the advice given, reevaluate and advise the caller to follow up with PCP, Clinic, or ED.

Z

Appendix A: Abbreviations

>	greater than	HIV	human immunodeficiency virus
<	less than	HTN	hypertension
AA	Alcoholics Anonymous	IUD	intrauterine device
AIDS	acquired immune deficiency syndrome	IV	intravenous
AMS	altered mental status	mg	milligram
bpm	beats per minute	mL	milliliter
°C	degrees Celsius	MMR	measles, mumps, rubella
CDC	Centers for Disease Control and Prevention	OTC	over-the-counter (medication)
CHF	congestive heart failure	PCP	primary care provider
COPD	chronic obstructive pulmonary disease	PID	pelvic inflammatory disease
CPR	cardiopulmonary resuscitation	RLQ	right lower quadrant
DPT	diphtheria, pertussis, and tetanus (immunization)	ROM	range of motion
		SARS	severe acute respiratory syndrome
DTs	delirium tremens	SOB	shortness of breath
ED	emergency department	STD	sexually transmitted disease
EMS	Emergency Medical Services	tbsp	tablespoon
ER	emergency room	tsp	teaspoon
°F	degrees Fahrenheit	UTI	urinary tract infection
GERD	gastroeshophageal reflux disease	VAC	vacuum assisted closure

Appendix B: Sample Telephone Triage Protocol Form

 Key Questions Name, Age, Onset, Cause, Medications, History, Pain Scale

Other Protocols to Consider

Reminder: Document caller response to advice, home care instructions, and when to call back.

ASSESSMENT	ACTION
A. Are any of the following present?	
	YES "Call ambulance" or "Seek emergency care now"
	NO Go to B
B. Are any of the following present?	
	YES "Seek medical care within 2 to 4 hours"
	NO Go to C
C. Are any of the following present?	
	YES "Seek medical care within 24 hours"
	NO Go to D
D. Are any of the following present?	
	YES "Call back or call PCP for appointment if no improvement" and Follow **Home Care Instructions**
	NO Follow **Home Care Instructions**

674

Home Care Instructions

-
-
-
-
-

Additional Instructions

_____

_____

_____

Report the Following Problems to Your PCP/Clinic/ED

-
-
-
-

Seek Emergency Care Immediately If Any of the Following Occur

-
-
-
-

If the caller agrees with the advice given, document the call and encourage the caller to call back or see PCP if the problem worsens. If the caller does not agree with the advice given, reevaluate and advise caller to follow up with PCP, Clinic, or ED.

Appendix C: Community Resources Telephone List

Emergency Services:

Ambulance _____ or 911

Fire _____ or 911

Police _____ or 911

County Sheriff _____

State Police Patrol _____

Poison Control _____

Local Hospitals

_____

_____

_____

_____

Public Health Clinic _____

Immunization Clinic _____

STD Clinics _____

Other Clinics _____

Local Pharmacies _____

_____

_____

_____

_____

Rape Crisis _____

STD Hotline _____

AIDS Hotline _____

Mental Health Crisis Line _____

Drug and Alcohol Crisis Line _____

Detox _____

Alcohol and Drug Treatment _____

Child Protective Services _____

Women's Shelter _____

Resources:

Animal Control _____

Handicapped/Senior Transport _____

Home Health _____

Medical Equipment Rental _____

Crutch Rental _____

Planned Parenthood _____

Mental Health Center _____

Physician Referral _____

Appendix D: Telephone Triage Quality Improvement Survey

Patient Name	Telephone #	Date and Time of Initial Call		
Question		Yes	No	Comments
1. Was the nurse courteous and professional?				
2. Were you comfortable with the advice given?				
3. Did you follow the advice given?				
4. Were you provided adequate referral information?				
5. Would you use our service again?				

Comments:

_____

_____

_____

_____

_____

_____

Follow-Up:

_____

_____

_____

_____

_____

_____

_____

Surveyor Name   Date and Time of Call

Appendix E1: Telephone Triage Documentation Form

Date: _____ Time: _____ Time Returned Call: _____

Name of patient: _____ Phone: _____

Name of caller: _____ Relationship: _____

Age of patient: _____ Sex: _____ Physician: _____

Has patient tried to contact physician? Yes_____ No_____

Presenting problem/symptoms:

_____

_____

_____

_____

Protocol used (list source, protocol name, and page number):

1. _____ Page #_____
2. _____ Page #_____
3. _____ Page #_____
4. Other:_____

Problem Emergent_____   Urgent_____   Semiurgent_____   Nonurgent_____

      (immediately)   (2 to 4 hours)   (within 24 hours)   (make appointment/home care)

1. Call 911 or ambulance for transport to nearest hospital.
2. Go to ED.
3. Call own physician; if unavailable, follow up with ED or Urgent Care Clinic.
4. See physician within 24 to 48 hours.
5. Call Mental Health Crisis Line @_____now.
6. Contact Health Department @_____.
7. Follow home care instructions:

_____

_____

_____

Additional Comments: _____

_____

_____

_____

Does caller agree with action taken? (circle) Yes No

Told caller to call back or be seen if problem worsens Yes No

Please review this taped conversation

Please call this person back for follow-up _____

Signature: _____

Appendix E2: Telephone Triage Log

Date and Time of Call	Patient Name/Age/Sex	Symptom or Concern and Onset	Protocol Used	Advice Given	Disposition and Caller Agreement	Nurse Name

Appendix F: Telephone Triage "Call Back" Log

Date of Call	Time of Call	Name	Phone #1	c/o	Treatment Location	Current Health Status				Signature	Date/Time
						I	S	W	Other		

Key: c/o, complaint; I, improved; S, same; W, worse.

Appendix G: Consulting Nurse Call Tape Review

Name of Consulting Nurse: _____ Date and Time of Call: _____

Name of Reviewer: _____ Date of Review: _____

	Yes	No	N/A
Did RN identify self as consulting nurse?			
Did RN inform caller that line is recorded?			
Did RN obtain patient's name?			
Did RN obtain caller's telephone number?			
Did RN obtain name of patient's PCP?			
Did RN determine whether caller had attempted to contact PCP?			
Did RN receive explanation of problem from caller?			
Did RN give appropriate information regarding problem?			
Did RN ask caller if he/she agrees with information given?			
Did RN instruct caller to call back as needed?			
Was RN courteous, respectful, polite?			

Comments:

_____

_____

_____

_____

_____

_____

_____

Appendix H: Consulting Nurse Call Documentation Review

Name of Consulting Nurse: _____ Date and Time of Call: _____

Name of Reviewer: _____ Date of Review: _____

	Yes	No	N/A
Signature of consulting nurse on form?			
Date and time of call recorded?			
Did RN record time call returned?			
Did RN record patient's name?			
Did RN record caller's telephone number?			
Did RN record relationship of patient to caller?			
Did RN record name of patient's PCP?			
Did RN record whether caller had attempted to contact PCP?			
Did RN record present problem/symptoms?			
Did RN record protocol used?			
Did RN record whether problem was urgent, emergent, or nonurgent?			
Did RN record action taken?			
Did RN record whether caller agreed with information given?			
Did RN record whether caller was instructed to call back prn?			

Comments:

_____

_____

_____

_____

_____

_____

Appendix I (1): Telephone Triage Training Outline

I. Overview
1. Program description
2. Evolution of telephone triage
3. Role of telephone triage in health care today
4. Medicolegal considerations

II. Operational Considerations
1. Policy and procedure review
2. Introduction to telephone triage program
3. Components of a call
4. Documentation
5. Call management
6. Community resources

III. Communication Skills
1. Uniqueness of telephone triage and management
2. Establishing rapport with the caller
3. Dealing with difficult calls

IV. Protocol Review and Practice
1. Review most common protocols
2. Review additional resources
3. Form triads to practice with scenarios
4. Written scavenger protocol hunt

V. Quallty Improvement Process
1. Review QI process and forms
2. Practice listening to actual calls

VI. Summary and Evaluation

Training and consultation services available on request.
Contact Julie Briggs at julie.briggs76@gmail.com

Appendix I (2)

Training Guidelines

Provide initial and ongoing training for all staff and identify how their roles are impacted by the triage process. Focus on interviewing the caller, protocol selection, application, and patient teaching. All staff should be alerted to community outbreaks such as a new widespread infestation of bedbugs or lice, or communicable diseases such as pertussis, or a new form of influenza. Post flyers from local health departments. Regularly review CDC guidelines for most current outbreaks, triage suggestions, isolation requirements, and treatment modalities.

Provide one-on-one, group training, or a combination of both. See Appendix I (**684**) for developing an in-house training program. Take advantage of outside training sessions and workshops or bring in a trainer for a more cost-effective and tailored program. In addition to formal training, staff training should include the following elements:

- Review the preface for key features of the book and to see how the protocols are structured.
- Review triage roles and responsibilities.
- Review Introduction chapter for protocol structure elements, using protocols safely, medical–legal safeguards, mental status challenges, documentation, training guidelines, and strategies to ensure quality.
- Review policies and procedures that address how calls should be handled. Policies should clearly outline roles and responsibilities of the triage nurse and other members of the team.
- Review the protocols that address the most frequent types of calls received in your setting.
- Most common adult and pediatric concerns:
  - Chest pain
  - Abdominal pain
  - Headache
  - Back pain
  - Fever
  - Vaginal bleeding
  - Sore throat
  - Gastrointestinal problems
  - Respiratory problems
  - Minor trauma
  - Skin and infectious disease problems
  - Earache
  - Immunization problems

- Review and become familiar with diseases that may result in a poor outcome if diagnosis is delayed:
  - Appendicitis
  - Meningitis
  - Pneumonia
  - Stroke
  - AMS
- Review and become familiar with Anatomical Table of Contents (xxi) to better understand how protocols address different body parts and systems.
- Review the emergency dispositions of the most common protocols.
- Review documentation standards and forms. (See Appendix E1 (**679**) for sample form.)
- Provide structured practice and feedback. See Appendix J (**687**): Guidelines for Scenario Practice; Appendix K (**691**): Difficult Caller Practice Scenario; and Appendix L (**693**): Skills Assessment and Exercise Form. Practice scenarios with one another to gain confidence and familiarity with using the protocols. It is important to the learning process to experience both the one asking the questions and being on the receiving end and providing answers. Assess understanding and provide feedback.
- Review Appendix Q (**707**): Teaching Self-Assessment. Practice with one another, asking the questions, performing the assessment techniques, and providing feedback.
- Review Appendices: M: Communicable Diseases (**696**); N: Sexually Transmitted Diseases (**700**); R: Abdominal Pain: Causes and Characteristics (**709**); S: Chest Pain: Causes and Characteristics (**712**); and T: Headache: Causes and Characteristics (**715**) to gain a better understanding of many of the potentially serious conditions a telephone triage nurse may encounter over the phone. Post in a convenient place for referral and review.
- Observe an experienced nurse providing telephone triage for at least 16 hours. There are devices available that enable two people to listen to the conversation at the same time.
- Provide supervised telephone triage for at least 24 hours.
- In a group setting, review and discuss examples of both calls that are well done and calls that could be improved. Play a recording of the call if available.
- Attend conferences, workshops, and continuing education seminars to increase your competency in telephone triage assessment and communication skills.

Appendix J: Guidelines for Scenario Practice

This exercise contains 10 different scenarios. If your organization does not treat pediatric patients, treat these scenarios as adults. There are no right or wrong answers. There are several different protocols that can be used to address the problems described in the scenarios. In general, it is best to choose a protocol that most closely matches the caller's greatest concern. This is strictly a learning experience to introduce you to the protocols and practice assessment and documentation of the telephone triage encounter. Read each scenario and indicate in the space provided:

- the protocol name and page number
- any additional information you want to know
- your disposition decision

   In addition, practice documenting the call using the documentation tool in Appendix E1 or your own organization's documentation tool.

1. Spend only about 5 to 6 minutes per scenario, as if you were on the phone talking with the caller. (This includes looking up the protocol and providing advice and all necessary documentation.) This exercise should take about an hour to complete.

2. Document the protocol used and page number on both the scenario and documentation form.

3. In the space provided for each scenario, describe additional information that would be important to manage the call appropriately. Not all scenarios provide adequate information to thoroughly assess the problem and to reach a disposition. Use this section to identify other questions that you would ask to complete a thorough assessment and choose an appropriate protocol. Based on the information provided, indicate your disposition decision.

4. Complete all 10 scenarios. Your supervisor will review your worksheets with you after you have completed this exercise. Remember, this is a learning opportunity. This exercise is designed to help you feel more comfortable with the protocols, applying your assessment skills and documenting the encounter.

Scenario Practice

1. Call received at 23:40 and returned at 23:50 hours. Jeff Smith called regarding his wife Linda. Phone number is 404-444-0202. Linda is 32 years old and a patient of Dr. Allen, who was not called prior to this call. Husband states that his wife has a wasp sting to the forearm that is badly swollen, about six across, and is warm and painful to the touch. She has pain in her arm and shoulder. There is no stinger. She has applied Benadryl lotion to the area. The incident occurred at 18:00 hours today. The wife denies any difficulty breathing, chest pain, rash, or other problems. Jeff wants to know what else can be done or if she should go to the ED.

Protocol Name/Page # _____

Additional Information Desired (what else is important to know in reaching a disposition):

Disposition Decision:

2. Call received at 20:20 hours. Patty Sing, a 25-year-old woman, is concerned about abdominal cramping and vaginal bleeding. Her phone number is 505-555-6767. Her PCP is Dr. Smitt, whom she has not tried to contact. She states that she is 1½ months pregnant and has abdominal cramping in her lower abdomen. She denies any other pain. She began having vaginal bleeding yesterday and has not passed any clots or tissue. She has saturated 2 to 3 pads this afternoon. She wants to know if she should be seen, as she is afraid she will lose her baby.

Protocol Name/Page # _____

Additional Information Desired (what else is important to know in reaching a disposition):

Disposition Decision:

3. Call received at 17:30 hours and returned at 18:05 hours. Lisa Kennedy, a 29-year-old woman, is concerned about her abdominal pain and vomiting. Her phone number is 808-845-2002. Dr. Shelby, her PCP, was not called because his office is closed. She states that she has had severe abdominal pain since noon today. The discomfort started as heavy bloating, then vomiting about 15 times this afternoon. No diarrhea or gas noted, but light-headed and dizzy for the past 45 minutes. She describes her pain as 8/10, with no relief after vomiting. Patient is asking what she can do at home. She does not want to come to the ER because she thinks that her health-care plan discourages ED use.

Protocol Name/Page # _____

Additional Information Desired (what else is important to know in reaching a disposition):

Disposition Decision:

4. Call received at 02:00 hours and returned at 02:05 hours. The caller is concerned about her 19-year-old daughter living away from home and attending a university. Her daughter's name is Marie Mason, and the caller's name is Jane Nelson. The phone number where she can be reached is 707-777-4242. Her daughter has no PCP. The mother states that her daughter has been sweating off and on since yesterday and has a cough. She developed small water blisters all over her body today and is nauseated. She has had a headache for 4 days and has been dizzy. She describes her rash as 20 to 30 red spots that are fleabite size with blisters in the middle. Some of the spots itch. She does not know if she has a fever, as she does not have a thermometer. There are no scabs. Mom cannot remember if this daughter ever had chickenpox. The daughter wants to know if she has chickenpox, if she should go home rather than continue at school, and if she should make an appointment to see a doctor.

Protocol Name/Page # _____

Additional Information Desired (what else is important to know in reaching a disposition):

Disposition Decision:

5. Call received at 12:00 hours and returned immediately. The caller's name is Paul, and he refuses to give his last name. He states that he does not have a phone, and he is calling from a friend's house and does not want to give out the number. He does not have a PCP because he does not have insurance, and he is unemployed at this time. Paul is 23 years old. He states that he was in a fight about 3 to 4 days ago in a bar. Now, his lower right arm is swollen and very sore. The other guy bit him twice just below the elbow. He has a reddened area about 3 × 6 that is very painful to the touch. There is pus in two areas, with fever of 102°F for 2 days. He describes the area on his arm as very warm to the touch and very painful.

Protocol Name/Page # _____

Additional Information Desired (what else is important to know in reaching a disposition):

Disposition Decision:

6. Call received at 02:00 hours. The caller's name is Barry Haines. He is calling about his 2-year-old daughter Rebecca. His phone number is 404-444-7272. Rebecca's PCP is Dr. Kneehigh, but he did not call him because he did not want to wake up the doctor. His daughter woke up at 01:00 hours, crying with ear pain. Barry gave her Tylenol 15 minutes ago and is asking what else he can do. His daughter is not crying at this time, but is lying on the couch holding her ear.

Protocol Name/Page # _____

Additional Information Desired (what else is important to know in reaching a disposition):

Disposition Decision:

7. Call received at 18:50 hours and returned at 19:03 hours. Peter Hammer is calling about his 3-year-old son, Derek Hammer. The phone number is 808-848-8080. The child does not have a PCP. The father stated that his son was running and fell, striking his head on a coffee table, and has a large abrasion to the forehead, approximately 1½ inch × 3 inch. The accident occurred about 30 minutes ago. Peter states that there was no loss of consciousness, and the child cried right away for a few minutes. His son is now playing quietly. The father is worried about a potential head injury and wants to know what he should do or observe.

Protocol Name/Page # _____

Additional Information Desired (what else is important to know in reaching a disposition):

Disposition Decision:

8. Call received at 20:20 hours and returned at 20:50 hours. Sue Shepard is calling about her niece Amanda, who is 2 months old. Her phone number is 444-454-0044. The child's PCP is Dr. Jollet, but she has not been called. The aunt states that the child has a fever of 102.5°F rectally and has not been eating or drinking much. She has a runny nose and cough. Further questioning reveals a very fussy baby who had a long nap earlier today. Sue cannot describe any other problems. The fever started last night. The child has been taking Tylenol every 4 to 6 hours, and the last dose was at 20:00 hours. Sue wants to know if she should take her niece to the ER or what else can be done.

Protocol Name/Page # _____

Additional Information Desired (what else is important to know in reaching a disposition):

Disposition Decision:

9. Call received at 18:42 hours and returned at 19:03. The caller's name is Jane Lambo, who is calling about her 6-month-old daughter, Jolyn Bosner. Her home phone number is 404-435-6789. The child does not have a pediatrician. The child has had a fever of up to 102°F for 2 days. Now the temperature is 102.4°F. Mom gave Tylenol at 7:30 this morning. The child is vomiting, "sleeping all the time today," and only waking up to cry or vomit. She has thrown up 6 times since noon and has had diarrhea 4 times. Her last wet diaper was around 11:00, but it was not very wet. Mom states that the child will not eat or drink anything. When questioned further, Mom states that Jolyn only drank 2 ounces of Pedialyte today and will not drink formula. Mom is concerned and wants to know what to do.

Protocol Name/Page # _____

Additional Information Desired (what else is important to know in reaching a disposition):

Disposition Decision:

10. Call received at 23:00 hours and returned at 23:40 hours. Jack Schmidt is calling about his son, John Simms, age 5. He states that his phone number is 310-444-5678 and that they are on vacation in Washington. He does not know his son's pediatrician's (Dr. Band) phone number by memory, so he has not called him. He states that his son has had a bad headache and a high fever. His temperature is now 102.6°F. Tylenol was given 1 hour ago. The child vomited once an hour ago and slept all day today, in addition to last night. Dad states that his son is lying on the couch holding his head. He has had a cold for the past few days with a runny nose. When asked, the child is unwilling to touch his chin to his chest when his dad shows him how and states that "it hurts too much." The dad is concerned and wants to know what he should do.

Protocol Name/Page # _____

Additional Information Desired (what else is important to know in reaching a disposition):

Disposition Decision:

Appendix K: Difficult Caller Practice Scenarios

This exercise is designed to help callers gain insight and experience in dealing with the difficult caller. Sometimes it is hard to figure out exactly what the caller wants and needs, which may influence your ability to select the correct protocol and disposition. Read each scenario and answer the questions for each one. This exercise requires the use of your critical thinking skills, experience, and communication skills.

Difficult Caller Practice Scenarios

1. A 45-year-old man c/o vomiting and diarrhea for 24 hours. Ate at Mudmart 2 days prior with three buddies. All have come down with the same symptoms plus stomach cramps. Wondering if they have food poisoning and what can be done. Also wondering if they can sue for this problem.

2. A 44-year-old man c/o headache, sinus problems, neck pain, back pain, and general aching all over. Had neck surgery 6 months prior. Was stabbed in the liver 2 months ago. He is angry that his doctors will not provide adequate pain relief. He was seen in the urgent care clinic yesterday and is unhappy with the prescription for muscle relaxants. He is obviously angry at the lack of concern for his multiple medical problems by his doctors and the health-care system.

3. A 65-year-old man's wife calls c/o husband with chest pain who refuses to go to the hospital. He had been working hard in the yard earlier in the day and now feels tired, has diffuse chest pain that is worse on the left side, which he believes is related to a fall when he lost his balance and tripped over a log. He is generally healthy but is a diabetic. Wife is concerned that he may be having a heart attack.

4. A 32-year-old woman c/o feeling overwhelmed and frightened. She states that she woke up in a strange apartment missing her undergarments. She remembers being in a bar the night before but believes she only had three to four drinks. She wonders if she has been drugged and sexually assaulted but is embarrassed to report it because she cannot remember many details. She wants to know if there is a test or what she should do.

5. A 26-year-old woman c/o feeling she cannot cope. Has had abdominal pain for 3 weeks. Her husband left her a month prior. She has four young children to care for and does not know how she is going to survive. She has constant headaches and feelings of hopelessness. She has suicidal thoughts but is worried about what will happen to her children if she dies. She begins sobbing and asks for help.

6. A 29-year-old man c/o back pain worsening over the past 2 months. He injured his back at work 6 months prior. He wants pain medication prescribed over the telephone. He becomes very angry and abusive when told that he needs to be evaluated by a physician/NP/PA before additional medication can be prescribed. He criticizes the health-care system and insists the only reason that they instruct him to see a physician is to make more money for the physician. He continues to use foul language in describing his concerns. He sounds intoxicated, using slurred words and repeating his concerns even after the nurse provides advice.

Questions

What does the caller need?

How can you help the caller?

What additional information do you need to help the caller?

What protocol would you use to address the caller's needs?

How would you handle this call?

In a worst-case scenario, what do you think could happen to this caller?

Appendix L: Quality Improvement Program

1. **Skill Assessment Form**—This form is versatile and can be used in a variety of ways to measure quality and competency.
- Initial competency review during training
- Competency performance review
- Ongoing quality review of adherence to standards and opportunities for improvement and education
- Training exercises

2. **For ongoing competency review and quality, see the following:**
- Telephone Triage Quality Improvement Survey—Appendix D
- Telephone Triage Documentation Form—Appendix E1
- Consulting Nurse Tape Review Form—Appendix G
- Consulting Nurse Documentation Review—Appendix H

3. **Mystery Caller Practice Exercise**

This exercise is designed to help the telephone nurse to gain experience with and insight into call management and to explore potential problems in soliciting accurate information to determine the appropriate disposition of a call.

It involves calling a telephone nurse within your organization or another facility (if the two facilities have agreed to participate). Staff should be notified that a mystery caller might be calling. You should participate as both the mystery caller and the telephone nurse receiving a call from the mystery caller.

1. Use the scenarios in Appendix K as a basis for your mystery call. Make up your own scenario if you feel it is more relevant to your practice. Write down the primary information before making the call. It helps to keep you on track and prevents the nurse from leading you down a different path than you had intended.

2. Use the "Telephone Triage Skills Assessment" form during the call to provide feedback to the telephone nurse. The mystery caller will use the same form to provide you with feedback during your practice calls.

3. At the completion of the call, inform the nurse that you are a mystery caller and thank the nurse for her or his participation. Feedback can be provided either at that time or in a review session at a later time.

4. Practice making and receiving three to five telephone calls.

5. Keep in mind that it is important to understand what it feels like to be a caller as well as the nurse receiving the call, to gain some understanding of the perceptions a caller may have of your telephone encounter.

Telephone Triage Skills Assessment Form

Greeting	Call Time:			All Time:		
	Yes	No	N/A	Yes	No	N/A
• Greets caller courteously.						
• Utilizes proper opening script (identifies self, services, RN, recorded line).						
• Clarifies accurately the type of call (triage, health info, other).						
• Gathers appropriate demographic data.						
• Comments:						
Protocol Utilization						
• Identifies emergency signs and symptoms.						
• Selects appropriate protocol.						
• Gathers appropriate patient history.						
• Upgrades caller to higher level of urgency as needed (child, confused adult, foreign speaking).						
• Makes acceptable recommendation and/or referral for care and time frame.						
• Offers appropriate medication recommendations/protocol.						
• Offers and documents interim care measures if not emergent.						
• Request caller feedback to evaluate understanding of information provided.						
• Documents appropriately, including assessment, advice given, protocol used, caller agreement with plan, and warning.						
• Comments:						
Communication Skills						
• Conveys a positive image of organization.						
• Maintains a courteous, calm, professional demeanor.						
• Exhibits ability to adapt to different personalities and emotions.						
• Assumes control of call: Listens attentively, interjects appropriately, and elicits necessary information.						
• Takes time with caller when appropriate; efficient without compromising quality.						
• Uses simple, direct language that caller understands.						
• Does not interrupt or interject for caller.						
• Speaks at a moderate rate with expressive modulation of tone.						
• Maintains control of call.						
• Comments:						

Closing Speech						
• Ends call efficiently.						
• Offers instructions to call back or seek medical care if condition worsens, new symptoms develop, or concern regarding condition.						
• Reviews recommendations and requests feedback to evaluate caller understanding and agreement with advice.						
• Disconnects last.						
• Comments:						

Appendix M: Communicable Diseases

DISEASE	MODE OF TRANSMISSION	INCUBATION PERIOD	CONTAGIOUS PERIOD
Acquired Immuno-deficiency Syndrome (AIDS)/HIV	Blood, breast milk, body tissues, fluids exchanged during sexual contact Other body fluids: saliva, urine, tears, bronchial secretions (especially if blood is present)	Variable incubation rates Virus exposure to sero-conversion (HIV+): ~1 to 3 months HIV+ to AIDS from <1 to 10 years	Although unknown, it is believed to begin just after onset of HIV and extend throughout life
Botulism	Contaminated food products	Within 12 to 36 hours of consumption, up to several days	Not contagious from secondary person-to-person contact
Bronchiolitis	Respiratory	4 to 6 days	Onset of cough until 7 days
Chancroid	Direct sexual contact with open or draining lesions	3 to 5 days up to 14 days	Until treated with antibiotic and lesions healed, usually about 1 to 2 weeks
Chickenpox (varicella) herpes zoster (shingles)	Direct person-to-person contact Respiratory droplet Soiled dressings or articles	Commonly 14 to 16 days Can be 2 to 3 weeks	1 to 5 days before the onset of rash, until all sores have crusted over, usually 10 to 21 days
Chlamydia	Sexual intercourse	Approximately 7 to 14 days	Unknown
"Cold," cough, croup	Respiratory	2 to 5 days	Onset of runny nose and/or cough until fever is gone
Conjunctivitis—Viral	Direct or indirect contact	1 to 12 days	4 to 14 days after onset of symptoms (minimally contagious)
Conjunctivitis—Bacterial	Direct contact with eye drainage	24 to 72 hours	Until treated with antibiotics
Fifth disease	Respiratory	Variable 4 to 20 days	7 days before rash develops, probably not communicable after rash starts
Giardia	Fecal contamination of food or water	3 to 25 days	Entire period of infection, often months

DISEASE	MODE OF TRANSMISSION	INCUBATION PERIOD	CONTAGIOUS PERIOD
Gonorrhea	Sexual contact	2 to 7 days	Continues until treatment begins
Hand, foot, and mouth disease (Coxsackie virus)	Direct contact with nasal or throat secretions, fecal Droplet	3 to 6 days	Onset of mouth ulcers until fever subsides, perhaps as long as several weeks with fecal contamination
Hepatitis A	Fecal–oral route Food contamination	15 to 50 days	During last half of incubation period until after first week of jaundice
Hepatitis B	Blood, saliva, semen, vaginal fluid	45 to 180 days	Infectious many weeks before onset of first symptom, until completion of acute clinical course of infection
Hepatitis C	Blood and plasma Percutaneous exposure	2 weeks to 6 months	From 1+ weeks before onset of symptoms; may persist indefinitely
Herpes simplex			
Type 1	Saliva	2 to 12 days	From onset of sores to 7 weeks after recovery from stomatitis
Type 2	Sexual contact (oral or genital)	2 to 12 days	7 to 12 days
Impetigo Staph Strep	Hand–skin contact Respiratory droplet Direct contact	4 to 10 days 1 to 3 days	Until draining lesions heal Untreated: weeks to months Treated: 24 hours on antibiotics
Influenza	Airborne Direct contact	1 to 3 days	Children: 7 days Adults: 3 to 5 days
Kawasaki	Unknown Seasonal variation	Unknown	Unknown
Legionnaire pneumonia	Airborne	2 to 10 days	Person to person: none
Lice Head/Body	Direct contact, indirect contact with objects	7 to 13 days Egg-to-egg cycle lasts 3 weeks	Continuous if alive, until first treatment Live off host for 7 to 21 days
Pubic (crabs)	Sexual contact		Live off host for 2 days
Lyme disease	Tick-borne	3 to 32 days	Person to person: none
Measles (rubeola)	Airborne Direct contact with nasal secretions	7 to 18 days	Before the onset of symptoms to 4 days after the appearance of rash

DISEASE	MODE OF TRANSMISSION	INCUBATION PERIOD	CONTAGIOUS PERIOD
Meningitis Bacterial: Meningococcal	Direct contact: respiratory droplet from nose and mouth	2 to 10 days	Usually after 24 hours on antibiotic therapy
Bacterial: *Haemophilus*	Droplet from nose and mouth	2 to 4 days	Noncommunicable within 24 to 48 hours on antibiotic therapy
Viral:	Varies with specific infectious agent	Varies with specific infectious agent	Variable, often approximately 7 days
Mononucleosis	Saliva	4 to 6 weeks	Prolonged, possibly a year
Pertussis	Direct contact Airborne droplet	6 to 20 days	Gradually decreases over 3 weeks
Pinworms	Direct transfer (anus to mouth) Indirect contact (infested bed, etc.)	2 to 6 weeks	As long as females are alive eggs survive for about 2 weeks

Rabies	Saliva
	  Direct contact (bite, scratch)
	  Indirect contact
		3 to 8 weeks	3 to 7 days before the onset of symptoms

Ringworm
  Tinea capitis
  (scalp)
	Direct skin-to-skin
	  Indirect contact (cloth seats, combs, etc.)
		10 to 14 days	Viable fungus may persist on contaminated articles for long periods of time

Tinea corporis (body)	Direct or indirect contact with infected people, articles, floors, benches, animals, shower stalls	4 to 10 days	While lesions are present and as long as viable fungus remains on articles
Rocky Mountain spotted fever	Tick-borne	3 to 14 days	Noncommunicable person to person Tick remains infectious for life, as long as 18 months
Roseola	Unknown Possibly saliva	10 to 15 days	Onset of fever until rash is gone

Rotavirus
  Rotaviral enteritis
	Fecal–oral route
	  Possibly respiratory
		24 to 72 hours	Average 4 to 6 days

Rubella	Direct contact, nasal secretions Droplet	14 to 23 days	1 week before to at least 4 days after onset of rash
Salmonella	Ingestion of contaminated food	6 to 72 hours	Throughout the course of infection
Scabies	Direct skin-to-skin contact	2 to 6 weeks	Until mites and eggs are destroyed
Scarlet fever	Large respiratory droplet Direct contact	1 to 3 days	Untreated: 10 to 21 days Treated: 24 hours of antibiotic therapy

DISEASE	MODE OF TRANSMISSION	INCUBATION PERIOD	CONTAGIOUS PERIOD
Shigella	Fecal–oral route Ingestion of contaminated food	12 to 96 hours	During acute infection until infectious agent no longer in feces (~4 weeks)
Sore throat			
Strep	Large respiratory droplet Direct contact	1 to 3 days	Untreated: 10 to 21 days Treated: after 24 hours of antibiotic therapy
Viral	Direct contact Inhalation of airborne droplet	1 to 5 days	Onset of sore throat until fever gone
Syphilis	Direct contact with moist lesions and body fluids	10 days to 3 months	Untreated: variable and indefinite Treated: after 24 to 48 hours of antibiotic therapy
Tetanus	Spores enter open wound	3 to 21 days	Noncommunicable from person to person
Trichomoniasis	Sexual contact through vaginal or urethral secretions	4 to 24 days	Untreated: may be symptom-free carrier for years
Tuberculosis	Airborne droplet	4 to 12 weeks	Degree of communicability depends on many factors Treated: within a few weeks Children with TB usually not infectious

Courtesy of Valerie Grossman. From Grossman, V. G. A. (2003). *Quick reference to triage* (2nd ed.). Philadelphia: Lippincott Williams & Wilkins.

Appendix N: Sexually Transmitted Diseases (STD)

DISEASE	CLINICAL PRESENTATION	COMPLICATIONS AND LONG-TERM RISKS
AIDS/HIV	May remain asymptomatic for many years Developing signs and symptoms include fatigue, fever, poor appetite, unexplained weight loss, generalized lymphadenopathy, persistent diarrhea, night sweats	Disease progression (from HIV to AIDS) is variable from a few months to 12 years Early intervention is essential in preserving and maintaining optimal health status
Chancroid	Painful genital ulceration(s) with tender inguinal adenopathy; ulcers may be necrotic or erosive	Chancroid has been associated with increased risk of acquiring HIV infection Should be tested for other infections that cause ulcers (e.g., syphilis)
Chlamydial cervicitis	Yellow mucopurulent cervical exudate May or may not be symptomatic Male sexual partner will likely have non-gonococcal urethritis	Untreated, may develop endometritis, salpingitis, ectopic pregnancy, and/or subsequent infertility High prevalence of coinfection with gonococcal infection Infection during pregnancy may lead to premature rupture of the membranes; pneumonia or conjunctivitis in the infant
Enteric infections	Sexually transmissible enteric infections, particularly among homosexual males Abdominal pain, fever, diarrhea, vomiting	Occurs frequently with oral–genital and oral–anal contact Infections can be life-threatening if they become systemic Organisms may be *Shigella*, hepatitis A, *Giardia*
Epididymitis	May or may not be transmitted sexually Can be asymptomatic Nonsexually transmitted, is associated with a urinary tract infection Unilateral testicular pain, swelling	Usually caused by gonorrhea or chlamydia May be caused by *Escherichia coli* after anal intercourse Must rule out a testicular torsion before making the diagnosis of epididymitis
Genital warts	Soft, fleshy, painless growth(s) around the anus, penis, vulvovaginal area, cervix, urethra, or perineum	Caused by the human papillomavirus Must rule out other causes of lesion(s), such as syphilis, etc. Lesions may cause tissue destruction Cervical warts are associated with neoplasia

DISEASE	CLINICAL PRESENTATION	COMPLICATIONS AND LONG-TERM RISKS
Gonorrhea	Males may have dysuria, urinary frequency, thin clear or yellow urethral discharge Females may have mucopurulent vaginal discharge, abnormal menses, dysuria, or may be asymptomatic	Untreated, risk of arthritis, dermatitis, bacteremia, meningitis, endocarditis At risk: males—epididymitis, infertility, urethral stricture, and sterility; females—pelvic inflammatory disease; newborns—ophthalmia neonatorum, pneumonia
Hepatitis B	Anorexia, malaise, nausea, vomiting, abdominal pain, jaundice, skin rash, arthralgias, arthritis	Chronic hepatitis, cirrhosis, liver cancer, liver failure, death Chronic carrier occurs in 6% to 10% of cases Infants born with hepatitis B are at high risk for developing chronic liver disease
Herpes genitalis Herpes simplex Type 2	Clustered vesicles that rupture, leaving painful, shallow genital ulcer(s) that eventually crust Initial outbreak lasts for 14 to 21 days; subsequent outbreaks are less severe and last 8 to 12 days	Other causes of genital ulcers (syphilis, chancroid, etc.) must be ruled out
Nongonococcal urethritis	Dysuria, urinary frequency, mucoid to purulent urethral discharge Some men may be asymptomatic Female sexual partners may have cervicitis or PID	Can be caused by chlamydia, mycoplasma, *Trichomonas*, or herpes simplex Can cause urethral strictures, prostatitis, epididymitis
Pelvic inflammatory disease (PID)	Lower abdominal pain, fever, cervical motion tenderness, dyspareunia, purulent vaginal discharge, dysuria, increased abdominal pain while walking	Must rule out appendicitis or ectopic pregnancy Risk for pelvic abscess, future ectopic pregnancy, infertility, pelvic adhesions
Proctitis	Sexually transmitted gastrointestinal illness Proctitis occurs with anal intercourse, resulting in inflammation of the rectum with anorectal pain, tenesmus, and rectal discharge	May be caused by chlamydia, gonorrhea, herpes simplex, and syphilis Among patients coinfected with HIV, herpes proctitis may be severe
Proctocolitis	Sexually transmitted gastrointestinal illness Proctocolitis occurs either with anal intercourse or with oral–fecal contact, resulting in symptoms of proctitis as well as diarrhea, abdominal cramps, and inflammation of the colonic mucosa	May be caused by *Campylobacter, Shigella,* or *Chlamydia* Other opportunistic infections may be involved among immunosuppressed HIV patients
Pubic lice	Slight discomfort to intense itching May have pruritic, erythematous macules, papules, or secondary excoriation in the genital area	Sexual partners within the last month should be treated May develop lymphadenitis or a secondary bacterial infection of the skin or hair follicle

DISEASE	CLINICAL PRESENTATION	COMPLICATIONS AND LONG-TERM RISKS
Scabies	The mite burrows under the skin of the fingers, penis, and wrists Scabies among adults may be sexually transmitted, while usually not sexually transmitted among children Itching (worse at night), papular eruptions, and excoriation of the skin	Sexual partners, household members, and close contacts within the past month should be examined and treated May develop a secondary infection, often with nephritogenic streptococci
Syphilis		
Primary syphilis	Painless, indurated, ulcer (chancre) at the site of infection approximately 10 days to 3 months after exposure	All genital ulcers should be suspected to be syphilitic Should be tested for HIV and retested again in 3 months
Secondary syphilis	Rash, mucocutaneous lesions, lymphadenopathy, condylomata lata Symptoms occur 4 to 6 weeks after exposure and resolve spontaneously within weeks to 12 months	At-risk sexual partners are those within the past 3 months plus duration of symptoms for primary syphilis, and 6 months plus duration of symptoms for secondary syphilis
Latent syphilis	Seroreactive yet asymptomatic Can be clinically latent for a period of weeks to years Latency sometimes lasts lifetime	Should be clinically evaluated for tertiary disease (i.e., aortitis, neurosyphilis, etc.) At-risk sexual partners are those within the past year for early latent syphilis
Tertiary/late syphilis	May have cardiac, neurologic, ophthalmic, auditory, or gummatous lesions	
Neurosyphilis	May see a variety of neurologic signs and symptoms, including ataxia, bladder problems, confusion, meningitis, uveitis May be asymptomatic	Diagnosis made based on a variety of tests, including reactive serologic test results, cerebrospinal fluid (CSF) protein or cell count abnormalities, positive VDRL on CSF
Congenital syphilis	Needs to be ruled out for infants born to mothers with untreated syphilis, mothers who received incomplete treatment, or insufficient follow-up of reported treated syphilis Serologic tests for mother and infant can be negative at delivery if mother was infected late in pregnancy	Syphilis frequently causes abortion, stillbirth, and complications of prematurity of infant Treated infants must be followed very closely and retested every 2 to 3 months Most infants are nonreactive by 6 months Infants with positive CSF should be retested every 6 months and be retreated if still abnormal at 2 years
Trichomoniasis vaginitis	Profuse, thin, foamy, greenish-yellow discharge with foul odor May be asymptomatic Male partners may have urethritis	Trichomoniasis often coexists with gonorrhea Perform a complete STD assessment if trichomoniasis is diagnosed

Courtesy of Valerie Grossman. From Grossman, V. G. A. (2003). *Quick reference to triage* (2nd ed.). Philadelphia: Lippincott Williams & Wilkins.

Appendix O: Temperature Conversion Chart

CELSIUS	FAHRENHEIT
43.0	109.4
42.0	107.6
41.0	105.8
40.5	104.9
40.0	104.0
39.5	103.1
39.0	102.2
38.5	101.3
38.0	100.4
37.5	99.5
37.0	98.6
36.5	97.7
36.0	96.8
35.0	95.0
34.0	93.2
33.0	91.4
32.0	89.6
31.0	87.8
30.0	86.0
29.0	84.2
28.0	82.4
27.0	80.6
26.0	78.8
25.0	77.0
24.0	75.2
23.0	73.4

CELSIUS	FAHRENHEIT
22.0	71.6
21.0	69.8
20.0	68.0
19.0	66.2
18.0	64.4

Formula for Fahrenheit to Celsius: $(1.8 \times$ Celsius reading$) + 32 =$ _____

Formula for Celsius to Fahrenheit: $0.55 \times$ (Fahrenheit reading $- 32) =$ _____

Appendix P: Weight Conversion Chart

POUND	KILOGRAM
1	0.45
2	0.5
3	1.35
4	1.8
5	2.25
6	2.7
8	3.6
10	4.5
11	5
22	10
33	15
44	20
55	25
66	30
77	35
88	40
99	45
110	50
121	55
132	60
143	65
154	70
165	75
176	80
187	85
198	90

209	95
220	100
231	105
242	110
253	115
264	120
275	125
286	130
297	135

Appendix Q: Teaching Self-Assessment

	INSTRUCTION	QUESTION
Ankle swelling	Using one finger, press over the bony part of the ankle for 2 seconds. Count 1001, 1002, and release.	Does the skin remain depressed or spring back into place?
Circulation	Squeeze the nail bed of your left middle finger between the first finger and thumb of your right hand. Count 1001, 1002, and release.	Does the color of the nail bed return immediately or is it sluggish? Repeat the action, and tell me the number of seconds it takes to return to normal. Count 1001, 1002, 1003, etc.
Dehydration	Pinch the skin over the top of the hand for 5 seconds. Count 1001, 1002, 1003, 1004, 1005, and release.	Does the skin remain raised like a tent, or does it spring back into place?
Extremity circulation	Expose both limbs (hands, feet, arms, legs). Using four fingers of one hand, touch the affected area for 2 seconds. Count 1001, 1002. Now touch the same area on the unaffected limb and count 1001, 1002.	Does one area feel cooler to touch than the area on the other limb? Is there a difference in color?
Extremity injury	Expose both limbs (hands, feet, arms, legs). Observe the area for swelling, discoloration, bone protrusion through the skin, or deformity.	Does one extremity look different from the other?
Infection	Using four fingers of one hand, touch the affected area for 2 seconds. Count 1001, 1002. Then move the hand and touch unaffected skin for 2 seconds. Observe the area and compare to surrounding skin.	Does one area feel warmer to touch than the other? Is the area red or swollen? Is there drainage? Are there red streaks? Is the area painful to touch?
Joint mobility	Bend and extend the affected joint to the extent possible. Move the joints above and below the affected area.	Does the movement cause or increase the pain? Is there difficulty moving the part?

	INSTRUCTION	QUESTION
Pain	Point to the location of the pain. Press on the painful area.	Describe the location of the pain. Can you locate the pain with one finger (localized pain)? Is the painful area larger than one finger? Describe the size of the painful area, i.e., size of a fist, one hand, or two hands (diffuse pain). Describe your pain on a scale of 1 to 10, 1 being minimal, and 10 being severe. Is the pain worse or the same when you press on the area? Does anything make the pain better or worse?
Postural	While in the presence of another adult, stand up from a sitting position.	Did any dizziness or light-headedness occur?
Pulse	Place two fingers (do not use your thumb) over the inner side of the wrist just below the base of the thumb. Feel the pulse. Count the number of beats for 30 seconds. Start counting when I say start and stop when I say stop.	How many beats did you feel? Did the beats feel even or regular?
Respirations	Remove clothing covering the chest. Observe the chest rising and falling. Count the number of times the chest rises for 15 seconds. Start counting when I say start and stop when I say stop.	Look at the fingernail beds, lips, earlobes, and skin. How many chest rises did you count? Are the respirations noisy? Is there a blue or gray discoloration in the fingernail beds, lips, or earlobes? Is the skin hot, cold, or moist? Is there excessive drooling in a child? Will the child eat or drink? What color is the sputum?
Swelling	Expose both limbs (hand, feet, arms, legs). Compare the limbs.	Is one area larger than the other?
Stroke symptoms	Ask person to: Smile Talk (repeat a four- to five-word sentence) Raise both arms in front of chest and hold at shoulder level Stick out tongue.	Possible stroke if any of these are positive: One side of smile is crooked Words are jumbled or unable to repeat One arm drifts down Tongue deviates to one side

Appendix R: Abdominal Pain: Causes and Characteristics

POSSIBLE DIAGNOSIS	SIGNS AND SYMPTOMS
Abdominal aortic aneurysm	• Asymptomatic until leakage or rupture occurs • Abrupt onset of severe back, flank, or abdominal pain • Pulsatile abdominal mass, mottling of lower extremities, signs of shock
Appendicitis	• Diffuse pain in epigastric or periumbilical area for 1 to 2 days • Localization of pain over the right lower quadrant between the umbilicus and right iliac crest • Anorexia, nausea/vomiting, fever, tachycardia, pallor, peritoneal signs • Increased pain with stairs, walking, etc.
Bowel obstruction	• Severe cramping or colicky abdominal pain • Vomiting, constipation, hypotension, tachycardia, abdominal distension, hyperactive bowel sounds, fever
Cholecystitis (inflammation of gallbladder)	• Colicky discomfort in the right upper quadrant midepigastric area • Pain radiating to the shoulders and back • Nausea/vomiting, fever, tachycardia, tachypnea, abdominal guarding, jaundice, malaise
Cholelithiasis (presence of gallstones)	• Severe, steady, or colicky pain in the upper abdominal quadrant, often right-sided • Pain usually begins 3 to 6 hours after a large meal • Pain radiating to scapula, back, or right shoulder • Nausea, vomiting, dyspepsia, mild to moderate jaundice
Constipation/fecal impaction	• Clinically defined as defecation less than 3 times per week • Each patient may interpret the symptoms differently • Fatigue, abdominal discomfort, headache, low back pain, anorexia, restlessness
Cystitis	• Dysuria, urinary frequency and urgency, fever, hematuria
Duodenal or ileojejunal hematoma	• Caused by a blow to the abdomen • Immediate bruising over upper quadrant of abdomen

POSSIBLE DIAGNOSIS	SIGNS AND SYMPTOMS
Epididymitis	• Infection or inflammation of the epididymis • Swelling, enlargement of the epididymis, sudden swelling of the spermatic cord, fever, dysuria, urethral discharge
Intussusception	• Paroxysms of acute abdominal pain, intermittent with episodes of being pain free • Currant jelly, mucous-type stools or rectal bleeding • Fever, lethargy, vomiting (food, mucus, fecal matter), dehydration
Orchitis	• Inflammation or infection of the testicle • Intense pain and swelling of the scrotum, dysuria, urethral discharge, fever, discomfort in the groin/lower abdomen, acutely ill
Pancreatitis	• Severe, constant upper quadrant midepigastric pain that radiates to the midback • Pain worsens when lying flat on back, relieved when lying on side with knees drawn up • Nausea, vomiting, fever, pallor, hypotension, tachycardia, tachypnea, restlessness, malaise, fatty or foul-smelling stools, abdominal distension, pulmonary crackles
Peritonitis	• Severe pain that gradually increases in intensity and worsens with movement • Riding in car, climbing stairs, or jumping on one foot greatly worsens pain • Radiation of pain to shoulder, back, or chest • Nausea, vomiting, fever, abdominal distension, rigidity, and tenderness
Prostatitis	• Perineal aching, low back pain • Urinary frequency, dysuria, fever, malaise, urethral discharge, prostatic swelling
Pyelonephritis	• Flank or back pain • Urinary frequency, dysuria, fever, malaise, nausea, vomiting, chills
Renal calculi	• Location of stone depicts associated pain: flank, lower abdominal quadrant, low back, groin, testicular, labial, or urethral meatus • Pain radiation varies on stone location • Nausea, vomiting, pale, diaphoretic, marked restlessness, dehydration
Ruptured ovarian cyst	• Sudden severe, unilateral lower quadrant abdominal pain associated with exercise or intercourse • Delayed or prolonged menstruation, vomiting, ascites, signs of peritonitis
Testicular torsion	• Sudden onset of severe, unilateral testicular pain and tenderness • Nausea, vomiting, fever, scrotal mass
Tubal pregnancy	• Intermittent diffuse abdominal pain • Radiation of pain to shoulder • Vaginal spotting/bleeding, syncope, dizziness, signs of peritonitis or shock

POSSIBLE DIAGNOSIS	SIGNS AND SYMPTOMS
Ulcer (gastric, duodenal, esophageal)	• Colicky, burning, squeezing pain in the epigastric or midback area • Pain intensity is variable; often begins 1 to 3 hours after meals, worsens at night • Nausea, vomiting, hematemesis, abdominal guarding, decreased or absent bowel sounds
Urinary tract infection	• Lower quadrant abdominal or pelvic pain • Urinary burning frequency, urgency, hematuria, foul-smelling urine, fever, bladder spasms

Courtesy of Valerie Grossman. From Grossman, V. G. A. (2003). *Quick reference to triage* (2nd ed.). Philadelphia: Lippincott Williams & Wilkins.

Appendix S: Chest Pain: Causes and Characteristics

SYSTEM	CAUSE	CHARACTERISTICS
Cardiovascular	Acute myocardial infarction	• Pain may be described as aching, pressure, squeezing, burning, tightness • Intensity: vague to severe • Location of pain may be substernal, epigastric, between the shoulder blades • Radiation of the pain to the neck, jaw, arm, back • Women may describe symptoms as nausea, fatigue, SOB • Diabetic neuropathy patients may have only vague pain
	Aneurysm	• Pain may be described as searing, continuous, severe • Radiation of pain to the back, neck, or shoulder(s) • Associated signs and symptoms: hypotension, diaphoresis, syncope
	Angina	• Pain may be described as squeezing, pressure, tightness relieved with rest or nitroglycerin • Pain may be persistent and intermittent • Occurs with activity, anxiety, sex, heavy meals, smoking, or at rest • Associated signs and symptoms: dyspnea, nausea, vomiting, diaphoresis, indigestion
	Cardiac contusion	• Cardiac compression between the sternum and vertebral column (falls, MVAs, blunt chest trauma, etc.) • May have EKG changes such as right bundle branch block, ST-T wave abnormalities, Q waves, atrial fibrillation, premature ventricular contractions, and A-V conduction disturbances
	Heart transplant	• Rejection may present with low-grade fever, fatigue, dyspnea, peripheral edema, pulmonary crackles, malaise, pericardial friction rub, arrhythmias, decreased EKG voltage, hypotension, increased jugular distention • Infection may be masked by use of immunosuppressive therapy—look for low-grade fever, cough, and malaise • Coronary heart disease is common in patients with heart transplants

SYSTEM	CAUSE	CHARACTERISTICS
	Pericarditis	• Pain may be described as severe, continuous, worse when lying on left side • Radiation of pain to shoulder or neck • History may include recent cardiac surgery, viral illness, or myocardial infarction • Diffuse ST elevation in multiple leads • PQ segment depression
	Tachydysrhythmias	• Pain may be described as severe, crushing, or generalized pain over chest • Associated signs and symptoms: anxiety, tachycardia, dizziness, impending doom
Gastrointestinal	Hiatal hernia	• Pain may be described as sharp, over the epigastrium • Occurs with heavy meals, bending over, lying down
	GERD	• Pain may be described as burning, heartburn, pressure • Nonradiating pain, not influenced by activity
Musculoskel-etal	Costochondritis	• Pain may be described as sharp or severe • Localized to affected area with tenderness on palpation • Associated signs and symptoms: cough, "cold"
	Muscle strain	• Pain may be described as aching • Occurs with increased use or exercise of upper body muscles • Pain is severe with localization over area of trauma • Pain worsens with palpations, movement, or cough • May have dyspnea
Pulmonary	Noxious fumes/ smoke inhalation	• Pain may be described as searing, sense of suffocation • History includes exposure to fire, pesticides, carbon monoxide, paint, chemicals • Associated signs and symptoms: dyspnea, hypoxia, cough, pallor, ashen skin, cyanosis, singed nasal hairs, soot in oropharynx, gray or black sputum, hoarseness, drooling • Carbon monoxide poisoning may additionally show nausea, headache, confusion, dizziness, irritability, decreased judgment, ataxia, collapse

SYSTEM	CAUSE	CHARACTERISTICS
	Pleural effusion	• May be described as sharp, localized, gradual onset yet pain is continuous • Dyspnea on exertion or at rest • Pain worsens with breathing, coughing, movement • Common in smokers
	Pneumonia	• Pain may be described as continuous dull discomfort to severe pain • Associated signs and symptoms: fever, SOB, tachycardia, malaise, cough, tachypnea • Children may complain of *abdominal pain instead of chest* pain
	Pneumothorax	• Pain may be described as sudden onset, sharp, severe • Associated signs and symptoms: SOB
	Pulmonary embolism	• Acute SOB • Risk factors include recent long bone fractures, surgery, smoking, use of oral contraceptives, sitting for long periods of time (i.e., long air travel)
Nervous	Anxiety	• Pain may be described as aching, stabbing • Associated with stressful event, anxiety • Associated signs and symptoms include hyperventilation, carpal spasms, palpitations, weakness, fear, or sense of impending doom

Courtesy of Valerie, G. (2003). *Quick reference to triage* (2nd ed.). Philadelphia: Lippincott Williams & Wilkins.

Appendix T: Headache: Causes and Characteristics

HEADACHE	CHARACTERISTICS
Cerebellar hemorrhage	Pain: • moderate to severe headache Associated signs and symptoms: • confusion • vomiting • altered gait
Cluster headaches	Pain: • very painful • knife-like • unilateral • over the eye Associated signs and symptoms: • excessive tearing • facial swelling • redness of the eye • diaphoresis
Increased intracranial pressure	Pain: • usually not excruciating Associated signs and symptoms: • nausea or vomiting • lethargy • diplopia • transient visual difficulty
Meningitis	Pain: • mild to severe headache • neck pain or stiffness Associated signs and symptoms: • fever • malaise • decreased appetite • irritability

HEADACHE	CHARACTERISTICS
Migraines	Pain: • periodic with gradual onset • throbbing, severe • frequently unilateral, may progress to bilateral • often above the eye(s) Associated signs and symptoms: • photophobia • sensitivity to sound • nausea • vomiting
Sinus headaches	Pain: • over the sinus areas (above the eyes, beside the nose, or over the cheekbone) Associated signs and symptoms: • fever • nasal drainage or congestion • ear pain • tenderness, swelling, or erythema of the sinus area
Subarachnoid Hemorrhage	Pain: • "worst headache of my life" Associated signs and symptoms: • with or without transient impairment of consciousness
Tension	Pain: • diffuse yet steady dull pain or pressure • "band-like" (back of head and neck, across forehead, and/or temporal areas)

Courtesy of Valerie Grossman. From Grossman, V. G. A. (2003). *Quick reference to triage* (2nd ed.). Philadelphia: Lippincott Williams & Wilkins.

Appendix U: Resources

Internet Resources by Topic

Anxiety

http://www.nimh.nih.gov/health/topics/anxiety-disorders/index.shtml

Bites, Animal

http://emedicine.medscape.com/article/768875-overview

http://www.cdc.gov/rabies/

Bites, Bedbug

http://emedicine.medscape.com/article/1088931-overview

Bites, Human

http://emedicine.medscape.com/article/768978-overview

Bites, Insect

http://www.cdc.gov/niosh/topics/insects/

http://emedicine.medscape.com/article/769067-overview

Bites, Snake

http://www.emedicine.com/med/topic2143.htm

Blood/Body Fluid Exposure; HIV Exposure

https://www.cdc.gov/hiv/risk/index.html—**Risks and precautions**

Common Cold Symptoms; Congestion, Avian Flu, Influenza

http://www.cdc.gov/flu/about/disease.htm

Diarrhea, Adult; Diarrhea, Child; Food Poisoning, Suspected

Ebola: http://www.cdc.gov/vhf/ebola/

https://wwwnc.cdc.gov/travel/page/travelers-diarrhea

Food Poisoning, Suspected

http://www.foodsafety.gov/poisoning/index.html

http://emedicine.medscape.com/article/175569-overview

Hepatitis

http://www.cdc.gov/ncidod/diseases/hepatitis/index/htm

Immunizations

www.cdc.gov/vaccines

Influenza

http://www.cdc.gov/flu/about/disease.htm

Lice

http://www.cdc.gov/parasites/lice/head/

Meningitis

http://www.cdc.gov/meningitis/about/faq.html

Mental Health Topics

http://health.nih.gov/

Neurological Disorders and Stroke

http://www.ninds.nih.gov/

Overdose; Poisoning, Suspected (link to poison control centers)

http://www.aapcc.org/

Posttraumatic Stress Disorder (PTSD)

https://www.mentalhealthameric.net/conditions/post-traumatic-stress-disorder

Scabies

http://www.cdc.gov/ncidod/dpd/parasites/scabies/default.htm

Severe Acute Respiratory Syndrome (SARS)

https://www.niaid.nih.gov/diseases-conditions/all?combine=SARS&disease_tid=All

Sexual Assault; Sexually Transmitted Disease

http://www.cdc.gov/std/general/

http://www.cdc.gov/ViolencePrevention/sexualviolence/index.html

Skin Lesions; Shingles

https://www.cdc.gov/shingles/about/overview.html

Stye

https://www.emedicinehealth.com/sty/article_em.htm

Suicide Attempt, Threat

https://emedicine.medscape.com/article/2013085-overview

Zika Virus

www.cdc.gov/zika

Standards and Professional Organization

American Academy of Ambulatory Care Nursing. (2018). *Scope and Standards of Practice for Professional Telehealth Nursing*, 6th Edition; Pitman, NJ: Anthony J. Jannetti.

American Academy of Ambulatory Care Nursing (AAACN). www.aaacn.org   800-AMB-NURS (800-262-6877)

American Accreditation Healthcare Commission (URAC). (2019). Health Call Center Standards V.3. Washington, DC. www.urac.org   202-216-9010

National Council of State Boards of Nursing (NCSBN). www.ncsbn.org

Appendix V: Mental Health Challenges in Telephone Triage

Telephone triage nurses play an important role in identifying and helping individuals with mental health problems. Nearly one in five American adults lives with a mental illness and 60% of those do not receive treatment for their symptoms. Telephone triage nurses are often the first point of contact for those trying to manage their mental illness and can help these individuals recognize the need for intervention. The role of the telephone triage nurse can include the following:

1. Provide accurate and timely triage.
2. Obtain an accurate medical history.
3. Assess the caller to rule out medical symptoms that need immediate attention.
4. Remove any biases that can affect the triage process.
5. Assess the caller's environment and available resources to determine the most appropriate plan for care.
6. Manage the uncertainty when callers have a difficult time articulating their concerns or condition. Are they coherent, answering questions appropriately, hallucinating, or delusional?
7. Focus on both the mental health issues and any medical concerns. Determine if there has been a recent new event, trauma, or medication noncompliance.
8. Serve as an advocate to help ensure the caller receives appropriate level of care in a timely fashion.
9. Provide a crisis line phone number or refer to the nearest emergency department.
10. Watch for red flag warnings of mental illness:
    a. Aggressive or violent behavior
    b. Delusions
    c. Hallucinations
    d. Paranoia
    e. Intentional or accidental ingestion
    f. Possession of a weapon is verbalized
    g. Expresses a desire or has a plan in place to harm self or others
    h. Disorganized speech pattern
    i. Sleeping difficulty
    j. Loss of job, home, or other financial stressors
    k. Excessive talking
    l. Unable to focus
11. Ask the caller "what can I do for you today?"
12. This encounter could be a life-changing event for the caller.

Altered Mental Status (AMS)

A complaint of altered mental status (AMS) is frequently only one of the concerns that compel someone to seek telephone advice. Often it is paired with fever, headache, anxiety, pain, vomiting, weakness, or some other somatic concern. However, the presence of AMS, combined with another physical concern, may be enough to push the disposition into the emergent category and should not be diminished or disregarded in the telephone triage process. For example, in the protocol Headache, if there is also confusion, the disposition is to "Seek emergency care now."

Signs of AMS may include confusion; irritability; less responsive to voice or touch; drowsiness; combative; uncooperative; nonsensical verbalizing; sudden change in behavior, thinking process, or ability to communicate; auditory (voices, buzzing, clicks), sensory (bug crawling), or visual hallucinations.

- AMS may be one of the first indicators of a urinary tract infection, dehydration, or a stroke in the elderly.
- In a child, AMS may be one of the first indicators of rapidly progressing meningitis or a head injury after trauma.
- New onset of paranoia or delusional thoughts may indicate a neurologic problem, electrolyte imbalance, or suicidal ideation.
- Remember that individuals with mental health issues also have serious health conditions, requiring prompt attention.

There have been a number of lawsuits that have alleged that the telephone triage nurse failed to recognize the significance of AMS and should have referred the caller to the ED. In one case, a child had a headache, congestion, and confusion and died from meningitis. In another case, a husband called concerned about his wife's new onset of strange behavior and paranoia. She was referred back to see her mental health provider but committed suicide before her appointment 2 days later. In both cases, there was a change in mental status. It is through listening, clarifying, and understanding that the nurse will be better equipped to apply the degree of AMS as it relates to other symptoms addressed in a protocol and reach an appropriate disposition.

Types of AMS

Paranoia: Often described as unfounded distrust in others and may be expressed as others are out to get them or are threatening harm to self or others. It is important to determine whether this is a new behavior, the person is under the influence of drugs or alcohol, taking a new medication, or has a history of mental illness.

Confusion: Mental state characterized by disorientation regarding time, place, person, or situation and can affect the person's ability to make decisions or perform activities of daily living. This becomes an emergency when associated with other symptoms, including fever >101°F, neck or body stiffness or rigidity, rash, head injury, flushing or dry skin, vomiting, fruity breath.

Delusion: Described as a false belief not shared by one's culture or incorrect beliefs not based on reality. A change from usual thinking process may indicate a more serious problem such as a stroke or other neurologic problem, substance abuse, withdrawal, poisoning, and requires further assessment and investigation.

Delirium: Sudden onset of confusion, disturbances in attention, disorganized thinking, or a decline in the level of consciousness occurring over a matter of hours to days. Requires emergency evaluation.

PTSD (Posttraumatic stress disorder): Most commonly known as a condition affecting military personnel, can affect anyone who has experienced or witnessed a traumatic event. The discussion on PTSD is not meant to diagnose PTSD, rather to help the nurse better understand PTSD and how the condition can have a profound impact on a person's life. PTSD symptoms can occur initially postevent, months or years after the traumatic event. Symptoms persist for at least a month and interfere with activities of daily living. Symptoms less than a month are categorized as an acute stress disorder. Manifestations of PTSD may include any of the following:

1. Reexperience the initial trauma through flashbacks or nightmares.
2. Avoidance of certain activities or places that evoke difficult emotions reminding the individual of the trauma.
3. Negative changes in thinking and mood, feelings of mistrust.
4. Feeling anxious, jumpy, irritable, frequent angry outbursts, difficulty sleeping, engaging in self-destructive behaviors (fast cars, alcohol or substance abuse). Panic attacks.
5. Frequent mood swings, difficulty concentrating, depression, isolating oneself from family and friends, apathy, hostility.
6. Changes in arousal, hyper-awareness, exaggerated startle response.
7. Constantly alert or on guard, preoccupied with staying safe, increase in physical problems such as constipation, diarrhea, rapid breathing, muscle tension, rapid heart rate, dizziness, nausea, headache, back pain, sweating.
8. Problems with daily living; work, school, social situations, relationship problems.
9. Suicidal thoughts.

Incidence of PTSD

1. Affects not only those experiencing the event, but also those witnessing or hearing the event such as post-9/11, terrorist attacks, school or event shootings.
2. Recently learned or experienced an unexpected or sudden death of a friend or relative.
3. Veterans who have returned to high-stress jobs such as law enforcement and firefighters.
4. First responders exposed to the aftermath of trauma.
5. Long-term abuse or life-threatening medical illness of a child or adult.
6. Loss of a job, home, spouse.
7. Actual or threatened death, serious injury, or sexual violence.
8. Violent personal assaults, natural or human-caused disasters.
9. Physical, sexual, or verbal abuse, severe emotional abuse or wartime violence.
10. Worst outcome of PTSD is suicide. The VA reports that greater than 6,000 suicides occur each year and are increasing 25.9% among veteran adults.
11. 4.4% of Americans are afflicted with PTSD.

PTSD in Children and Adolescents: Manifestations of PTSD in children and adolescents may be related to a traumatic event and include any of the following:

1. Agitation or confused behavior, intense fear, helplessness, anger, sadness, horror, and denial.
2. Repeated trauma may result in emotional numbing.
3. Nightmares, flashbacks.

4. Avoidance of situations or places that remind the person of the event, resulting in social isolation or withdrawal.
5. Develop repeated physical or emotional symptoms when reminded of the event such as headaches and stomach aches.
6. Worry about dying at an early age.
7. Acting younger than their age (clingy or whiny behavior, thumb-sucking or bed wetting).

Treatment of PTSD: The most common treatment modalities include:

1. Connect and network with support groups and people who have had similar experiences (trauma, violence, disasters, abuse).
2. Cognitive behavioral therapy is considered a front-line treatment for PTSD and helps the person change thought patterns that interfere with overcoming one's anxiety.
3. Help the person to focus on their response to memories and the feelings those events trigger.
4. Medications that can help to treat symptoms of PTSD; lower anxiety, minimize depression, and assist with sleeping disorders.
5. Medications such as Ketamine infusions have proven to be effective.
6. Connecting with family and friends.
7. Exercise.
8. Keep a journal.
9. Avoid drugs, alcohol, and caffeine.
10. Practicing meditation and mindfulness such as woodworking, repetitive motion activities like sewing and restoring cars.
11. If no treatment is provided, symptoms will continue.
    - May have difficulty functioning at home, work, school, and in relationships.
    - May lose a job due to irritability, anxiety, or numbness.
    - Heightened suicide risk.

Suicide Prevention

The telephone triage nurse can play a critical role in the prevention of suicide. They are frequently the first point of contact for a person needing immediate assistance or attention. Nurses who are knowledgeable about mental health issues are better prepared to intervene in a time of crisis. Approximately 123 Americans die by suicide every day and this number seems to be rapidly increasing. Telephone triage nurses can help people with warning signs of potential suicidal events by recognizing the warning signs and talking with the person about their thoughts and feelings. The telephone triage nurse can play a pivotal role saving lives one call at a time.

Most Common Warning Signs of Suicidal Risk

1. Expressed desire to die or kill oneself.
2. Exploring ways to commit suicide.

3. Talking about feelings of hopelessness.

4. Expressing a feeling of being trapped or unbearable pain.

5. A sense of being a burden to others.

6. A drastic change in behavior or extreme mood swings.

7. Giving away prized possessions.

8. Increased use of drugs or alcohol.

9. Demonstrating anxiousness, agitation, or recklessness.

10. Expressing or demonstrating feelings of isolation or withdrawal from friends or family.

11. Rage or plans to seek revenge.

Suicide Prevention Interventions

1. Deescalate the suicidal crisis and provide assistance for help.

2. Don't be afraid to discuss suicide, treat the person like any other person in crisis such as the person with chest pain or difficulty breathing.

3. Identify local emergency assistance contact numbers and request a welfare check as needed.

4. Involve all resources to assist person from harming self. This could be a family member, law enforcement, 911, crisis personnel.

5. Show empathy and nonjudgmental and accepting behavior to assist the caller in feeling safe.

6. Provide reassurance to the person that you want to help address their call for help.

7. Apply clinical judgment and emotional support to assess the caller's condition and possible mental health issues.

8. Be aware that not all callers are able to accurately describe their condition, history, and feelings. It is imperative that the nurse be able to skillfully deal with the ambiguous caller and ask appropriate questions to ensure caller safety and treatment as necessary.

9. There will be times when the caller will need emergency treatment and other times when all the caller wants and needs is a safe place to talk through their concern about life, loneliness, and difficult life situations.

10. Provide the national suicide prevention lifeline phone number—1-800-273-TALK (1-800-273-8255).

Appendix W: Emergency Preparedness

Over the past few years there have been a number of devastating mass casualty events causing widespread damage, injuries, and death. Hurricanes, flooding, fires, severe weather, and violent events have challenged health-care workers to provide health-care services to the community in a time of great need. Often the first people mobilized to help in dangerous and deadly situations are nurses. Multiple states have issued temporary licenses to out-of-state nurses to assist in relief efforts from hospitals to shelters. Telephone triage nurses can play a valuable role in the preparation for and management of catastrophic events.

A disaster is considered a serious disruption of the functioning of a community due to hazardous events, conditions of exposure, vulnerability, and capacity limitations leading to human, material, economic, and environmental losses. It is important to understand the type of disaster most commonly occurring in your community so that planning efforts and preparation are as efficient and inclusive as possible. Challenges in emergency preparedness planning include:

- Protecting the practice through mitigation activities before a disaster strikes
- Ensuring that staff's personal and professional needs are met
- Ensuring that patients have access to health care in a time of need
- Anticipate power outages
  - Portable rechargers for tablets and phones
  - Keep solar-powered flashlights and wind-up radios
  - Anticipate running out of supplies including soaps and linens—plan alternatives
  - Consider keeping a change of clothes and personal effects on hand in case the situation worsens and returning back home that day is no longer possible
- Plan for a contaminated water supply and mold postevent
- Anticipate a disruption in infrastructure and property damage
  - Plan for establishing an alternative site to provide services
- Establish a relationship with county Emergency Management leadership
  - Communicate your practice needs and how you can serve the public during and after a disaster as a strategy to help reduce the surge on emergency departments
  - Ask for assistance in spreading the word to the public of options for securing medical needs during and after a disaster strikes
  - Utilize social media and the radio for keeping the public informed
- Plan for staff being both victims and responders when disaster strikes. Staff member availability may be impacted for the first several days following a disaster. Staff may have lost homes, cars, pets, or family members.
- Communicate with patients when current location must be closed due to power outage, floods, fire, etc. Consider using practice website, social media, front-door signage, and office phone outgoing message to relay current situation and where to seek medical assistance.
- Consider the fact that during a disastrous event many people may stay home or evacuate, reducing the need for available services during the initial event.

Natural Disasters

- Earthquakes, landslides, tsunamis
- Avalanches, floods, lightning strikes, forest fires
- Extreme temperatures, drought, wildfires
- Cyclones, storms, wave surges, hurricanes, tornados
- Disease epidemics, animal plagues

Man-Made Disasters

- War
- Industrial accidents
- Famine
- Transportation crashes
- Active shooters
- Terrorist activities

There have been countless catastrophic events over the past few years, some natural and others man-made. With each disaster, lessons are learned and help organizations to plan for future events. In most of these events, nurses played a key role in helping to save lives and direct patients to an appropriate level of care in a timely fashion. In some cases when the infrastructure is impaired due to power outages or structural damage rendering facilities unusable for a period of time, telephone triage nurses have been able to establish alternative sites to provide triage and care using their telephone triage protocols. This approach helps to reduce the surge on emergency departments so those whose conditions are serious and require a higher level of care can be seen in the emergency department.

Pandemics: A statewide Nurse Triage Line was established in Minnesota during the 2009 H1N1 Influenza pandemic. Approximately 27,300 calls were received; 11,000 unnecessary health-care facility visits were avoided. Lessons learned include:

1. The public needs timely, accurate information of when and where to seek medical care.
2. Public flyers, e-mails, and newscasts helped to communicate the availability of the service.
3. Available resources for care included clinics and medical offices to help reduce the surge on emergency departments.
4. Crowded conditions can cause a delay in seeing a provider and receiving antiviral treatment.
5. When planning for a severe pandemic, it is important to mitigate medical facility surge.
6. Explore ways to reduce face-to-face provider encounters.
7. When appropriate, utilize protocols and standing orders approved by the provider to provide antiviral prescriptions.

Campfire: Paradise Calif required the evacuation of the city and local hospital as the fire quickly spread and engulfed the city.

1. Approximately 70 deaths occurred.
2. Chico, California, served as the primary evacuation destination for the city of Paradise.

3. Several shelters were established for the evacuees. The shelters included 3 RNs and a paramedic to help triage health conditions as they occurred.

4. Local health-care resources were at capacity with the addition of 20,000 residents now residing in Chico and the evacuation of Feather River Hospital.

Las Vegas Shooting: Took place at an outdoor concert. 58 Individuals were killed and 500 were injured. Lessons Learned:

1. First responders helped to save countless lives, especially with rapid transport to hospitals by cars, SUVs, and pick-up trucks.

2. Use of prehospital tourniquets provided additional life-saving measures.

Boston Marathon Bombing and the Pulse Nightclub Shooting in Orlando Florida: Lesson Learned:

1. Many lives were saved using combat application tourniquets and improvised tourniquets including a small chain.

START Method Triage: Simple Triage and Rapid Treatment is used when a mass casualty incident occurs and resources are overwhelmed or limited. This process of triage is used to quickly determine who needs immediate treatment and who can wait. The triage process takes about 30 seconds and evaluates respirations, perfusion, and mental status. Color-coded tags are used to signify the category of the victim and indicate who should be moved to a treatment area first or is safe to remain waiting until the most critical have been taken for treatment. Start Categories include:

- Deceased (black tags)—the person is not breathing and does not improve with repositioning the airway.
- Immediate (red tags)—the person has serious injuries but is not at high risk for early death. Their condition may be due to shock from blood loss or a head injury. Respirations are greater than 30 per minute, radial pulse absent or capillary refill >2 seconds, or unable to follow simple commands.
- Delayed (yellow tag)—the person has serious injuries but is not at high risk for early death. Frequently reassess and reprioritize as needed.
- Minor (green tag)—the person is considered the walking wounded with minor injuries that do not require immediate attention.
- Uninjured—does not require medical attention.

Active Shooter Incidents: The increased incidence of active shooter events has grown significantly in the past few years and has occurred not only in schools and emergency departments, but also in malls, large public events, bars, clinics, and airports. It is important for nurses to understand how to prevent active shooter events, what to do during a shooting event to stay safe, and what to do after the shooting stops.

Prevention

- Ensure only authorized personnel are allowed to enter patient care areas.
- Encourage everyone to report suspicious activity.
- Locked doors should remain locked and secure.
- Practice what to do in the event of a shooting incident.
- Observe for signs of a potentially violent situation.
  - Concealed weapon usually in the waistband or pocket
  - Hands in constant motion, quick movements, may have hand on weapon or tucked inside shirt or jacket

○ Walks through a crowd sideways to avoid a face-to-face encounter
○ Inappropriate clothing for the season

- Discuss with others what to do to be safe when faced with an active shooter.
- Know where unlocked exits are.
- Ensure staff know safe places to hide if necessary.

Actions to Take During the Incident: "Run, Hide, Fight"

- Run away from the area/facility in a zigzag pattern.
- Unless personal belongings are readily available and portable, leave behind. If possible keep a cell phone handy to alert police or family of the situation.
- Avoid escalators and elevators that have limited exit points.
- People generally need direction during a time of crisis, instruct others to follow you out and away from the building.
- Call 911 when safe to do so.
- If unable to run from the building, hide in an area with few to no windows and greater protection. Lock and barricade doors and windows. Pull blinds and darken the room. Silence cell phones, pagers, and other electronic devices.
- Fight if running and hiding are not safe options. Try to disrupt the shooter using blunt force objects such as tables, chairs, fire extinguishers.

Actions to Take After the Incident

- Hemorrhage control has proven to help save lives.
  ○ Apply direct pressure with both hands until additional help arrives.
  ○ Apply pressure with a pressure dressing or bleeding control gauze if available.
  ○ If unable to control the bleeding with direct pressure, apply a tourniquet to the extremity, if available and trained in its application. Apply 2 to 3 inches above the wound. If unable to control the bleeding, may apply a second tourniquet 2 to 4 inches above the first tourniquet. Label the tourniquet with time of application. Do not loosen tourniquet. Once patient is safely in a care facility that can take definitive action, that is, surgery, they will loosen or remove the tourniquet. Commercial tourniquets are safer to use. Avoid using improvised tourniquets unless properly trained in the type of material to use and application. Tourniquets can be safely applied (if direct pressure is ineffective in controlling the bleeding) for 2 hours before risk of tissue damage.
  ○ Hemorrhage control kits are preferable and now are readily available and accessible. Some facilities and businesses secure hemorrhage control kits with fire extinguishers or automated external defibrillators. Kits may include gloves, chest seals, commercial tourniquets, bleeding control gauze, trauma bandages for packing wounds, marking pen for labeling with time applied, instructions for tourniquet application. Kits should be sufficient to treat 20 people.

Bibliography

American Academy of Ambulatory Nursing. (1997). *Telephone nursing practice administration and practice standards*. Pitman, NJ: Anthony J. Jannetti.

American Health Consultants. (2000, March). Bite wounds: Don't let patients leave with the wrong impression. *ED Legal Letter, 2*(3), 21–32.

American Health Consultants. (2005a, March). Are elderly patients undertriaged? Don't miss life-threatening conditions. *ED Nursing, 8*(5), 49–51.

American Health Consultants. (2005b, March). Tips to teach nurses to do neuro assessments. *ED Nursing*, 54.

American Health Consultants. (2005c, September). EDs aren't following heart attack guidelines: Revamp protocols now. *ED Nursing, 8*(11), 121.

American Health Consultants. (2005d, October). Sickle cell: Learn how to help patients in severe pain. *ED Nursing*, 136.

American Health Consultants. (2005e, October). Use this protocol for sickle cell patients in your ED. *ED Nursing*, 137.

American Heart Association. (2006). *Healthcare provider's manual for basic life support*. Dallas, TX: Author.

Brennan, M. (1992). Nursing process in telephone advice. *Nursing Management, 23*(5), 62–66.

Briggs, J., & Grossman, V. (2005). *Emergency nursing: 5-tier triage protocols*. Philadelphia, PA: Lippincott Williams & Wilkins.

Briggs, J. K. (2016). *Telephone triage protocols for nurses* (5th ed.). Philadelphia, PA: Wolters Kluwer.

Briggs, J. K. (2019). *Triage protocols for aging adults*. Philadelphia, PA: Wolters Kluwer.

Briggs, J. K., & Meadows-Oliver, M. (2018). *Telephone triage protocols for pediatrics*. Philadelphia, PA: Wolters Kluwer.

Brown, J. L. (2005). *Pediatric telephone medicine: Principles, triage, and advice* (2nd ed.). Philadelphia, PA: Lippincott Williams & Wilkins.

Buppert, C. (2009). Guidelines for telephone triage. *Dermatology Nursing, 21*(1), 40–41.

Clayman, C. B., & Curry, R. H. (1992). *The American Medical Association guide to your family's symptoms*. New York, NY: Random House.

Davis, M. A. (1999). *Signs and symptoms in emergency medicine*. St. Louis, MO: Mosby.

Domino, F. J., Balder, R. A., Golding, J., & Grimes, A., (2014). *The 5-minute clinical consult standard*. Philadelphia, PA: Wolters Kluwer.

Dunn, J. (1985, August). Giving telephone advice is hazardous to your professional health. *Nursing, 15*(8), 40–41.

Editors of Prevention. (2002). *The doctor's book of home remedies*. New York, NY: Rodale Books.

Ferri, F. F. (2004). *Ferri's clinical advisor: Instant diagnosis and treatment*. St. Louis, MO: Mosby-Year Book.

Gorbach, S. L., Fatagas, M., Mylonakis, E., & Stone, D. R. (2001). *The 5-minute infectious disease consultant*. Philadelphia, PA: Lippincott Williams & Wilkins.

Greensher, A., Roemer, H., & Siemering, K. (1984). *Ambulatory protocols for emergency care*. Bowie, MD: Robert J. Brady.

Griffith, W. H. (1985). *Complete guide to symptoms, illness, and surgery*. Los Angeles, CA: The Body Press.

Grossman, V. G. A. (2003). *Quick reference to triage* (2nd ed.). Philadelphia, PA: Lippincott Williams & Wilkins.

Group Health Cooperative of Puget Sound. (1984). *Nurses' guide to telephone triage and health care*. Pacific Palisades, CA: Nurseco.

Hoare, K., Lacoste, J., Haro, K., & Conyers, C. (1999, October). Exploring indicators of telephone nursing quality. *Journal of Nursing Care Quality, 14*(1), 38–46.

Jenkins, J. L., & Loscalzo, J. (1990). *Manual of emergency medicine*. Boston, MA: Little, Brown and Company.

Katz, H. P. (1990). *Telephone medicine: Triage and training*. Philadelphia, PA: F. A. Davis.

Kemper, D. W. (1995). *Healthwise handbook: A self-care manual* (12th ed.). Boise, ID: Healthwise Publications.

Long, V. E., & McMullen, P. C. (2019). *Telephone triage for obstetrics & gynecology* (3rd ed.). Philadelphia, PA: Wolters Kluwer Health.

Mayo, A. M. (1998, November/December). The role of the telephone advice/triage nurse. *AAACN Viewpoint, 20*(6), 9.

McGear, R., & Price-Simms, J. (1988). *Telephone triage and management: A nursing process approach*. Philadelphia, PA: WB Saunders.

729

Miller, H. S., McEvers, J., & Griffith, J. A. (1997). *Instructions for obstetric and gynecologic patients* (2nd ed.). Philadelphia, PA: WB Saunders.

Narayan, M. C., Tennant, J. K., Benedict, L., Morrison, K. L., & Peyton, C. (1998). *Telephone triage for home care.* Gaithersburg, MD: Aspen.

Perlman, M. D., & Tintinalli, J. E. (Eds.). (1998). *Emergency care of the woman.* New York, NY: McGraw-Hill.

Perry, K. (1993, January). Answering the phone: Risks and rewards. *Nursing Management, 24*(1), 77–79.

Physicians' Desk Reference. (1996). *Physicians' desk reference for nonprescription drugs.* Montvale, NJ: Medical Economics.

Pool, S. R. (2004). *The complete guide: Providing telephone triage and advice in a family practice—During office hours and/or after hours.* Elk Grove Village, IL: American Academy of Pediatrics.

Porretto-Loehrke, A., Cassandra, S., & Szekeres, M. (2016). Clinical manual assessment of the wrist. *Journal of Hand Therapy, 29*(2), 123–135. doi:10.1016/j.jht.2016.02.008

Proehl, J. A., & Jones, L. M. (1998). *Mosby's emergency department patient teaching guide.* St. Louis, MO: C. V. Mosby.

Protocols help staff give appropriate telephone advice. (1994, January). *ED Management,* 8–12.

Reisinger, P. B. (1997, September/October). Telephone triage and child abuse assessment. *AAACN Viewpoint, 19*(5), 16–17.

Robinson, D. L., Anderson, M., & Eipenbeck, P. (1997, March). Telephone advice: New solutions for old problems. *Nurse Practitioner, 22*(3), 170–192.

Rosenthal, B. (Ed.). (2000). *A comprehensive resource guide to medical call centers: Players, implementation, and strategies. Directory of medical call centers.* New York, NY: Falkner & Gray.

Rouzier, P. (1999). *The sports medicine patient advisor.* San Francisco, CA: SportsMedPress.

Rutenberg, C. (2000, March). Telephone triage: When the only thing connecting you to your patient is the telephone. *American Journal of Nursing, 100*(3), 77–81.

Schaider, J. J., Hayden, S. R., Wolfe, R. E., Barkin, R. M., & Rosen, P. (2007). *Rosen and Barkin's 5-minute emergency medicine consult* (3rd ed.). Philadelphia, PA: Lippincott Williams & Wilkins.

Schwartz, W. M. (Ed.). (2005). *The 5-minute pediatric consult* (4th ed.). Philadelphia, PA: Lippincott Williams & Wilkins.

Schweitzer, P. B. (2000, March/April). Depression in primary care: The personal and social consequences of under treatment. *AAACN Viewpoint, 22*(2), 1.

Shealy, C. N. (2002). *The illustrated encyclopedia of healing remedies.* New York, NY: Thorsons/Element.

Sheehy, S. B., & Lenehan, G. P. (1999). *Manual of emergency care* (5th ed.). St. Louis, MO: Mosby.

Springhouse. (1999). *Nursing 99 drug handbook.* Springhouse, PA: Author.

Telephone advice lines. Worth the risk? (1996, April). *ED Management, 8*(4), 44–47.

Tintinalli, J. E. (Ed.). (1996). *Emergency medicine: A comprehensive study guide* (4th ed.). New York, NY: McGraw-Hill.

Tscheschlog, B. A., & Jauch, A. (2015). *Emergency nursing made incredibly easy* (2nd ed.). Philadelphia, PA: Wolters Kluwer.

Vickery, D. M., & Fries, J. F. (1993). *Take care of yourself* (5th ed.). Menlo Park, CA: Addison Wesley.

Visser, L., & Montejano, A. (2018a). *Fast facts for the triage nurse.* New York, NY: Springer Publishing Company.

Visser, L., & Montejano, A. (2018b). *Rapid access guide for triage and emergency nurses.* New York, NY: Springer Publishing Company.

Weinstein, A. (2002). Topical treatment of common superficial tinea infections. *American Family Physician, 65*(10), 2095–2102.

Wheeler, S. Q. (1993). *Telephone triage, theory, and protocol development.* Albany, NY: Delmar Publishers.

Wheeler, S. Q. (1994, May). Telephone triage: Sidestepping the pitfalls. *Nursing, 24*(5), 32LL–32OO.

Wheeler, S. Q. (1997). Calling all nurses: How to perform telephone triage. *Nursing, 27*(7), 37–41.

Wheeler, S. Q. (2009). *Telephone triage protocols for adult populations.* New York, NY: McGraw-Hill.

Wicking, K. H. (1999, September/October). Telephone triage: Surviving the storm. *AAACN Viewpoint, 21*(5), 12–19.

Woodke, D. (1995). *Telephone triage protocols for primary care centers.* Indianapolis, IN: HealthNet Community Health Centers and Methodist Hospital of Indiana.

Internet Resources

2017   ACC/AHA/AAPA/ABC/ACPM/AGS/APhA/ASH/ASPC/NMA/PCNA guideline for the prevention, detection, evaluation, and management of high blood pressure in adults. *J Am Coll Cardiol.* Retrieved from https://doi.org/10.1016/j.jacc.2017.11.006

American College of Cardiology. (2017). *New ACC/AHA high blood pressure guidelines lower definition of hypertension.* Retrieved from https://www.acc.org/latest-in-cardiology/articles/2017/11/08/11/47/mon-5pm-bp-guideline-aha-2017

American Lung Association. (2011). Retrieved from http://www.lungusa.org

Arthritis. Retrieved from https://www.emedicinehealth.com/arthritis/article_em.htm

Body piercing aftercare guidelines. (2011). Retrieved from http://www.safepiercing.org

Centers for Disease Control and Prevention. (2011a). *Acute public health consequences of methamphetamine laboratories*. Retrieved from http://www.cdc.gov/mmwr/preview/mmwrhtml/mm5414a3.htm

Centers for Disease Control and Prevention. (2011b). *Avian flu*. Retrieved from https://www.cdc.gov/flu/avianflu/

Centers for Disease Control and Prevention. (2011c). *Influenza*. Retrieved from http://www.cdc.gov/flu

Centers for Disease Control and Prevention. (2011d). *Public health consequences among first responders to emergency events associated with illicit methamphetamine laboratories*. Retrieved from https://www.cdc.gov/vaccines/vpd/mmr/public/index.html

Centers for Disease Control and Prevention. (2011e). *SARS*. Retrieved from http://www.cdc.gov/ncidod/sars/factsheetcc.htm

Centers for Disease Control and Prevention. (2011f). *Swine flu (H1N1 virus)*. Retrieved from http://www.cdc.gov/h1n1flu

Centers for Disease Control and Prevention. (2011g). *West Nile virus*. Retrieved from http://www.cdc.gov/ncidod/dvbid/westnile/

Centers for Disease Control and Prevention. (2014a). *Pertussis*. Retrieved from https://www.cdc.gov/pertussis/clinical/index.html

Centers for Disease Control and Prevention. (2014b). *Vaccines & immunizations*. Retrieved from http://www.cdc.gov/vaccines

Centers for Disease Control and Prevention—Injury Center. (2014). *Older adults falls—Home and recreational safety*. Retrieved from www.cdc.gov

Chest pain: "Women & heart disease." Retrieved from https://www.womenshealth.gov/heart-disease-and-stroke/heart-disease

Cooper, M. A. (2014). Lightning injuries. *eMedicine*. Retrieved from http://www.emedicine.com/emerg/topic299.htm

Dehydration in adults. (2014). Retrieved from http://www.emedicinehealth.com/dehydration_in_adults/article_em.htm

Delirium in the older person: A medical emergency (2014). Retrieved from https://www.islandhealth.ca/sites/default/files/2018-05/delirium-decision-tree.pdf

Disaster strikes—What's the plan for your urgent care center. (2019). *Journal of Urgent Care Medicine*. Retrieved from https://www.jucm.com/disaster-strikes-whats-plan-urgent-care-center/

Dryden-Edwards, R. (2014). *Anxiety disorders*. Retrieved from http://www.emedicinehealth.com/anxiety-health/article_em.htm

Ebola (Ebola virus disease). (2014). Retrieved from http://www.cdc.gov/vhf/ebola/index.html

Ebola virus disease (EVD) information for clinicians in U.S. healthcare settings. (2014). Retrieved from http://www.cdc.gov/vhf/ebola/hcp/clinician-information-us-healthcare-settings.html

Emergency 'MacGyver' tips for physicians. (2018, December 03). *Medscape*. Retrieved from https://www.medscape.com/viewarticle/905376

Environmental emergencies. (2013). Retrieved from https://www.slideshare.net/troypenn/environmental-emergencies-29362048

Frostbite. (2014). Retrieved from http://www.webmd.com/first-aid/undestanding_frostbite-treatment

Helman, A. (2012). *Emergency medicine cases: Low back pain emergencies*. Retrieved from https://emergencymedicinecases.com/episode-26-low-back-pain-emergencies/

Howley, E. K. *PTSD*. National Institute of Mental Health-Medline Plus

Hypothermic. Retrieved from https://www.emedicinehealth.com/hypothermia/article_em.htm

National Center for Injury Prevention & Control. *Check for safety: A home fall prevention checklist for older adults*. Retrieved from https://www.cdc.gov/HomeandRecreationalSafety/Falls/index.html

National Heart, Lung, and Blood Institute. (2014). *Asthma*. Retrieved from https://www.nhlbi.nih.gov/health-topics/asthma

National Institute of Allergy and Infectious Diseases. (2014). Retrieved from http://www.niaid.nih.gov

Phantom pain. Retrieved from https://www.mayoclinic.org/diseases-conditions/phantom-pain/symptoms-causes/syc-20376272

Poison Control Center. (web based). Retrieved from https://www.webpoisoncontrol.org/

Howley, E. K. *PTSD*. Retrieved from https://medlineplus.gov/posttraumaticstressdisorder.html

Public spaces should stock bleeding-control kits for mass casualties, experts say. (2019). *Medscape*. Retrieved from https://www.medscape.com/viewarticle/907573

Ringworm. (2011). Retrieved from https://www.mayoclinic.org/diseases-conditions/phantom-pain/symptoms-causes/syc-20376272

RN responders: Understanding disaster nursing. (2017, November 29). Retrieved from https://online.alvernia.edu/articles/category/nursing/

Staggs, S. (2017). Posttraumatic stress disorder (PTSD) symptoms. *PsychCentral*. Retrieved from https://psychcentral.com/ptsd/posttraumatic-stress-disorder-ptsd-symptoms/

"Stop the bleed" kits—Preparing everyone for mass casualties. (2019, January 10). *Medscape*. Retrieved from https://www.medscape.com/viewarticle/907187

Tattoos. (2011). Retrieved from https://www.mayoclinic.org/healthy-lifestyle/adult-health/in-depth/tattoos-and-piercings/art-20045067

Update policy. Retrieved from https://doi.org/10.1016/elsevier_cm_policy

U.S. Department of Health and Human Services. (2006, January). *Pandemic influenza planning: A guide for individuals and families*. Retrieved from http://www.pandemicflu.gov

U.S. Drug Enforcement Administration. (2011). *Methamphetamine*. Retrieved from https://www.cdc.gov/mmwr/preview/mmwrhtml/mm5414a3.htm

Wright, R. K. (2005, March 4). Electrical injuries. *eMedicine*. Retrieved from http://www.emedicine.com/emerg/topicl62.htm

Index

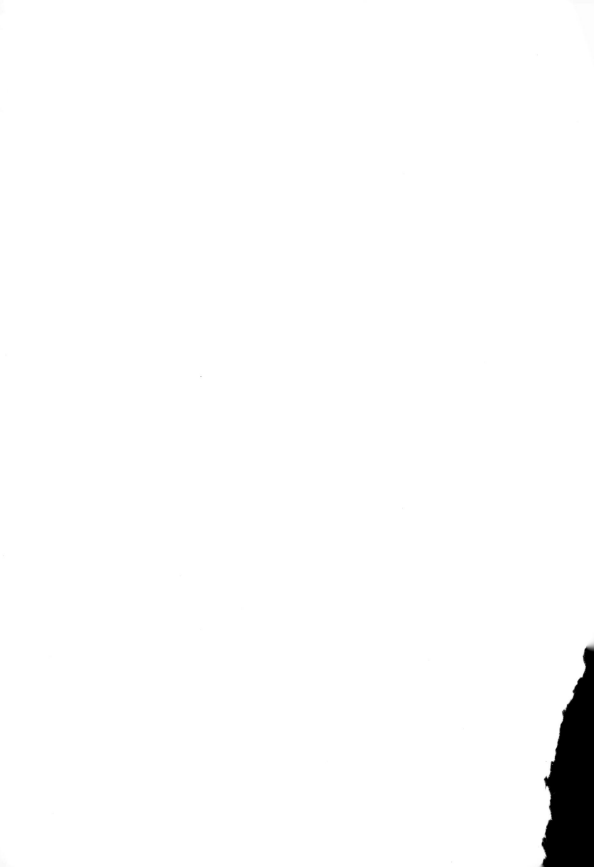

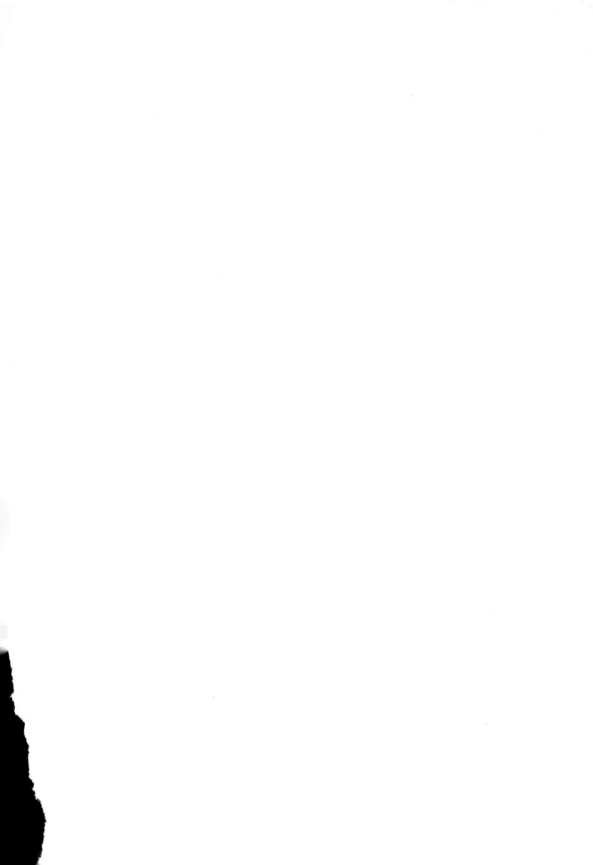